An Aid to the MRCP PACES
VOLUME 1
STATIONS 1 AND 3

'MRCP; Member of the Royal College of Physicians . . .
They only give that to crowned heads of Europe'.
From *The Citadel* by A.J. Cronin

Dear Reader of *An Aid to the MRCP PACES*

Please help us with the next edition of these books by filling in the survey on our website for every sitting of PACES that you attend. It does not matter if you pass or fail or pass well or fail badly. We need information from all these situations. These books are only as they are because of candidates in the past who filled in the surveys. Please do your bit for the candidates of the future.

The website where you can fill in the survey is **www.ryder-mrcp.org.uk**

Good luck on the day.

Best wishes,
Bob Ryder
Afzal Mir
Anne Freeman

An Aid to the MRCP PACES

FOURTH EDITION
VOLUME 1
STATIONS 1 AND 3

**R.E.J. Ryder, M.A. Mir
and E.A. Freeman**

*Departments of Medicine, City Hospital, Birmingham,
University Hospital of Wales and
University of Wales College of Medicine, Cardiff
and Department of Integrated Medicine,
Royal Gwent Hospital, Newport*

⊛WILEY-BLACKWELL
A John Wiley & Sons, Ltd., Publication

One-third of the royalties from this book will be donated to the Missionaries of Charity of Mother Teresa of Calcutta.

This edition first published 2012, © 1986, 1999, 2003 by Blackwell Publishing Ltd, 2012 by John Wiley & Sons Ltd.

Wiley-Blackwell is an imprint of John Wiley & Sons, formed by the merger of Wiley's global Scientific, Technical and Medical business with Blackwell Publishing.

Registered office: John Wiley & Sons, Ltd, The Atrium, Southern Gate, Chichester, West Sussex, PO19 8SQ, UK

Editorial offices: 9600 Garsington Road, Oxford, OX4 2DQ, UK
The Atrium, Southern Gate, Chichester, West Sussex, PO19 8SQ, UK
111 River Street, Hoboken, NJ07030-5774, USA

For details of our global editorial offices, for customer services and for information about how to apply for permission to reuse the copyright material in this book please see our website at www.wiley.com/wiley-blackwell

Library of Congress Cataloging-in-Publication Data

An aid to the MRCP PACES. – 4th ed. p. ; cm. Aid to the Membership of the Royal College of Physicians Practical Assessment of Clinical Examination Skills includes bibliographical references and index. Summary: "The first volume in this revised suite of the best-selling MRCP PACES revision guides is now fully updated. It reflects both feedback from PACES candidates as to which cases frequently appear in each station. Also taken into account is the new marking system introduced in which the former four-point marking scale has been changed to a three-point scale and candidates are now marked explicitly on between four and seven separate clinical skills"–Provided by publisher. ISBN 978-0-470-65509-2 (v. 1 : pbk. : alk. paper) – ISBN 978-0-470-65518-4 (v. 2 : pbk. : alk. paper) – ISBN 978-1-118-34805-5 (v. 3 : pbk. : alk. paper) I. Wiley-Blackwell (Firm) II. Title: Aid to the Membership of the Royal College of Physicians Practical Assessment of Clinical Examination Skills. [DNLM: 1. Physical Examination–Great Britain–Examination Questions. 2. Ethics, Clinical–Great Britain–Examination Questions. WB 18.2]610.76–dc232012020848

A catalogue record for this book is available from the British Library.

Wiley also publishes its books in a variety of electronic formats. Some content that appears in print may not be available in electronic books.

Cover image: © Wiley-Blackwell
Cover design by Sarah Dickinson

Set in 8.75 on 11.5 pt Minion by Toppan Best-set Premedia Limited

Contents

Preface

'MRCP; Member of the Royal College of Physicians...They only give that to crowned heads of Europe.'*

A short history of *An Aid to the MRCP PACES*

'Remember when you were young, you shone like the sun . . . .'†

At the beginning of the 1980s, Bob Ryder, an SHO working in South Wales, failed the MRCP short cases three times.‡ On each occasion I passed the long case and the viva which constituted the other parts of the MRCP clinical exam in those days but each time failed the short cases. Colleagues from the year below who had been house physicians, with me the SHO, came through and passed§ while I was left humiliated and without this essential qualification for progression in hospital medicine. The battle to overcome this obstacle became a two or more year epic that took over my life. I transformed from green and inexperienced¶ to complete expert in everything to do with the MRCP short cases as viewed from the point of view of the candidate. I experienced every manifestation of disaster (and eventually triumph) recorded by others in Volume 2, Section F. By the time of the third attempt I was so knowledgeable that I was out of tune with the examiner on a neurology case simply because I was thinking so widely on the case concerned.|| I believed at the time that I came close to passing at that attempt, although one never really knows and it was, after all, the occasion where I failed to feel for a collapsing pulse!** This was an important moment in the story because it was from this failure, along with the experience in the neurology case in my second attempt¶ that the examination *routines* and *checklists,* which are so central to this book, emerged. I finally passed on the fourth attempt whilst working as a registrar.†† During the journey, various consultants, senior registrars and colleague registrars tried to help in their various ways and amongst these one of the consultants in my hospital, Afzal Mir, offered the advice that I should make a list of all the likely short cases and make notes on each and learn them off by heart. His exact advice was to 'put them on your shaving mirror'. An important point should be made at this juncture. In order to be able to achieve this, one needed to attain the insight that it was indeed possible to do this. In those days there was no textbook for the exam, like the one you are reading, and there was no syllabus. Things had perhaps improved a little since the quote at the top of this Preface from A.J. Cronin,* but nevertheless MRCP did carry with it an awe, a high failure rate and an aura that the exam was indeed one consisting of cases you had not seen before and questions you did not know the answer to. Indeed, many of us sitting it at the time would have found this a reasonable definition of the MRCP short cases. A crucial part of my two or more years, four-attempt, journey that formed the seed that eventually grew into the first edition of this book, was the realization that, in fact, behind the mystique the reality was that the same old cases were indeed appearing in the exam over and over again, that there was a finite list and, indeed, from that list some cases occurred very frequently indeed.‡‡ The realization of this led me to do exactly what Afzal Mir had advised (without the shaving mirror bit!). At the time there was a free, monthly journal that we all received called *Hospital Update* and it had a regular feature dedicated to helping candidates with MRCP. In one issue the writer listed 70 cases which he reckoned were the likely short cases to appear in the exam and an eye-balling of this suggested it was fairly comprehensive.

And so I studied each of these 70 cases in the textbooks and made notes which were distilled into their classical features and other things that seemed important to remember and I wrote out an index card for each of the 70. Thus, the original drafts of the main short case *records* were penned whilst I was still sitting MRCP.

Another major contributor to my final success with the exam was junior doctor colleague, Anne Freeman. She had been on the Whipps Cross MRCP course with me prior to our first sittings of the exam and she passed where I had failed. Until that point, I think we would have considered ourselves equals in knowledge, ability and likelihood of passing.‡ I would describe Anne as being like Hermione Granger.§§ In her highly organized manner she had written down the likely instructions that might be given in the short cases exam and under each had recorded exactly what she would do and in what order should she get that instruction. She then practised over and over again on her spouse until she could do it perfectly without thought or mistake or missing something out, even in the stress of the exam.** I, on the other hand, was not like Hermione Granger. I could examine a whole patient perfectly in ordinary clinical life but had not actually thought through exactly what I would do, and in what order, when confronted with an instruction such as 'examine this patients legs' until it actually occurred in the exam.¶ And so eventually I did what Anne Freeman had done and the first versions of the *checklists* (for which I am especially grateful to my wife, Anne Ryder, who wrote them out tidily and then ticked off each point as I practised the examining, pointing out whenever I missed something out!) and primitive versions of the examination *routines* were born, again whilst I was still sitting MRCP.

Having finally passed the exam, it seemed a shame to waste all the insights into the exam and the experience I had gained, and all the work creating the 70 short case index cards and the examination *routine checklists* I had created and practised and honed so laboriously – and so I conceived the idea of putting them in a book for others to have the benefit without having to do so much of the work or, perhaps, to go through the ordeal of failing through poor preparation as I had done. I shortlisted what seemed to be the four major publishers of the moment and on a day in 1982 was sitting in the library of the University Hospital of Wales penning a draft letter to them. At a certain moment I got stuck over something – I have long since forgotten what – and on an impulse went down to Afzal Mir's office to ask him something to do with whatever it was I was stuck over. It was a defining moment in the history of these volumes. When I exited Afzal Mir's office the project had changed irrevocably. I was a registrar, he was a consultant. He was extremely interested in the subject himself and my consultation with him ended up with the project being one with both of us involved and me with a list of instructions (consultant to registrar!) as to what to do next!

And so an extremely forceful and creative relationship began, which led to *An Aid to the MRCP Short Cases*. It was not that we worked as a peaceful collaborative team – rather the thing came into existence through creativity on a battleground occupied by two equally creative and forceful (in very different ways) people with very different talents and approaches. There are famous examples of this type of creative force, e.g. Lennon and McCartney or Waters and Gilmour.¶¶ Looking back, there is no doubt that without the involvement of myself and Afzal working together, an entirely different and inferior book would have emerged (probably the short 100-page pocket book desired by Churchill Livingstone – see below) but at the time I did not realize this and only thought that I was losing control of my project through the consultant-registrar hierarchy! My response was to bring in Anne Freeman, who I am sure would be very happy to be thought of as the Harrison/Starr or the Wright/Mason of the band!¶¶

Anne and I, in fact, also became a highly creative force through the development of the idea of surveying successful MRCP candidates to find out exactly what happened in the exam. It started off with me interviewing colleagues and this led to the development of a questionnaire to find out what instruction they had been given, what their findings were, what they thought the diagnosis was and their confidence in this, what supplementary questions they were asked, and their comments on the experience of that sitting. I distributed it to everyone I could find in mine and neighbouring hospitals, whilst Anne took on, with tremendous response, the immense task of tracking down every successful candidate at one MRCP sitting and getting a questionnaire to them! We asked all to report on both their pass and previous fail experiences.

Our overture to the publishers resulted in offers to publish from Churchill Livingstone (now owned by Elsevier Ltd) and Blackwell Scientific Publications (now owned by John Wiley & Sons) with the former coming in first and so we signed up with them. They were thinking of a 100-page small pocket book (70 brief short cases – a few examination routines, hardly any illustrations) sold at a price that would mean the purchaser would buy without thinking. The actual book however created itself once we got down to it and its size could not be controlled by our initial thoughts or the publisher's aspirations. We based the book on the, by now, extensive surveys of candidates who had sat the exam and told us exactly what happened in it – the length and the breadth. This information turned the list of 70 cases into 150 and from the surveys also emerged the 20 examination *routines* required to cover most of the short cases which occurred. As to what should be included with each short case, that was determined by ensuring that we gave everything that the candidate might need to know according to what they told us in the surveys. We were determined to cover everything that the surveys dictated might occur or be asked. It was also clear that pictures would help. We battled obsessively over every word and checked and polished it until it was as near perfect as possible. By the time it was finished three years later, the 100-page pocket book had turned into a monster manuscript full of pictures.

I took it to Churchill Livingstone who demanded that it be shrunk down to the size in the original agreement or at least some sort of compromise size. We were absolutely certain that what we had created was what the MRCP short case-sitting candidates wanted and we refused to be persuaded. And so we were rejected by Churchill Livingstone. This was a very depressing eventuality! I resurrected the original three-year-old offer letter from Blackwell Scientific Publications and made an appointment to see the Editorial director – Peter Saugman. I turned up at his office carrying the massive manuscript and told him the tale. Wearing his very experienced publisher hat he instantly and completely understood the Churchill Livingstone reaction but also understood something from my passion and certainty about the market for the book. He explained that he was breaking every publishing rule but that he was senior enough to do that and that he would go ahead and publish it in full on a hunch. In 1986, he was rewarded by the appearance of a 400-page textbook-sized book, which rapidly became one bought and studied by almost every MRCP candidate. Indeed, that original red and blue edition can be found on the bookshelves either at home or in their offices of nearly every medical specialty consultant in the UK.

After this, our first and best, we all pursued solo careers with Afzal making clinical videos of patients depicting how to examine them, and writing other books such as *An Atlas of Clinical Diagnosis* (Saunders Ltd, 2nd edition, 2003), Anne developing services for the elderly and people with stroke in Gwent, and me pursuing diabetes clinical research in various areas. Meanwhile, Anne in particular continued to accumulate survey data and in the second half of the 1990s we came together again to make the second, blue and yellow, edition of the book (1999). The surveys (which by this stage were very extensive indeed) had uncovered a further 50 short cases that needed to be included and the original material all needed updating.

Then, in 2001, the Royal Colleges changed the clinical exam to PACES. Until then the short cases exam had been a room full of patients of all different kinds with the can-

didate being led round them at random – according to the examiners whim – for exactly 30 minutes. Anything from 4 to 11 patients might be seen. This was now transformed into Stations 1, 3 and 5 of the PACES exam, each 20 minutes long, thus doubling the time spent with short cases and ensuring that patients from all the main medical specialty areas were seen by every candidate. Hence, *An Aid to the MRCP Short Cases* was transformed into *An Aid to the MRCP PACES Volume 1* with the short cases divided into sections according to the Stations. Specialists helped us more than ever with the updating and by now surveys had revealed that there were 20 respiratory cases that might occur, 19 abdominal cases, 27 cardiovascular cases, 52 central nervous system cases, 51 skin cases, 19 locomotor cases, 18 endocrine cases, 21 eye cases and 8 'other' cases. The long case and viva sections of the old clinical exam were replaced by Stations 2 (History taking) and 4 (Communications and ethics). To help us with these we recruited new blood – a bright and enthusiastic young physician who had recently passed MRCP – Dev Banerjee, and he led on the Volume 2 project and finally in 2003 the third edition was published in silver and gold.

After many years intending to do this, we also created a medical student version of the short cases book on the grounds that medical student short cases exams are essentially the same as MRCP in that it is the same pool of patients and the examiners are all MRCP trained so that is how they think. However, whilst most MRCP candidates continue to use our books, most medical students have not discovered their version – it has the wrong title – medical students no longer have short cases exams – they have OSCEs! Those who have discovered it report that they have found it useful for their OSCEs.

And now the Royal Colleges have changed the exam again. And so *An Aid to the MRCP PACES* has become a trilogy. Stations 1 and 3 remain roughly the same and hence Volume 1 covers Stations 1 and 3 and Volume 3 has been created to deal with the new style of Station 5. Each short case has been checked and updated by one or more specialist(s) and these are now acknowledged at the start of the station concerned against the short case they have taken responsibility for. The same applies to the short cases in Station 5. Nevertheless, I have personally checked every suggestion and update and took final editorial responsibility, changing and amending as I thought fit. The order of short cases was again changed according to new surveys (now done online) and yet again a few more new short cases were found from surveys – only four for Volume 1 – kyphoscoliosis and collapsed lung for Respiratory, PEG tube for Abdominal and Ebstein's anomaly for Cardiovascular. New young blood has again been recruited – a further two bright, young and enthusiastic physicians. The updating of Volume 2 covering Stations 2 (History taking) and 4 (Communications and ethics) has been led by Nithya Sukumar. Volume 3, covering the new Station 5, has had major input from Ed Fogden.

We are grateful to the specialists, now listed in the appropriate sections, who have checked and updated the cases in their specialties, and especially grateful for the enthusiasm with which they have done this despite the considerable workload involved. We are grateful to Mrs Jane Price, patient representative and advocate at the

Royal Gwent Hospital, for her input into Volume 2, Station 4. Our surveys have always dictated the content of the books and so we are especially grateful to all the PACES candidates who have taken the trouble to fill in the on-line MRCP PACES survey at www.ryder-mrcp.org.uk. Finally, we are particularly grateful to our colleagues for their support in the ongoing project, which is a considerable undertaking, and we reiterate the deep thanks to our families expressed in the previous prefaces.

Bob Ryder
2012

---

*From *The Citadel* by A.J. Cronin.

†From the song *Shine on You Crazy Diamond* by Pink Floyd from the album *Wish You Were Here*.

‡'The result comes as a particular shock when you have been sitting exams for many years *without* failing them.' Vol. 2, Section F, Quotation 374.

§See Vol. 2, Section F, Experience 108.

¶See Vol. 2, Section F, Experience 109.

‖ See Vol. 2, Section F, Experience 145.

**See Vol. 2, Section F, Experience 144.

††See Vol. 2, Section F, Experience 175. I measured my pulse just before going into start this, my final attempt at MRCP clinical, and the rate I remember is 140 beats/minute, but in retrospect I feel it must have magnified in my mind through the years –

nevertheless whatever it was it was very high. It is clear though that stress remains a major component of the exam – see Vol. 2, Section F, Experience 15.

‡‡See Vol. 2, Section F, Useful tip 328 and Quotations 349 and 411–415.

§§A prominent character in the Harry Potter books by J.K. Rowling. Highly organised; expert at preparing for and passing exams.

¶¶Lennon and McCartney were the writing partnership of the Beatles with Harrison and Starr as the other members of the band. Similarly Waters and Gilmore for Pink Floyd with Wright and Mason as the other band members. In both cases it is believed that there was a special creativity through the coming together of the different talents of the individuals concerned, though the relationship was sometimes adversarial.

Preface to the third edition

The second edition of *An Aid to the MRCP Short Cases* comprehensively dealt with the old MRCP short cases exam. Stations 1, 3 and 5 of the MRCP PACES exam (Practical Assessment of Clinical Examination) have replaced this exam. Though the new exam is more structured and potentially more fair in several important ways, it is, in its essence, fundamentally the same exam, testing the same things. The skills and experience required to pass it remain the same, as do the many ways of failing it. Thus, the third edition of *An Aid to the MRCP Short Cases* has become *An Aid to the MRCP PACES*, Vol. 1 and we have been able to focus all that was helpful in the first two editions on the new format of the exam. This book deals with Stations 1, 3 and 5 of the MRCP PACES exam.

At the time of writing the exam remains relatively new, but we have already been able to undertake an initial survey. As with our previous editions this forms the basis of the book. Though smaller than previous surveys, candidates were again aware of our book and poured out information to us. On reflection, it is not surprising that we have found that the same old short cases continue to occur with frequencies that are not dissimilar. This is inevitable because the same patient pools are being tapped and the same patients lend themselves to testing the clinical skills that the College wishes to assess. In terms of frequency of occurrence, there are some notable exceptions. For example, the wider and earlier use of cardiac surgery has led to 'prosthetic valves' becoming the most common cardiac case, with 'mitral stenosis', which was the most common at the time of our first survey in the 1980s, now relegated to sixth most common as patients with this condition get fewer and are operated on earlier.

The new format of the exam has also had its effect. For example, the fact that there 'must be' a 'skin' case in Station 5 has meant that the majority of the small number of new short cases we have had to create for the new edition are 'skin' cases. Nevertheless, we have yet again found from the feedback from candidates in our survey that overall the cases seen, mistakes made or avoided, accounts of triumphs, tragedies and downward spirals remain remarkably constant as each sitting comes and goes.

We have during the first year of PACES been able to amass enough questionnaires from candidates to update the 'frequency of occurrence' figures and apply them to each of the subsections of Stations 1, 3 and 5. Because the new survey is as yet not great enough to cover all the less common short cases, we have adapted the figures from earlier surveys where there were inadequate data from the new surveys. In acknowledgement of the creation of Station 5, Locomotor, in PACES, we have created for this new edition two new examination *routines*: 'Examine this patient's knee' and 'Examine this patient's hip'.

In the guide notes for host examination centres, the College states: 'The patients attending the clinical stations should exhibit mainstream medical conditions. Patients with esoteric conditions are not suitable'. There is a problem, however, as to what constitutes an 'esoteric' condition. One physician's esoteric condition is another's extremely interesting and important one. Our survey suggests that the spectrum of patients being selected remains unchanged. Presumably the more there is a tendency to a consensus that a condition tends towards the esoteric end of things, the less likely such a patient is to be selected. On the other hand, less likely does not necessarily mean never, and this is reflected in the frequency of occurrence rates, which are sometimes very low indeed. Our own view remains that it would be a shame if clinical awareness of uncommon conditions was extinguished from the physicians of the future just because these conditions are rare or considered by some to be esoteric. What about the patient with an 'esoteric' condition? Would he/she not be horrified to learn that there was a policy that his/her condition no longer had to be studied and recognized in the way it had been by physicians in the past? We maintain our belief that failure to recognize a rare condition would never be an important pass/fail factor. On all types of cases, both 'easy' and 'hard', observation shows that some candidates perform well and others badly and all types of case can act as discriminators in one way or another. There is potential, with rarities, to show a breadth of clinical diagnostic skills which may distinguish a candidate from his/her peers.

Before coming to terms with rarities, however, you should ensure you can perform well with the more commonly occurring short cases. As our overriding principle remains to translate the standards set by the Colleges, we have covered them all in this book – the common and rare with rates of frequency of appearance in the clinical exam given so that you can ensure that you establish your priorities appropriately.

Stations 2 and 4 are dealt with in a new book *An Aid to the MRCP PACES*, Vol. 2. The PACES survey has enabled us to further expand our collection of experiences and anecdotes that are now presented in Vol. 2. We have been able to present a number of hardly edited complete PACES accounts written in the first person. At the same time the similarity of Stations 1, 3 and 5 to the old short cases exam has meant that most of our older collection of experiences and anecdotes from our previous editions are as valuable now as ever and they have been retained.

Medical Short Cases for Medical Students

In previous editions we encouraged medical students to use this book and many did. We have therefore written a medical student version. *Medical Short Cases for Medical Students*. We invite all of you who find this book useful to draw the attention of your medical students to the medical student version, to help with their clinical exams, whether OSCE or the traditional short case format.

Acknowledgements

We are extremely grateful to the following for reviewing some or all of the second edition short cases and/or examination routines related to their speciality. Many of these devoted a considerable amount of their valuable time to this task for no reward other than the accolade of 'Speciality advisor to *An Aid to the MRCP PACES*, Volume 1'. We should stress that we did not necessarily always take the advice given but we hope the errors of fact are minimal. They are acknowledged in order according to the number of short cases they dealt with: S. Sturman (neurology), C. Tan (dermatology), T. Millane (cardiology), D. Banerjee (respiratory), S. Jones (endocrinology), D. Carruthers (rheumatology), P. Wilson (gastroenterology), P. Dodson (medical ophthalmology), J. Wright (haematology) and T. Pankhurst (renal). We are grateful to D. Banerjee who wrote the first drafts of two of the new short cases – stridor and lung transplant – and to D. Carruthers who wrote the first drafts of the new examination *routines*, 'Examine this patient's knee' and 'Examine this patient's hip'.

We are grateful to so many candidates for their encouragement and enthusiasm and especially the many who have filled in questionnaires and to colleagues for their tolerance and support. Finally, we once again reinforce the gratitude, expressed at the end of previous prefaces, to our long-suffering families without whose forbearance and help the whole venture would never have happened.

Bob Ryder
Afzal Mir
Anne Freeman
2003

Preface to the second edition

Following publication of the first edition, my co-authors continued making surveys of candidates and accumulated an overwhelming number of questionnaires finding that many candidates, now aware of our book, poured out information to us. These greatly reinforced the information found in our original surveys and presented in the first edition. We found another 50 short cases which we present in this new edition, yet overall the cases seen, mistakes made or avoided, accounts of triumphs, tragedies and downward spirals remain remarkably constant as each sitting comes and goes. Our much more limited time, now that I have also become a consultant, meant that we were not able to analyse the new surveys to anything like the same extent as in the original edition. Therefore we have not altered the 'frequency of occurrence' figures used in the first edition for the 150 short cases of that edition as we do not believe that a more superficial analysis of the new surveys would be as accurate. It is possible that, for instance, 'old tuberculosis' is occurring in the exam less often than it did as fewer patients who had a thoracoplasty all those years ago are still available (patients with similar signs due to partial or complete pneumonectomy may appear instead, however, and indeed this is one of the new short cases); similarly Fallot's tetralogy with a Blalock shunt. Nevertheless, the vast majority of cases seem to maintain a remarkably constant rate of occurrence.

We were able to assign an approximate occurrence rate for each of the additional 50 short cases so that they could be merged in with the original 150. One of the new short cases has come into existence since the first edition because of new College guidelines ('Resuscitation Annie') and one because of the spread of a new condition ('AIDS related'). Some of the new cases are relative rarities which appear in the exam just occasionally. We do not believe that such cases should be excluded from the exam. It would be a shame if clinical awareness of uncommon conditions were extinguished from the physicians of the future just because these conditions are rare. At the same time we do not believe that failure to recognize a rare condition would ever be an important pass/fail factor in the MRCP short cases. A candidate seeing such a case is also likely to see a number of other more usual cases on which the main pass/fail decisions would be made.

Nevertheless, there is potential, with rarities, to show a breadth of clinical diagnostic skills which may distinguish a candidate from his/her peers. Before coming to terms with rarities, however, you should ensure you can perform well with the more commonly occurring short cases. In this book we cover them all – the common and rare with rates of frequency of appearance in the clinical exam so that you can ensure that you establish your priorities appropriately. The new surveys have enabled us to considerably expand the experiences and anecdotes in Section 4 and because candidates often 'knew what they were writing for', we have been able to present a number of hardly edited accounts written in the first person.

Acknowledgements

We are grateful to the following for reviewing some or all of the first edition short cases and/or examination routines related to their speciality. We should stress that we did not necessarily always take the advice given but we hope the errors of fact are minimal. G.S. Venables (neurology), S. Sturman (also neurology), K.S. Channer (cardiology), E.E. Kritzinger (medical ophthalmology), P. Stewart (endocrinology), C. Tan (dermatology), D. Honeybourne (respiratory medicine), T. Iqbal (gastroenterology), M. El Nahas (renal medicine), D. Situnayke (rheumatology), D. Bareford (haematology), P. Harper (medical genetics), K.G. Taylor (lipids) and E. McLoskey (Paget's disease). There was also a contribution from A. Jackowski (neurosurgeon). We thank C. Tan for Figs 3.114b and c, and C. Ellis for Fig. 3.156b.

I am particularly grateful to my co-authors for their tolerance with regard to my contribution to the tardiness of the new edition; to colleagues, in particular Ken Taylor and Sharon Jones for their support; to Anne's family, Pete, Lizzie and Jonathan Williams for what they have had to put up with; similarly to Lynda, Farooq, Deborah and Joanne Mir (especially for their wonderful hospitality during some crucial sessions over several days at Afzal's house); similarly and more so to my children Bobby and Anna for what they have had to put up with, but most of all sincere thanks to my wife Anne, without whose support and tolerance, well beyond the call of duty, none of it could ever have happened.

Bob Ryder
1999

Preface to the first edition

The short cases part of the examination for the Membership of the Royal College of Physicians (MRCP) is, by tradition, considered to be the most critical test of bedside behaviour and diagnostic competence. It forms an important milestone in the development of practising physicians. There is, however, no formal syllabus or tutoring and, despite the high failure rate, there is a notable lack of books specifically written to help candidates with this test.

The spectrum of clinical conditions used in the short cases examination is determined by a variety of interchanging factors such as the availability of patients with demonstrable physical signs, the prejudice of the doctors choosing the cases, that of the examiners taking part in the examination and, occasionally, the speciality bias of the examination centre. The cases chosen by the examiners from those assembled on the day in turn determine the problems presented to the candidates and the clinical skills required of them. For this reason we decided to build this book around an extensive survey conducted amongst successful candidates. Our questionnaires yielded information about the cases presented, the questions asked, answers given and the reactions of the examiners. We have thus been able to identify the chief difficulties of candidates in dealing with this practical examination and have attempted to help with these. The advice in Section 1 on how to prepare for the short cases is based on, and illustrated by, the comments received from the candidates. Section 2 is written around the clinical instructions given by the examiners to the candidates, the likely diagnoses under each instruction as revealed in the survey, and details of the examination steps suitable for each command. Section 3 forms the bulk of the book and presents the clinical features of 150 short cases in order of the frequency of their occurrence in the examination as derived from our survey. Thus, priorities are sorted out for the candidates preparing for the examination. In the final section we pass on the experiences and advice of some of the candidates in our survey which we felt would be of interest.

In fulfilling our main task of helping candidates to improve their performance in clinical examinations, we have used three learning techniques which are rather novel to this field. Firstly, the iterative approach which exploits the retentive potential of reinforcement by repeating the main clinical features of a number of conditions whenever any reference to these is made. It is hoped that this method will not only reinforce, but will also alert the candidates to other diagnostic possibilities when looking at a related condition. Secondly, in the examination methods suggested by us we have individualized the inspection to the examination of each subsystem, and have provided a *visual survey* to note the features most likely to be present. This enriches the usual advice to look for everything which often accomplishes nothing unless a specific sign is being looked for. Thirdly, we have reduced our suggested clinical methods to simple steps (*checklists*) which, if practised, may become spontaneous clinical habits, easy to recall and execute.

In the age of superspecialization, the task of summarizing and streamlining a subject as vast and diverse as general medicine to the needs of the short cases examinee has been formidable. We are in no doubt that our attempt will have its inadequacies and would be pleased if you would write to us (c/o Blackwell Scientific Publications) about any errors of fact, or with any suggestions which might be helpful for a future edition, or indeed with any other comments. We would also be interested to hear of any short cases which have occurred in the examination and which are not included on our lists (please give us an idea of your confidence that the case was indeed the condition concerned and why – clinical details, invigilator's confirmation, etc.) or of any Membership experiences which might be of interest.

Medical student note

Although this book has concentrated exclusively on the needs of MRCP candidates, it is noteworthy that the cases included in undergraduate medical short cases examinations are drawn from the same pool as those used in the MRCP examination. Furthermore, physicians are all MRCP trained and tend to use the MRCP style in these examinations. Though clearly the required standard of performance is lower, we feel that medical students preparing for their short cases examinations would also benefit from using this book. It would be a supplement to information gained from more comprehensive textbooks (we assume much basic knowledge) and an aid to practice on the wards.

Acknowledgements

We are indebted to the late Dr Ralph Marshall and his team (especially Paul Crompton, Keith Bellamy, Steve Young and Adrian Shaw) in the Department of Medical Illustration at the University Hospital of Wales, and Nigel Pearce and Steve Cashmore at the Department of Medical Illustration at the Royal Gwent Hospital. A large proportion of the photographs in the book are from the archives of these departments.

We are grateful to all the patients who gave their consent to the publication of the photographs depicting their medical conditions. Our thanks are due to many colleagues who have allowed us to use photographs from their own collections and photographs of their patients including: T.M. Hayes, the late C.E.C. Wells, M.S.J. Pathy, R. Marks, the late R. Hall, J.G. Graham, B.H. Davies, P.J.A. Holt, J. Jessop, M.H. Pritchard, N.W.D. Walshaw, I.S. Petheram, J.M. Swithenbank, M.D. Mishra, B.D. Williams, I.N.F. McQueen, P.E. Hutchinson, J. Rhodes, C.A.R. Pippen, A.J. Birtwell, P.M. Smith, A.G. Knight, S. Richards, A.G. Karseras, J.P. Thomas, C.N.A. Matthews, P.J. Sykes, M.L. Insley, P.I. Williams, B.S.D. Sastry, J.H. Jones, M.Y. Khan, the late J.D. Spillane, K. Tayton, G.M. Tinker, A. Compston, B.A. Thomas, H.J. Lloyd, G.B. Leitch, the late B. Calcraft, O.M. Gibby, G.O. Thomas, E. Graham Jones, Byron Evans, D.J. Fisher, G.S. Kilpatrick, L.E. Hughes, P. Harper, G. Griffiths, A.D. Holt-Wilson, D.B. Foster, D.L.T. Webster, J.H. Lazarus, D. Beckingham, J.E. Cawdery, R. Prosser, M.F. Scanlon, M. Wiles, I.A. Hughes, the late O.P. Gray, E. Waddington and L. Beck. Figure 3.42b has already been published in *An Atlas of Clinical Neurology* by Spillane and Spillane (Oxford University Press) and Figs 3.97b and 3.114 from the UHW Medical Illustration archives are also published in *A Picture Quiz in Medicine* by Ebden, Peiras and Dew (Lloyd-Luke Medical Books Ltd). Figures 3.115a (i) and (ii) are published with the permission of the Department of Medical Photography, Leicester Royal Infirmary and Fig. 3.110 with the permission of the University of Newcastle upon Tyne, holders of the copyright.

Our thanks go to colleagues who advised us on points of uncertainty in their fields of interest; especially A.C., B.H.D., M.J.D., L.G.D., R.H., T.M.H., M.H., T.P.K., I.N.F.M., M.D.M., M.F.S., H.S., P.M.S., S.S. and B.D.W.

We are obliged to: Andrea Hill for typing and retyping the manuscript; Janet Roberts for secretarial help with the survey; Jill Manfield for telephoning, chasing and writing again in pursuit of patient consents and for numerous minor secretarial chores; Alan Peiras for some nifty detective work in Edinburgh during the survey; Steve Young for the cover photograph for the book; and to certain pharmaceutical companies for financial assistance (including Astra Pharmaceuticals Ltd, CIBA Laboratories, May and Baker Ltd, Roche Products Ltd, Merck Sharp and Dohme Ltd and Thomas Morson Pharmaceuticals). Our particular thanks to Bayer UK Ltd for sponsoring the colour photographs.

Most of all we thank our long-suffering families without whose forbearance and help the book would never have been finished.

Bob Ryder
Afzal Mir
Anne Freeman
1986

Introduction

*'The result comes as a particular shock when you have been sitting exams for many years without failing them.'**

From June 2001, the Royal College of Physicians replaced the traditional MRCP 'clinical' examination, consisting of 30 minutes of short cases, a long case lasting 1 hour and 20 minutes and a viva lasting 20 minutes, with the MRCP PACES exam (Practical Assessment of Clinical Examination). In Autumn 2009, the College changed the format of Station 5 of this exam. The candidate who reaches the MRCP PACES examination has already demonstrated considerable knowledge of medicine by passing the MRCP Part I and MRCP Part II written examinations. The PACES exam is divided into five stations, each of which is timed for precise periods of 20 minutes. Stations 1 and 3 are divided into two substations of 10 minutes each. The stations are:

Station 1	Respiratory system
	Abdominal system
Station 2	History-taking skills
Station 3	Cardiovascular system
	Central nervous system
Station 4	Communication skills and ethics
Station 5	Integrated clinical assessment

Stations 2 and 4 are dealt with in Volume 2 of *An Aid to the MRCP PACES*. For this new edition of *An Aid to the MRCP PACES*, a third volume has been added to deal with the new Station 5. Stations 1 and 3 represent a more structured version of the old MRCP short cases exam that we dealt with in the first two editions of *An Aid to the MRCP Short Cases* and are dealt with in Volume 1.

The marking system for PACES is subject to change and you should study it at www.mrcpuk.org. At the time of writing, marking was being done in the skills of:

- Physical examination
- Identifying physical signs
- Clinical communication
- Differential diagnosis
- Clinical judgement
- Managing patient concerns
- Managing patient welfare.

The following table shows, at the time of writing, the stations at which each of these skills are tested.

Skill	Station 1: Respiratory	Station 1: Abdominal	Station 2	Station 3: Cardiovascular	Station 3: Neurological	Station 4	Station 5: Brief clinical consultation 1	Station 5: Brief clinical consultation 2
Physical examination	✓	✓	✗	✓	✓	✗	✓	✓
Identifying physical signs	✓	✓	✗	✓	✓	✗	✓	✓
Clinical communication	✗	✗	✓	✗	✗	✓	✓	✓
Differential diagnosis	✓	✓	✓	✓	✓	✗	✓	✓
Clinical judgement	✓	✓	✓	✓	✓	✓	✓	✓
Managing patient concerns	✗	✗	✓	✗	✗	✓	✓	✓
Managing patient welfare	✓	✓	✓	✓	✓	✓	✓	✓

*Vol. 2, Section F, Quotation 374.

At the time of writing the system is that, on the mark sheet, the examiner in the station concerned gives for each skill being tested in that station one of the following marks:

Satisfactory   mark = 2
Borderline   mark = 1
Unsatisfactory   mark = 0

If you study the marking system, and you can be bothered to do the analysis, you will be able to work out the minimum number of scores of 2 that you need assuming all other scores are 1. However, in practice this is probably of limited use because undoubtedly you will be trying to get a score of 2 in everything regardless. Two things are important however.

1. At the time of writing the College states on its website that:

'The onus is on the candidate to demonstrate each of the skills noted on the marksheet for each encounter (see above table) and, in the event that any one examiner decides that a skill was not demonstrated by a candidate in any one particular task, an unsatisfactory mark (score = 0) will be awarded for this skill.'

Thus, it is important to always be aware of the station that you are in and to be proactive, in as far as you can, in ensuring that you attempt to demonstrate your abilities in each of the headings concerned – the ones that are relevant to that station according to the above table. For example, with regard to Station 1 and 3, with only 10 minutes, it may easily occur that the bell has gone signalling the end of the 10 minutes before all of Physical examination, Identifying physical signs, Differential diagnosis, Clinical judgement and Managing patient welfare have been addressed. If you are still addressing differential diagnosis as the time is coming to an end it may be that you could deliberately move on to discussing management relevant to the patient concerned to demonstrate some knowledge in the area to give the opportunity to the examiner to give a score under the heading of clinical judgement other than zero.

2. It is essential to remember as you move from station to station that all 10 examiners mark independently and as you go into the next station the examiners have no idea how you did in the station you have just left so essentially you start with a blank sheet with them. If you have done badly in a station and fear you have scored some zeros these can be compensated for by scoring more 2s in other stations. In the five minutes between stations it is crucial to recharge yourself psy-

chologically, forget what has just happened in the station you have left and give yourself a complete fresh start – see 'Getting psyched up' in Section A.

Over the years, all have been agreed that the short cases examination is the major hurdle in MRCP Part II and with the advent of PACES the cases appearing remain as challenging as ever. For many who do fail, it is the first examination they have ever failed and it may also be the only examination they have taken that does not have some form of syllabus.

The exam is a practical test which assesses various facets of clinical competence in many subtle ways. Although it is generally accepted that clinical competence cannot be acquired from textbooks, a book such as this can provide indirect help towards that objective. We hope that the examination *routines* (Section B) together with the *checklists* (Appendix 1) may assist candidates in developing a keen sense of clinical search and detection. The short case *records* (Section C, Volume 1 and Section I, Volume 3) should provide the framework, i.e. the main clinical features, the discipline of how to look for them, how to differentiate the diagnostic from the incidental or associated findings, and how and when to be alert to other possibilities. By basing our book on the results of surveys of MRCP candidates (see below) we have *created a form of syllabus*, which we hope will be of value to future candidates. Not only do the results of the surveys advise as to what you are required to know and do, but they also grade these requirements in order of importance.

The examination in Stations 1 and 3

'I am sure they assess you very quickly…and decide whether they would like you to be in charge of their patients.'*

Two examiners will each take you for half of each 20-minute station. They each record a separate mark. At each case you will be given a written instruction, for example, 'This 48-year-old man has had a heart valve operation. He complains of recent shortness of breath on exertion but not at rest. Examine the cardiovascular system to see if you can establish the cause.' Nevertheless it is clear from our PACES survey that candidates translate the instruction into the traditional one: 'Examine this patient's heart'. We would counsel you to be careful on this point. Sometimes there is an important clue in the instruction. For example, one candidate in our survey (see Vol. 2, Section F, Experience 26) was asked to look at the patient and then listen to the heart. The

*Vol. 2, Section F, Quotation 423.

diagnosis was Marfan's syndrome with a prosthetic heart valve and the clue in the instruction was that the candidate was specifically asked to look before examining. In the case of the patient with acromegaly and homonymous hemianopia described on the second page of Section B, the candidates were given the written instruction to inspect the patient and then undertake a visual field assessment. Many undertook their visual field examination without spotting the acromegaly and then got into difficulty putting the whole thing together accordingly.

During the examination the examiners are constantly testing your ability to *elicit and interpret physical signs*. Many examiners say that, in the final analysis, whether a candidate will pass or fail depends very much on the general air of competence or incompetence which prevails during his/her clinical performance. Many candidates who fail feel that the exam is unfair in one way or another (see Vol. 2, Section F, Experience 237). However, candidates are not in a good position to judge their performance. A candidate who diagnosed a patient with aortic stenosis (which the last three candidates before him all diagnosed correctly) as having mitral stenosis may never know of his error. Furthermore, it is more than just a question of getting the right diagnosis. One candidate who failed complained that he knew, because he had a contact at the examination centre, that he had got the right diagnosis in all except two of the cases he saw. He was reporting this during the feedback session of a subsequent mock exam which he had also failed. During that mock exam, after examining the wasted legs of a patient with myotonic dystrophy, his first suggestion as to the cause of the signs in the legs was 'cauda equina lesion'. He eventually got to the correct diagnosis but his initial responses left a poor impression on the mock examiners, especially since other candidates in the same mock exam noticed, at once and without prompting, that the patient had gross generalized wasting, indicating that the problem was not one confined to the legs. In similar ways he had performed poorly on many of the other cases in the mock exam and as a mock examiner one could easily see how he had failed in the real exam whilst he thought he was getting the right diagnosis. Most agree that the move to PACES has increased the fairness of the exam, in particular because of the break between stations followed by 'starting again' with two new examiners who are not influenced by what occurred in the previous station. It is clear from our survey that this may have interrupted in some cases what may otherwise have gone on to become a 'downward spiral' disaster (see Vol. 2, Section F, Experiences 18, 20 and 28). Nevertheless, some continue to feel unfairly treated (see Vol. 2, Section F, Experiences 24 and 31). However, experience suggests, as one senior membership examiner put it, that the MRCP will usually pick out those who should fail; it will also usually pick out those who should pass – but not necessarily on the current attempt! Given the importance of clinical competence and the fact that this can only be assessed through a clinical exam (and clinical exams by their very nature will always have some in-built inadequacies), it seems unlikely that one could ever improve on this situation. In the old short cases exam the mark for each case was out of 12. As testimony to the precision of the marking system, it was an impressive fact that examiners, though marking independently, rarely differed by more than one mark in the scores out of 12 that they gave. The degree to which, generally, the examiners' marks concur suggests that the exam is probably as good as it can be. Our aim in this book, if you are one of those who should pass, is to try to help you to let the examiners know this on the current attempt or the next, rather than on the next attempt or the one after!

The surveys of MRCP short cases

'Certain "favourite" topics seem to recur. Make sure you know these.'*

First edition

This survey has been introduced in the Preface to the first edition. In the first part of this survey, questionnaires were obtained from a number of doctors who had gained the MRCP during the previous 10 years. In the second part all the successful candidates at a single sitting were circulated. The questionnaires obtained in the two parts of the survey included both the pass and the previous fail attempts of those candidates. Altogether we collected accounts of 248 attempts at the MRCP short cases, covering over 1300 'main focus' short cases as well as over 500 'additional' short cases (a short case could have a main focus, e.g. exophthalmos, and additional features, e.g. goitre and pretibial myoedema). The diagnoses given by these candidates were graded according to the confidence each candidate had in his retrospective assessment. Pass attempt diagnoses were given more weight than fail attempt ones. As a result we hoped that the rather complex analysis performed produced a picture which was as near to the

*Vol. 2, Section F, Quotation 351.

truth as possible. Analysis of the first part of the survey covering candidates' attempts over several years was essentially the same as the analysis of the second part. This suggested that the cases used and the skills tested tend to remain constant. This comparison also gave some support to the accuracy of our method of analysis. The figures are used wherever they may be helpful throughout this volume. Apart from figures, the organization of our suggested examination *routines* (Section B) and the contents of our short case *records* (Volume 1, Section C and Volume 3, Section I) have been closely guided by this original, as well as subsequent, surveys. For light entertainment, but with ingrained lessons, a number of Experiences, Anecdotes and Quotations from the survey are given in Volume 2, Section F of *An Aid to the MRCP PACES*.

Second edition

As discussed in the Preface to the second edition, the original surveys were embellished for the second edition with several surveys conducted between the two editions. We collected accounts of a further 379 attempts covering nearly 2300 additional 'main focus' short cases. Although the second edition surveys were more extensive than those for the first edition, the analysis of them was more superficial and, therefore, the analysis from the first edition surveys remained the bedrock of the book.

Third (first PACES) edition

As discussed in the Preface to the third edition, we were able to undertake a small initial PACES survey which

provided, despite its size, considerable valuable information for us to modify our book accordingly. We used for the survey the first 50 PACES questionnaires that we received during the first 12 months. This gave us accounts of 400 short cases – 200 from Stations 1 and 3 and 200 from Station 5. The questionnaires gave accounts from the first three PACES sittings with one questionnaire from the fourth sitting. Wherever the data from this survey was sufficient to supersede that from previous surveys, it was thus used. We were also able to give a number of complete PACES Experiences written in the first person at the end of Volume 2 of *An Aid to the MRCP PACES*.

Current (second PACES) edition

For the current edition, we were able to enhance the data from previous surveys with the data from about 100 online questionnaires submitted at www.ryder-mrcp.org.uk from recent PACES experiences. Some before, and some after, the changes to Station 5 in Autumn 2009. Using this, we have been able to update the examination frequencies for the short cases in the current volume, as well as adding four new ones (see Preface) and to provide some recent full PACES Experiences (since Autumn 2009) written in the first person at the end of Volume 2, Section F of *An Aid to the MRCP PACES*. By studying these, the first-timer, in particular, can be given considerable insight into what the exam is actually like.

Section A
Preparation

'Expressionless and without comment they led me away.'*

These books exist as they are because of many previous candidates who, over the years, have completed our surveys and given us invaluable insight into the candidate experience. Please give something back by doing the same for the candidates of the future. For all of your sittings, whether it be a triumphant pass or a disastrous fail . . .

Remember to fill in the survey at www.ryder-mrcp.org.uk

THANK YOU

The clinical skills required for the MRCP examination, particularly in relation to the short cases, can only be acquired by thoughtful preparation, experience and purposeful practice. Tutors and examiners alike agree that it is more important to spend time examining patients than reading textbooks. The examiners are not looking for encyclopaedic knowledge – they are just anxious to ascertain that you can be trusted to carry out an adequate clinical examination and make a competent clinical assessment. This book aims to help you organize your overall preparation to meet that objective. We have provided preparatory aids including examination *routines* and short case *records* (see below). We also aim to give you some insight into what most candidates experience in the examination and we hope to help you prepare psychologically. We would like to stress that although the written examination may appear a formidable hurdle, it often turns out to be less of an obstacle than the PACES. You would be wise to err on the side of safety and prepare for the PACES before, during and after your preparations for the written exam. Thus, we begin with some basic principles of practice and preparations at work.

Clinical experience in everyday work

'Imagine you are seeing the cases in a clinic and carrying out a routine examination.'*

The intention of the College in the examination is to gain a reflection of your usual working-day clinical competence for the examiners to judge. In arriving at their final verdict, the examiners may take particular note of factors such as your approach to the patient, your examination technique, spontaneity of shifting from system to system in pursuit of relevant clinical signs, fluidity in giving a coherent account of all the findings and conclusions, and your composure throughout. Though you can acquire all this for the day only, as some successful candidates do who are experts at passing examinations, it would be preferable if you could adopt many of these good habits into your everyday clinical approach. In either event, a long, diligent and disciplined practice is required if your aim is to be able to perform a smooth and polished clinical examination, to display the subtle confidence of a skilled performer, and to suppress signs of anxiety.

One simple approach to the task is that, whatever your job, you should consider all the patients you see as PACES patients from one station or another. Such a practice should not only improve your readiness for the

examination but also improve your standard of patient care – the primary objective of every clinician. Look out for all the 'good signs' passing through your hospital and use as many of these as possible as practice short cases. Ask your colleagues to let you know of every heart murmur, every abnormal fundus, every case with abnormal neurology, etc. If you are in, or can get to, a teaching hospital, make regular trips not only to clinical meetings and demonstrations but also, more importantly, to *visit the specialist wards* – neurology, cardiology, chest, rheumatology, dermatology, etc. It is useful to study the signs and conditions even when you know the diagnosis in order to further familiarize yourself with them. It is also a good practice to see cases 'blind' to the diagnosis and to try to simulate the examination situation. Imagine that two examiners are standing over you and there is a need to complete an efficient, once-only examination followed by an immediate response to the anticipated questions: 'What are your findings?' 'What is the diagnosis?' or 'How would you manage this patient?'.

Simulated examination practice

'I had a lot of practice presenting short cases to a "hawk" of a senior registrar. This experience was invaluable.'†

If a constant effort is made to improve your clinical skills by seeing as many cases as possible, there is no reason why the spontaneity and competence so acquired should not show up on the day. As with all examinations, however, much can be learned about the deficiencies requiring special attention when you put your composite clinical ability to the test in 'mock' examinations. In most district general, and all teaching, hospitals, the local postgraduate clinical tutors organize Membership teaching and 'mock' examination sessions, and you should find out about, and join in, as many of these as you can manage. Unfortunately, a lot of these, though useful, tend to teach in groups and discuss management or look at X-rays, rather than provide the intensive 'on-the-spot' practice on patients that is the ideal preparation for PACES. It is, therefore, advisable to supplement these sessions with simulated examination practice arranged by yourself. This requires the cooperation of a 'mock' examiner (consultant, experienced registrar and, on occasion, a fellow examinee) on a *one-to-one basis*. If you can practise with a variety of 'mock' examiners, you will not only broaden the assessment of your imperfections but also learn to respond to the varied approaches of different examiners.

---

*Vol. 2, Section F, Quotation 428.

†Vol. 2, Section F, Quotation 356.

Examination *routines*

'The most important point is to look professional – as if you have done it a hundred times before.'*

The short cases are a very important part of the Membership examination because they are designed to test critically two major areas of clinical competence. The first and more important of these is your ability to detect abnormal physical signs, interpret them correctly and put them together into a reasonable diagnosis or differential diagnosis. The second is your competence in conducting a professional and efficient clinical examination (see Vol. 2, Section F, Experience 142). As said above, these are generally considered to arise from day-to-day work and your conduct in the examination will reflect your experience in performing clinical tasks, presenting your assessments of patients to your seniors and getting their constant constructive criticism. If you are lucky enough to have worked with a good teacher, you may have acquired a firm foundation upon which you could build a structured clinical examination for all systems. As most candidates are engaged in busy clinical jobs and their seniors are often overburdened by administrative chores, etc., useful clinical dialogue between them may be limited. As a result, there may be little improvement in the weaknesses acquired during the undergraduate years.

The enormous task of preparing for the Membership examination provides an ideal opportunity to remedy any deficiencies in one's clinical methods. We would suggest that you work out the exact number and sequence of clinical steps for the examination of each subsystem, particularly those you would need to take in response to a particular command from the examiner, then practise going through these steps. Practise them over and over again† on your spouse, or any other willing person, until all the steps become as automatic as driving a car. Practise them on patients until you are confident of being able to pick up or demonstrate any abnormal physical signs. You should be able to maintain the same sequence and run through it rapidly and comprehensively in a way that is second nature to you. The sequence of clinical steps required for the examination of each system or subsystem is collectively referred to as the examination *routine* in this book. In Section B we suggest various examination *routines* (which you may wish to adopt or adapt) for you to practise in

response to particular commands. In Appendix 1 we provide *checklists* which summarize the major points in each examination *routine*. The *checklists* are designed to help in practising the *routines*.

Short case *records*

'The more practice at presenting short cases the better.'‡

A knowledge of the possible short cases that may be used in the examination is important so that you can become familiar with the physical signs associated with each, and know what you are looking for as you work through the examination *routine*. Having a good grasp of the clinical features of the case may enable you to score extra marks by looking for additional signs that may be present. Such extra marks distinguish the above-average candidate from the average ones. Furthermore, by becoming acquainted with descriptions of typical cases, you will find it easier to present the case to the examiner using acceptable descriptive terms. In this book, under each short case, we have presented the typical clinical features for you to remember, and to 'regurgitate' what you see (hence the descriptive term *record*), omit what you do not find and add what you find new. Thus, when confronted with the face of a man with Parkinson's disease which you diagnose at once on seeing his tremor, instead of stuttering and stumbling as you try to think of the right words to describe his face, the terms depressed, expressionless, unblinking, drooling and titubation will immediately surface for you to use. In Section C, under the headings of each PACES substation, we have covered the overwhelming majority of cases which could occur and we have put them in order of priority according to the likelihood of occurrence as assessed from our surveys.

Getting 'psyched up'

'Do not be distracted by mistakes made (or imagined) in preceding cases or the examiners' mannerisms or approach (I was and suffered for it). Being very nervous does not necessarily fail you and one bad case should not put you off.'§

It is common to hear candidates agonizing over their feeling that they failed to give a performance commensurate with their actual capabilities, simply because they were discouraged by the 'examination ordeal'. Though it is true that knowledge and competence tend to generate

---

*Vol. 2, Section F, Quotation 352.
†MRCP = Methods Require Constant Practice.

‡Vol. 2, Section F, Quotation 355.
§Vol. 2, Section F, Quotation 382; see also Quotations 384–391 and 418.

confidence and capability, it is also true that extreme anxiety can seriously impair the performance of even the most knowledgeable and competent candidate.

The downward spiral syndrome[*]

'After the first case there was a long pause as if they were waiting for me to say more – I went to pieces after this.'[†]
The candidate, an otherwise able and experienced doctor, enters the PACES examination room extremely anxious and lacking in confidence. He is just hovering on the edge of despair and the slightest upset is going to push him over. On one or more of the cases, he convinces himself that he is doing badly (whether or not he actually is) and over the edge he goes. The first stage of a rapid 'downward spiral' sets in, the dispirited candidate gets worse and worse and actually gives up before the end in the certainty that he has failed. Months of intensive bookwork and bedside practice, not to mention the examination fee, go to waste because of *inadequate psychological preparation*. To avoid this, there are four basic rules that are well worth noting.

1 You never know you have failed until the list is published

'Don't be put off if you get a few things wrong. I made a lot of mistakes that I know of and still passed.'[‡]
In the same way as it is said of the greatest saints that they considered themselves to be the greatest sinners, many successful candidates leave the examination centre feeling certain that they have failed. Good candidates may have a heightened awareness of the imperfections of their performance and thereby may exaggerate the impact of their mistakes on the examiner. Furthermore, the 'hawk' examiner may make you feel that you are doing badly, or you may deduce it from his mannerism, regardless of your performance. By the same token, the newcomer may slide through the stations unaware of any errors and with the examiners acting benignly, and then express great surprise as the inevitable 'thin' envelope arrives. It is not really important whether or not you think you have failed during the days between the examination and the arrival of the result. However, if you become convinced that you are

failing while you are still sitting the examination, the thought can be disastrous and impair your performance to the extent that your conviction becomes a reality (e.g. see Vol. 2, Section F, Experiences 108 and 109, Anecdote 271 and Quotation 389).

2 Do not be put off by the examiners or their reactions

'The most off-putting aspect of each case is the lack of feedback from the examiners as to whether you are right or wrong. This is much more disconcerting than outright criticism.'[§]
Many first-timers, despite excellent clinical experience, are stunned by the sombre and restrained atmosphere of the examination, which is unlike anything in their past experience (except perhaps the driving test!). It is as well, therefore, to be aware that the examiners tend to wear a 'poker face' and usually give no feedback or encouragement. The 'hostile hawk' may appear dissatisfied with everything you do and say, but this is not necessarily a guide as to whether you are doing badly or not. A positive atmosphere is no guide either: the smiling ('smiling death'!) and pleasant ('deadly dove'!) examiner (and the apparently uninterested one) can be as deadly as a black widow spider if you get yourself into a diagnostic maze! Bear in mind that 'hawks' and 'doves' tend to have similar rates of passing and failing candidates. Disregard the atmosphere and concentrate on what the examiner asks you to do rather than on what he looks like, and recall and use your *routines* and *records*.

3 The cases are easy and you have seen it all before

'My cases were more straightforward than I had been led to believe. Nothing was particularly rare.'[¶]
The psychological scenario of the examination is such that many candidates enter it with the distorted view that behind every case and every question there will be some catch, some clever trap, something never seen before or

---

[*]It should be noted that the downward spiral syndrome is not the absolute rock bottom. Candidates have experienced even worse – see Vol. 2, Section F, Anecdote 107.
[†]Vol. 2, Section F, Quotation 386; see also Vol. 2, Section F, Experience 19.
[‡]Vol. 2, Section F, Quotation 381.

[§]Vol. 2, Section F, Quotation 397. This quotation refers to the 'poker-face' examiner (see also Vol. 2, Section F, Quotation 344). The candidates in our survey give similar warnings regarding the 'hawk' ('The examiners may appear irritable and unsympathetic – don't worry') and the 'dove' ('Don't be fooled by the apparent relaxed nature of the examiners'). Remember, 'if your examiner challenges, don't assume it means you have said something wrong'.
[¶]Vol. 2, Section F, Quotation 411.

a diagnosis never heard of. In fact, these suspicions are rarely justified. The *vast majority* of cases and questions are straightforward and a realization of this is likely to produce a confident, straightforward answer from the start instead of the hesitancy born of a mind filled with suspicion and struggling to solve the hidden catch. A study of Membership short cases* reveals that there are two broad groups. The first group includes common conditions which you are well used to seeing in everyday clinical practice such as rheumatic heart disease, cirrhosis of the liver, rheumatoid hands and so on. These should surely present little difficulty (especially if you have tailor-made *routines* and *records*). In the second broad group are the rarities with good physical signs such as Osler–Weber–Rendu syndrome, pseudoxanthoma elasticum, Peutz–Jeghers syndrome, etc. You should be well used to these from the study of colour atlases, etc. that you will have done in preparation for the MRCP written examination. These too, therefore, should be easy (once you recognize the condition, all you have to do is 'play the *record*'!).

4 You have already passed and you have just got to keep it that way

'It's like skating on thin ice – if you keep going and don't fall through, you make it.'†

Confidence in one's ability is a very important ingredient in any form of competition. As you go into the examination, imagine that you have a clean sheet with a 100% mark and that you just have to keep it that way as the examiners show you cases that you are perfectly capable of coping with as you pass through the various stations. Such an attitude should replace the more usual 'Everybody fails this examination; it's too difficult; how can I possibly pass?'. The examination on clinical short cases for the MRCP has been well described (Royal Northern course) as 'like walking up a path full of puddles without stepping in the puddles; and you make the puddles yourself'. Remember the way to success is '*Readiness, Routines, Records* and *Right frame of mind*'.

*The cases covered in these volumes form a list far more comprehensive than you probably need in order to pass. If you have studied all the cases it would be excessively rare for you to be surprised by a condition not met before.

†Vol. 2, Section F, Quotation 396.

Section B
Examination *Routines*

*'Work out the best method for examination and practise it until it is second nature to you.'**

*Vol. 2, Section F, Quotation 348.

These books exist as they are because of many previous candidates who, over the years, have completed our surveys and given us invaluable insight into the candidate experience. Please give something back by doing the same for the candidates of the future. For all of your sittings, whether it be a triumphant pass or a disastrous fail . . .

Remember to fill in the survey at www.ryder-mrcp.org.uk

THANK YOU

In this chapter *routines* are suggested for the clinical assessment of various subsystems. These are readily adaptable to your individual methods. The subsystems are arranged according to the examiners' standard instructions (e.g. examine the heart, abdomen, hands, etc.). We have retained the original choice of subsystems, which was governed by our first edition surveys, except for the addition of 'Examine this patient's knee' and 'Examine this patient's hip', when PACES was first introduced. Examples of variations of the instruction are given both from our original survey and from our original PACES survey. Even though Station 5 is now covered in Volume 3, we have kept all the examination *routines* together in this volume as we believe they represent 'a whole'. They have, in more or less unchanged form, prepared the candidates for MRCP for over a quarter of a century and, on the grounds that *'if it ain't broke, don't fix it'**, we have left them relatively undisturbed. It is accepted that with the new Station 5, Spot Diagnosis *routines* (e.g. 'What is the diagnosis') are likely to be overtly called upon less often. Nevertheless, the conditions lending themselves to spot diagnosis will undoubtedly continue to appear and although the instruction from the examiner may be different, you will still be expected to 'spot' the diagnostic clues in your *visual survey*. The *routines* as a whole prepare you for the challenge of being able to examine anything wherever that challenge comes in PACES. Under each subsystem a list of the possible short cases is presented in order of their occurrence based on our surveys that led up to the third edition. We have not felt any merit in making any changes for the fourth edition. The percentages given represent our estimate of your chances of each diagnosis being present when you hear the particular instruction.† These lists of diagnoses have guided our suggested *routines*. The latter are broken down into numbered constituents to aid memory and *checklists* are given in Appendix 1 which match up to the numbered points in the examination *routine*. The *checklists* are to help your practice with each subsystem.

The idea is to develop a controlled, spontaneous and flawless technique of examination for each subsystem, so that you do not have to keep pausing and thinking what to do next and so that you do not miss out important steps (see Vol. 2, Section F, Experience 144). Often you will not need the complete sequence in the examination (for example, with regard to the 'Examine this patient's chest' *routine*, often the examiner will ask you to only examine 'the back of this patient's chest') but it will certainly increase your confidence if you enter the examination armed with the complete *routines* so that you can adapt them as necessary. The examination methods are supplemented with appropriate hints to avoid common pitfalls and to simplify the diagnostic maze.

The *routines* are presented in a single section without necessarily being associated with a particular station because our PACES survey has confirmed that many of the routines may be called upon in more than one station. For example, assessment of visual fields may be required in Station 3 for a patient with a hemiplegia who might

---

*Accredited to Bert Lance, American businessman, 1977.

†As with all our survey analyses, we graded the confidence of each candidate in his retrospective diagnosis of each short case seen. The percentages are not meant to add up to 100% because: (i) there are always missing percentages representing those short cases we could not be certain about; (ii) sometimes more than one diagnosis was considered worth counting for one instruction (for example, in order to give you the percentage of 'heart' cases with clubbing, when clubbing was present it was counted as well as the underlying cardiac condition). The figures are best used to give an index of the *relative importance* of the different conditions in terms of frequency of occurrence when you hear a given instruction.

have homonymous hemianopia, or Station 5 for a patient with acromegaly who might have a bitemporal hemianopia. It is essential that you bear in mind the station you are in when you are given the particular instruction and adapt it accordingly, but you also need to be wary of jumping to conclusions. For example, we are aware of the anecdote from a PACES pilot, hosted by Dr Ryder at City Hospital for the Royal Colleges, of a patient with acromegaly who had had a cerebrovascular accident secondary to acromegalic hypertension; her visual fields were required to be examined in Station 5 and showed homonymous hemianopia! Similarly, the only radial nerve palsy patient to occur in any of our surveys since the 1980s turned up in Station 5, Locomotor, of a PACES sitting. In Vol. 2, Section F, Experience 27 and Anecdote 88, accounts are given of patients with Marfan's syndrome appearing in Station 1, Respiratory, so it is important to remain open to many possibilities whilst taking into account the station you are in.

Before dealing with the individual subsystems, we would make some general points. You should avoid repeating the instruction or echoing the last part of it. Refrain from asking questions like: 'Would you like me to give you a running commentary or give the findings at the end?'. Such a response wastes invaluable seconds which could be used running through the *checklist* and completing your *visual survey*. It is like a batsman asking a bowler in a cricket match whether he would like his ball hit for a six or played defensively! You must do what you are best at and hope that the examiner does not ask you to do otherwise. As suggested below, a well-rehearsed procedure suited to each subsystem should make it possible for you to start purposefully without delay.

Your approach to the patient is of great importance. You should introduce yourself to him and ask his permission to examine him.* Permission should also be sought for various manoeuvres, such as adjusting the backrest when examining the heart or before removing any clothing. These polite exchanges will not only please most examiners and patients, but will also provide you with an opportunity to calm your nerves, collect your thoughts and recall the appropriate *checklist*.

Although we have continually emphasized the value of looking for signs peripheral to the examiner's instruction (e.g. examine this patient's heart, abdomen, chest), we would also like to emphasize that *dithering* may be counterproductive. In the *visual survey*, you should be scanning the patient rapidly and purposefully with a trained eye, not gazing helplessly at him for a long period while you try to decide what to do next. While you are feeling the pulse (heart) or settling the patient lying flat (abdomen), a quick look at the hands should establish whether there are any abnormalities or not. Pondering over normal hands from all angles at great length looks as unprofessional as, indeed, it is. It is of paramount importance to be gentle with the patient. Rough handling (e.g. roughly and abruptly digging deep into the patient's abdomen so that he winces with pain) has always been a behaviour to bring you instantly to the pass/fail borderline or below it (see Vol. 2, Section F, Experience 192). The new PACES marking system is now formally seeking to confirm that all the candidates who pass achieve near perfection under the heading 'Managing Patient Welfare'. At the time of writing, the marking system requires a score of at least 90% under this heading to ensure a pass. Make sure that you cover the patient up when you have finished examining him, and thank him.

*Throughout the book we often use him/his for brevity when we are talking about patients, examiners or candidates, when of course we mean him/her or his/hers.

1 | 'Examine this patient's pulse'

Variations of instruction from our original survey
Feel this pulse.
Examine this patient's pulse – look for the cause.
Examine this patient's pulses.

Diagnoses from our original survey in order of frequency
1 Irregular pulse 44%
2 Slow pulse 12%
3 Graves' disease (Vol. 3, Station 5, Endocrine, Case 3) 12%
4 Aortic stenosis 9%
5 Complete heart block 9%
6 Brachial artery aneurysm 9%
7 Impalpable radial pulses due to low output cardiac failure 9%
8 Tachycardia 6%
9 Takayasu's disease (Vol. 3, Station 5, Other, Case 3) 3%
10 Hypothyroidism (Vol. 3, Station 5, Endocrine, Case 5) 3%
11 Fallot's tetralogy with a Blalock shunt 3%

Examination *routine*

As you approach the patient from the right and ask for his permission to examine him you should:

1 look at his **face** for a *malar flush* (mitral stenosis, myxoedema) or for any signs of *hyper-* or *hypothyroidism*. As you take the arm to examine the right radial pulse, continue the *survey* of the patient by looking at

2 the **neck** (Corrigan's pulse, raised JVP, thyroidectomy scar, goitre) and then the *chest* (thoracotomy scar). Quickly run your eyes down the body to complete the *survey* (ascites, clubbing, pretibial myxoedema, ankle oedema, etc.) and then concentrate on

3 the **pulse** and note

4 its **rate** (count for at least 15 sec), volume and

5 its **rhythm.** A common diagnostic problem is presented by *slow atrial fibrillation* which may be mistaken for a regular pulse. To avoid this, concentrate on the *length of the pause* from one beat to another and see if each pause is equal to the succeeding one (see also Station 3, Cardiovascular, Case 8). This method will reveal that the pauses are variable from beat to beat in controlled slow atrial fibrillation.

6 Assess whether the **character** (waveform) of the pulse (information to be gained from radial, brachial and carotid) is normal, *collapsing, slow rising* or jerky. To determine whether there is a collapsing quality, put the palmar aspect of the four fingers of your left hand on the patient's wrist just below where you can easily feel the radial pulse. Press gently with your palm, lift the patient's hand above his head and then place your right palm over the patient's axillary artery. If the pulse has a *water-hammer* character you will experience a flick (a sharp and tall upstroke and an abrupt downstroke) which will *run* across all four fingers and at the same time you may also feel a flick of the axillary artery against your right palm. The pulse does not

merely become palpable when the hand is lifted but its character changes and it imparts a sharp knock. This is classic of the pulse that is present in haemodynamically significant aortic incompetence and in patent ductus arteriosus. If the pulse has a collapsing character but is not of a frank water-hammer type then the flick runs across only two or three fingers (moderate degree of aortic incompetence or patent ductus arteriosus, thyrotoxicosis, fever, pregnancy, moderately severe mitral incompetence, anaemia, atherosclerosis). A *slow rising* pulse can best be assessed by palpating the brachial pulse with your left thumb and, as you press *gently*, you may feel the anacrotic notch (you will need practice to appreciate this) on the upstroke against the pulp of your thumb. In mixed aortic valve disease, the combination of plateau and collapsing effects can produce a bisferiens pulse. Whilst feeling the brachial pulse, look for any catheterization *scars* (indicating valvular or ischaemic heart disease).

7 Proceed to feel the **carotid** where either a slow rising or a collapsing pulse can be confirmed.

8 Feel the **opposite radial pulse** and determine if both radials are the same (e.g. Fallot's with a Blalock shunt; see Station 3, Cardiovascular, Case 23), and then feel

9 the **right femoral pulse** checking for any *radiofemoral delay* (coarctation of the aorta). If you are asked to examine the pulses (as opposed to the pulse), you should continue to examine

10 all the other **peripheral pulses**. It is unlikely that the examiner will allow you to continue beyond what he thinks is a reasonable time to spot the diagnosis that he has in mind. However, should he not interrupt, continue to look for

11 **additional diagnostic clues**. Thus, in a patient with atrial fibrillation and features suggestive of thyrotoxicosis, you should examine the thyroid and/or eyes. In a patient with atrial fibrillation and hemiplegia or atrial fibrillation and a mitral valvotomy scar, proceed to examine the heart.

See Appendix 1, Checklist 1, Pulse.

2 | 'Examine this patient's heart'

Variations of instruction in initial PACES survey (resultant diagnoses in brackets)
Examine this patient's heart (mitral stenosis)

Examine this patient's cardiovascular system (mitral valve disease and aortic regurgitation; mitral valve disease; mixed aortic valve disease; prosthetic valves; aortic stenosis; atrial fibrillation and prosthetic mitral valve; corrected Fallot's tetralogy)

Examine this gentleman's heart. He has been complaining of palpitations (atrial fibrillation and mitral stenosis)

The GP has referred this 72-year-old lady with a murmur. Please examine her (mitral regurgitation)

This patient has been having palpitations – can you find a cause? (atrial fibrillation and mitral stenosis)

This patient is short of breath. Please examine the heart (mixed aortic valve disease)

You are seeing this elderly lady in the cardiology clinic which she has been attending for some time (prosthetic valve)

This young lady presented with increasing shortness of breath on exertion. Examine the cardiovascular system (aortic incompetence)

This lady has a heart murmur. Please examine her cardiovascular system (mitral stenosis and cerebrovascular accident)

This patient had a myocardial infarct 1 year ago. Please examine the cardiovascular system (aortic stenosis)

This man has been complaining of chest pain and palpitations. Please examine the cardiovascular system (aortic stenosis)

This patient has had an acute episode of breathlessness. Please examine the cardiovascular system (aortic stenosis)

This patient presented with shortness of breath. Please examine the cardiovascular system (mixed mitral valve disease and atrial fibrillation; aortic incompetence)

This gentleman came in on the take 2 days ago and he was breathless. Examine his cardiovascular system (atrial fibrillation and mitral regurgitation)

This man has just returned from the ITU. Please examine his cardiovascular system (prosthetic valves)

This woman, who is about 60 years of age, is becoming increasingly breathless. Can you examine her cardiovascular system and see if you can find a reason? (atrial fibrillation and mitral stenosis)

Look at this patient and describe what you see. Then listen to the heart (Marfan's syndrome and prosthetic aortic valve)

The GP has noted a murmur – can you tell me what you think?(mixed aortic valve disease)

This man has a heart murmur. Please examine him (mitral regurgitation)

Examine the cardiovascular system (hypertrophic cardiomyopathy)

Diagnoses from survey in order of frequency

1 Prosthetic valves 17%
2 Mitral incompetence (lone) 13%
3 Mixed aortic valve disease 9%
4 Mixed mitral valve disease 9%
5 Other combinations of mitral and aortic valve disease 8%
6 Mitral stenosis (lone) 7%
7 Aortic stenosis (lone) 7%
8 Aortic incompetence (lone) 5%
9 Ventricular septal defect 3%
10 Irregular pulse 2%
11 HOCM 2%
12 Marfan's syndrome (Vol. 3, Station 5, Locomotor, Case 9) 2%
13 Eisenmenger's syndrome 2%
14 Mitral valve prolapse 2%
15 Patent ductus arteriosus 2%
16 Tricuspid incompetence 2%
17 Fallot's tetralogy/Blalock shunt 0.9%
18 Raised jugular venous pressure 0.9%

19 Coarctation of the aorta 0.9%

20 Slow pulse 0.9%

21 Dextrocardia 0.5%

22 Pulmonary stenosis 0.5%

23 Cannon waves 0.5%

24 Subclavian-steal syndrome 0.3%

25 Pulmonary incompetence 0.3%

26 Infective endocarditis 0.3%

27 Atrial septal defect 0.1%

Other diagnoses were: chronic liver disease due to tricuspid incompetence (<1%), pulmonary stenosis (<1%), cor pulmonale (<1%), complete heart block (<1%), transposition of the great vessels (<1%), repaired thoracic aortic aneurysm (<1%) and left ventricular aneurysm (<1%).

Examination *routine*
When asked to 'examine this patient's heart', candidates are often uncertain as to whether they should start with the pulse or go straight to look at the heart. On the one hand, it would be absurd to feel all the pulses in the body and leave the object of the examiner's interest to the last minute, whilst on the other hand it would be impetuous to palpate the praecordium straight away. Repeating the examiner's question in the hope that he might clarify it, or asking for a clarification, does nothing but communicate your dilemma to the examiner. You should not waste any time. Bear in mind that our survey has confirmed that the diagnosis is usually mitral and/ or aortic valve disease. Approach the right-hand side of the patient and adjust the backrest so that he reclines at 45° to the mattress. If the patient is wearing a shirt, you should ask him to remove it so that the chest and neck are exposed. *Meanwhile*, you should complete a *quick:*

1 *visual survey*. Observe whether the patient is

(a) breathless,

(b) *cyanosed*,

(c) pale, or

(d) whether he has a *malar flush* (mitral stenosis).

Look briefly at the earlobes for creases* and then at the *neck* for *pulsations:*

(e) forceful carotid pulsations (Corrigan's sign in aortic incompetence; vigorous pulsation in coarctation of the aorta), or

(f) tall, sinuous venous pulsations (congestive cardiac failure, tricuspid incompetence, pulmonary hypertension, etc.).

Run your eyes down onto the chest looking for:

(g) a *left thoracotomy scar* (mitral stenosis†) or a *midline sternal scar* (valve replacement‡), and then down to the feet looking for:

---

*Frank's sign: a diagonal crease in the lobule of the auricle: grade 3 = a deep cleft across the whole earlobe; grade 2A = crease more than halfway across the lobe; grade 2B = crease across the whole lobe but superficial; grade 1 = lesser degrees of wrinkling. Earlobe creases are associated statistically with coronary artery disease in most population groups.

†NB: Vol. 2, Section F, Experiences 111 and 114.
‡Other scars may also be noted during your *visual survey* – those of previous cardiac catheterizations may be visible over the brachial arteries.

(**h**) ankle oedema. As you take the arm to feel the pulse, complete your *visual survey* by looking at the hands (a quick look; don't be ponderous) for

(**i**) clubbing of the fingers (cyanotic congenital heart disease, subacute bacterial endocarditis) and splinter haemorrhages (infective endocarditis).

If the examiner does not want you to feel the pulse he may intervene at this stage – otherwise you should proceed to

2 note the *rate* and *rhythm* of the **pulse**.

3 Quickly ascertain whether the pulse is **collapsing** (particularly if it is a large-volume pulse) or not (make sure you are seen lifting the arm up; see Vol. 2, Section F, Experience 144).

Next may be an opportune time to look for

4 **radiofemoral delay** (coarctation of the aorta), though this can be left until after auscultation if you prefer and if you are sure you will not forget it (see Vol. 2, Section F, Experience 108).

5 Feel the brachial pulse followed by the carotid pulses to see if the pulse is a **slow rising** one, especially if the volume (the upstroke) is small.

If the pulsations in the neck present any interesting features you may have already noted these during your initial *visual survey*. You should now proceed to confirm some of these impressions. The Corrigan's sign in the neck (forceful rise and quick fall of the carotid pulsation) may already have been reinforced by the discovery of a collapsing radial pulse. The individual waves of a large venous pulse can now be timed by palpating the opposite carotid. A large *v* wave, which sometimes oscillates the earlobe, suggests tricuspid incompetence and you should later on demonstrate peripheral oedema and the pulsatile liver using the bimanual technique. If the venous wave comes before the carotid pulsation, it is an *a* wave suggestive of pulmonary hypertension (mitral valve disease, cor pulmonale) or pulmonary stenosis (rare). After

6 assessing the height of the **venous pressure** in centimetres vertically above the sternal angle, you should move to the praecordium* and

7 localize the **apex beat** with respect to the mid-clavicular line and ribspaces, firstly by inspection for visible pulsation and secondly by *palpation*. If the apex beat is vigorous you should stand the index finger on it, to localize the point of maximum impulse, and *assess* the extent of its thrust. The impulse can be graded as just palpable, lifting (diastolic overload, i.e. mitral or aortic incompetence), thrusting (stronger than lifting) or heaving (outflow obstruction).

8 Palpation with your hand placed from the lower left sternal edge to the apex will detect a tapping impulse (left atrial 'knock' in mitral stenosis) or *thrills* over the mitral area (mitral valve disease), if present.

9 Continue palpation by feeling the **right ventricular lift** (left parasternal heave). To do this, place the flat of your right palm parasternally over the right ventricular area and apply *sustained* and gentle pressure. If right ventricular hypertrophy is present, you will feel the heel of your hand lifted by its force (pulmonary hypertension).

10 Next, you should **palpate** the pulmonary area for a *palpable second sound* (pulmonary hypertension), and the aortic area for a palpable *thrill* (aortic stenosis).†

---

*The *visual survey* and the examination steps 2–6 should be completed *quickly* and efficiently, particularly if you have been asked to examine the *heart*.

†The thrill of aortic stenosis is best felt if the patient leans forwards with his breath held after expiration.

If you feel a strong right ventricular lift, quickly recall, and sometimes recheck, whether there is a giant *a* wave (pulmonary hypertension, pulmonary stenosis) or *v* wave (tricuspid incompetence, congestive cardiac failure) in the neck. A palpable thrill over the mitral area (mitral valve disease) or palpable pulmonary second sound over the pulmonary area (pulmonary hypertension) should make you think of, and check for, the other complementary signs. You should by now have a fair idea of what you will hear on auscultation of the heart but you should keep an open mind for any unexpected discovery.

11 The next step will be **auscultation** and you should only stray away from the heart (examiner's command) if you have a strong expectation of being able to demonstrate an interesting and relevant sign (such as a pulsatile liver to underpin the diagnosis of tricuspid incompetence). *Time* the first heart sound with either the apex beat, if this is palpable, or by feeling the carotid pulse (see Vol. 2, Section F, Experience 188). It is important to listen to the expected murmurs in the most favourable positions. For example, mitral diastolic murmurs are best heard by turning the patient *onto the left side*, and the early diastolic murmur of aortic incompetence is made more promi-nent by asking the patient to *lean forwards* with his breath held after expiration.* For low-pitched sounds (mid-diastolic murmur of mitral stenosis, heart sounds), use the bell of your chest-piece but do not press hard or else you will be listening through a diaphragm formed by the stretched skin! The high-pitched early diastolic murmur of aortic incompetence is very easily missed (see Vol. 2, Section F, Anecdote 276). Make sure you specifically listen for it.

If the venous pressure is raised you should check for

12 sacral oedema and, if covered, expose the feet to demonstrate any *ankle oedema*. Auscultation over

13 the **lung bases** for inspiratory crepitations (left ventricular failure), though an essential part of the routine assessment of the cardiovascular system, is seldom required in the examination. You may make a special effort to do this in certain relevant situations such as a breathless patient, aortic stenosis with a displaced point of maximum impulse or if there are any signs of left heart failure (orthopnoea, pulsus alternans, gallop rhythm, etc.). Similarly, after examination of the heart itself it may (on rare occasions only) be necessary to

14 palpate the **liver**, especially if you have seen a large *v* wave and heard a pansystolic murmur over the tricuspid area. In such cases you may be able to demonstrate a *pulsatile* liver by placing your left palm posteriorly and the right palm anteriorly over the enlarged liver.† Finally, you should offer to

15 measure the **blood pressure**. This is particularly relevant in patients with aortic stenosis (low systolic and narrow pulse pressure), and aortic incompetence (wide pulse pressure).

See Appendix 1, Checklist 2, Heart.

---

*With the diaphragm of your chest-piece *ready* in position: 'Take a deep breath in; now out; hold it'. Listen intently for the absence of silence in early diastole. Ask the patient to repeat the exercise if necessary.

†An alternative and useful way of demonstrating a pulsatile liver is to place the knuckles of your closed right fist against the inferior border of the liver in the right hypochondrium (warn the patient beforehand!). Your fist will oscillate with each pulsation of the liver.

3 | 'Examine this patient's chest'

Variations of instruction in initial PACES survey (resultant diagnoses in brackets)

Examine this patient's chest (bronchiectasis; pleural effusion with chest drain; pleural effusion; bilateral lower lobectomy and fibrosis)

This gentleman is breathless on climbing stairs. Examine his respiratory system (chronic obstructive pulmonary disease)

Examine this patient's respiratory system (lung transplant and bronchiolitis obliterans; lung cancer)

This gentleman presented with a cough and shortness of breath. Please examine his respiratory system (pleural effusion)

This is a 56-year-old lady who has been dyspnoeic for a long time. Examine her respiratory system (Marfan's syndrome and pulmonary fibrosis)

This patient is complaining of shortness of breath. Please examine the chest (pleural effusion)

Examine this man's chest from the back (reduced expansion with reduced breath sounds and increased vocal resonance)

This patient presented with worsening shortness of breath. Please examine his chest (pulmonary fibrosis)

This lady is short of breath, please examine her respiratory system (pulmonary fibrosis)

This man has a long history of breathlessness. Please examine his respiratory system (pulmonary fibrosis)

Examine this lady's respiratory system from the front. About half a minute later I was asked to examine her chest from the back (carcinoma of the lung)

This gentleman has been getting more breathless in recent months. Please examine his chest (thoracotomy)

This lady is breathless. Please examine her chest (emphysema)

This man has noisy breathing. Please examine his chest to find out why (upper airways obstruction)

This man has developed a productive cough. Please examine his chest and suggest a cause (aspergillosis and old tuberculosis)

Examine this patient's respiratory system and comment on positive findings as you go (pulmonary fibrosis)

This young man is breathless. Please examine his chest (chronic obstructive pulmonary disease and α1-antitrypsin deficiency)

This man has a cough. Please examine his chest (bronchiectasis)

This man has been becoming increasingly breathless over the past 2 years. He is a non-smoker. Please examine his respiratory system to determine a cause (no diagnosis reached)

This man complains of shortness of breath. Examine him and find out why (no diagnosis reached)

Diagnoses from survey in order of frequency
 1 Interstitial lung disease (fibrosing alveolitis) 21%
 2 Pneumonectomy/lobectomy 16%

3 Bronchiectasis 12%

4 Dullness at the lung bases 10%

5 Chronic bronchitis and emphysema 8%

6 Rheumatoid lung 8%

7 Old tuberculosis 6%

8 Stridor 4%

9 Superior vena cava obstruction 3%

10 Kartagener's syndrome 2%

11 Marfan's syndrome (Vol. 3, Station 5, Locomotor, Case 9) 2%

12 Lung transplant 2%

13 Cor pulmonale 2%

14 Chest infection/consolidation/pneumonia 1%

15 Obesity/Pickwickian syndrome 1%

16 Tuberculosis/apical consolidation 1%

17 Carcinoma of the bronchus <1%

18 Pneumothorax <1%

19 Cystic fibrosis <1%

Examination *routine*

While approaching the patient, asking for his permission to examine him and settling him reclining at 45° to the bed with his chest bare, you should observe from the end of the bed

  1 his **general appearance**. Note any evidence of *weight loss*. The features of conditions such as superior vena cava obstruction (see Station 1, Respiratory, Case 22), systemic sclerosis (see Vol. 3, Station 5, Locomotor, Case 3) and lupus pernio (see Vol. 3, Station 5, Skin, Case 9) may be readily apparent as should be severe kyphoscoliosis. However, *ankylosing spondylitis* is easily missed with the patient lying down (see Vol. 2, Section F, Experiences 110 and 139). Observe specifically whether the patient

  2 is **breathless** at rest or from the effort of removing his clothes,

  3 **purses** his lips (chronic small airways obstruction), or

  4 has central **cyanosis*** (cor pulmonale, fibrosing alveolitis, bronchiectasis). Central cyanosis may be difficult to recognize; it is always preferable to look at the oral mucous membranes (see below). Observe

  5 if the **accessory muscles** are being used during breathing (chronic small airways obstruction, pleural effusion, pneumothorax, etc.),

  6 if there is generalized **indrawing** of the intercostal muscles or supraclavicular fossae (hyperinflation) or if there is indrawing of the lower ribs on inspiration (due to low, flat diaphragms in emphysema). Localized indrawing of the intercostal muscles suggests bronchial obstruction.

---

*Occurs with mean capillary concentration of ≥4g dL^{-1} of deoxygenated haemoglobin (or 0.5g dL^{-1} methaemoglobin). Alternatively, the presence of cyanosis may be supported by demonstrating a low arterial oxygen saturation (<85%) non-invasively with an ear oximeter applied to the antihelix of the ear. Central cyanosis is more readily detected in patients with polycythaemia than in those with anaemia – because of the low haemoglobin, patients with anaemia require a much lower oxygen saturation to have 4g dL^{-1} of unsaturated haemoglobin in capillary blood.

Listen to the breathing with unaided ears whilst you observe the chest wall and hands (but do not dither). This will allow a dual input whereby a combination of what you hear and what you see may help you form a diagnostic impression. You should listen to whether *expiration* is more *prolonged* than inspiration (normally the reverse), and difficult (chronic airways obstruction), whether it is *noisy* (breathlessness) and if there are any additional noises such as *wheezes* or *clicks*. Difficult and noisy inspiration is usually caused by obstruction in the major bronchi (mediastinal masses, retrosternal thyroid, bronchial carcinoma, etc.) while the more prolonged, noisy and often wheezy expiration is caused by chronic small airways obstruction (asthma, chronic bronchitis). Note the character of any cough, whether it is productive (?bronchiectasis) or dry. While you are listening, observe

7 the *movement* of the **chest wall**. It may be mainly *upwards* (emphysema) or *asymmetrical* (fibrosis, collapse, pneumonectomy, pleural effusion, pneumothorax). In the context of the examination, it is particularly important to look for localized *apical flattening* suggestive of underlying fibrosis due to old tuberculosis (see Station 1, Respiratory, Case 7) or pneumonectomy (see Station 1, Respiratory, Case 2). You may also note a thoracotomy or thoracoplasty *scar* (see Station 1, Respiratory, Cases 2 and 7) or the presence of *radiotherapy field markings* (Indian ink marks) or radiation *burns* on the chest (intrathoracic malignancy; see Vol. 3, Station 5, Skin, Case 31).

Before touching the patient, ensure that you have looked for any peripheral clues, such as sputum pots for haemoptysis or purulent sputum, nebulizer therapy, inhaler therapy, oxygen (what rate per minute?), temperature chart, peak flow chart or transplant pagers.

Check the hands for

8 **clubbing** (see Vol. 3, Station 5, Skin, Case 17), *tobacco staining*, coal dust tattoos or other conditions which affect the hands and may be associated with lung disease such as rheumatoid arthritis (nodules; see Vol. 3, Station 5, Locomotor, Case 1) or systemic sclerosis (see Vol. 3, Station 5, Locomotor, Case 3).

9 Feel the **pulse** and if it is bounding, or if the patient is cyanosed, check for a *flapping tremor* of the hands (CO_2 retention) or a fine tremor due to β-agonist therapy (salbutamol or terbutaline). If there is doubt about the presence of cyanosis, you could at this point check the tongue and the buccal mucous membranes over the premolar teeth before moving to the neck to look for

10 **raised venous pressure** (cor pulmonale) or fixed distension of the neck veins (superior vena cava obstruction). Next examine

11 the **trachea**. Place the index and ring fingers on the manubrium sternae over the prominent points on either side. Use the middle finger as the exploring finger to gently feel the tracheal rings to detect either *deviation* or a *tracheal tug* (i.e. the middle finger being pushed upwards against the trachea by the upward movement of the chest wall). Check the *notch–cricoid* distance.*

12 Feel for **lymphadenopathy** (carcinoma, tuberculosis, lymphoma, sarcoidosis) in the cervical region and axillae. As the right hand returns from the left axilla, look for

---

*The length of trachea from the suprasternal notch to the cricoid cartilage is normally three or more finger breadths. Shortening of this distance is a sign of hyperinflation.

13 the **apex beat** (difficult to localize if the chest is hyperinflated) which in conjunction with tracheal deviation may give you evidence of mediastinal displacement (collapse, fibrosis, pneumonectomy, effusion, scoliosis).

14 To look for **asymmetry**, rest one hand lightly on either side of the front of the chest to see if there is any diminution of movement (effusion, fibrosis, pneumonectomy, collapse, pneumothorax). Next grip the chest symmetrically with the fingertips in the ribspaces on either side and approximate the thumbs to meet in the middle in a straight horizontal line in order to

15 assess **expansion** first in the inframammary and then in the supramammary regions. Note the distance between each thumb and the midline (may give further information about asymmetry of movement) and between both thumbs and try to express the expansion in centimetres (it is better to produce a tape measure for a more accurate assessment of the expansion in centimetres). Comparing both sides at each level,

16 **percuss** the chest from above downwards starting with the supraclavicular fossae and over the clavicles* and do not forget to percuss over the axillae. Few clinicians now regularly map out the area of cardiac dullness. In healthy people there is dullness behind the lower left quarter of the sternum which is lost together with normal liver dullness in hyperinflation. Complete palpation by checking for

17 **tactile vocal fremitus** with the ulnar aspect of the hand applied to the chest.

18 Auscultation of the **breath sounds** should start *high* at the apices and you should remember to listen in the *axillae*. You are advised to cover both lung fields first with the bell† before using the diaphragm (if for no other reason than that this allows you a chance to check the findings without appearing to backtrack!). In the nervousness of the examination, harsh breathing heard with the diaphragm near a major bronchus (over the second intercostal space anteriorly or below the scapula near the mid-line posteriorly) may give an impression of bronchial breathing, particularly in thin people. Compare corresponding points on opposite sides of the chest. Ensure that the patient breathes with the mouth open, regularly and deeply, but not noisily (see Vol. 2, Section F, Experience 162). Auscultation is completed by checking

19 **vocal resonance‡** in all areas; **if** you have found an area of bronchial breathing (the sounds may resound close to your ears – aegophony), check also for whispering pectoriloquy. The classic timings of crackles/crepitations of various origins are:

    (a) *early inspiratory*: chronic bronchitis, asthma,

    (b) *early and mid-inspiratory and recurring in expiration*: bronchiectasis (altered by coughing),

    (c) *mid/late inspiratory*: restrictive lung disease (e.g. fibrosing alveolitis§) and pulmonary oedema.

20 **To examine the back** of the chest, sit the patient forward (it may help to cross the arms in front of the patient to pull the scapulae further apart) and repeat steps 14–19. You may wish to start the examination of the back by palpating for cervical

---

*Percussion on the bare clavicle may cause discomfort to the patient.

†Many physicians prefer to use the diaphragm in their routine examination of the chest, though purists believe that as the respiratory auscultatory sounds are usually of low pitch, the bell is preferable.

‡See Footnote, Station 1, Respiratory, Case 21.

§In fibrosing alveolitis, late inspiratory crackles may become reduced if the patient is made to lean forward; thereby the compressed dependent alveoli (which crackle-open in late inspiration) are relieved of the pressure of the lungs.

nodes from behind (particularly the scalene nodes between the two heads of the sternomastoid).

Though with sufficient practice this whole procedure can be performed rapidly without loss of efficiency, often in the examination you will only be asked to perform some of it – usually 'examine the back of the chest'. As always when forced to perform only part of the complete *routine*, be sure that the partial examination is no less thorough and professional. Be prepared to put on your 'wide-angled lenses' so as not to miss other related signs (see Vol. 2, Section F, Experience 108 and Anecdotes 254 and 255).

Though by now you will usually have sufficient information to present your findings, occasionally you will wish to check other features on the basis of the findings so far. Commonly, you will wish to inspect the ankles for oedema and, if relevant and available, the peak flow chart and temperature chart. Further purposeful examination gives an impression of confidence but it should not be overdone. For example, looking for evidence of Horner's syndrome or wasting of the muscles of one hand* in a patient with apical dullness and a deviated trachea will suggest professional keenness whereas routinely looking at the eyes and hands after completion of the examination may only suggest to the examiner that you do not have the diagnosis and are hoping for inspiration! If you suspect airways obstruction, the examiner may be impressed if you perform a bedside respiratory function test – the *forced expiratory time* (FET).†

See Appendix 1, Checklist 3, Chest.

4 | 'Examine this patient's abdomen'

Variations of instruction in initial PACES survey (resultant diagnoses in brackets)
Examine this patient's abdomen (transplanted kidney; hepatomegaly and lymph nodes; ascites and chronic liver disease; ascites and hepatosplenomegaly)
This gentleman was found collapsed. Examine his abdomen and give a differential as to the cause of his collapse (alcoholic liver disease)
This gentleman has lost weight and is experiencing fullness in his abdomen. Please examine the abdomen (hepatosplenomegaly and axillary lymph nodes)

*A good *visual survey* may reveal such signs at the beginning.
†Ask the patient to take a deep breath in and then, on your command (timed with the second hand of your watch), to breathe out as hard and as fast as he can until his lungs are completely empty. A normal person will empty his lungs in less than 6 sec (1 sec for every decade of age, e.g. a normal 30-year-old will do it in 3 seconds). An FET of >6 sec is evidence of airways obstruction. You need to practise this test with patients if it is to

be slick. As with peak flow rate (PFR) and forced expiratory volume in 1 second (FEV$_1$), etc., it is important to make sure that certain patients, particularly females, *are* blowing as hard and as fast as they can ('don't worry about what you look like – give it everything you've got – like this' and give a demonstration) and empty their lungs completely ('keep going, keep going . . . keep going, well done!').

This lady has thrombocytopenia. Examine her abdomen and come up with a likely diagnosis (splenomegaly)

This patient is complaining of tiredness, examine his abdomen (hepatosplenomegaly and rheumatoid hands)

Examine this gentleman's abdomen (alcoholic liver disease, tender hepatomegaly and encephalopathy)

This man has pain on walking. Please examine his abdomen (hepatosplenomegaly and polycythaemia rubra vera)

This patient's abdomen has shown intermittent swelling – what could one cause be? (alcoholic liver disease)

Examine this abdomen (jaundice, parotid swelling and palpable liver; hepat-osplenomegaly and ascites; hepatosplenomegaly and Dupuytren's contracture)

This patient has been referred from the cardiology clinic with sweats and a mass in the abdomen. Please examine (infective endocarditis)

Please examine this gentleman's abdominal system and comment on the findings (alcoholic liver disease)

I was given some haematology results which were suggestive that the patient might have a spleen palpable. Examine the abdomen (splenomegaly)

This patient attends the renal clinic with hypertension. Please examine his abdominal system (transplanted kidney)

This 62-year-old man has a lymphocytosis. Please examine his abdomen (splenomegaly)

This lady has been having abdominal pain. Please examine and suggest a cause (polycystic kidneys and polycystic liver)

Examine this man's abdomen, commenting on what you are doing (hepatosplenomegaly)

Please examine the abdomen of this man who is complaining of pruritus (polycystic kidneys)

This man has high blood pressure. Please examine his abdomen (heart transplant and dialysis fistula)

This 43-year-old man failed a routine medical examination for insurance purposes. Please examine the abdomen and suggest if you can find a reason why (hepatomegaly)

Examine this man's abdomen and tell me what you find (chronic liver disease)

Diagnoses from survey in order of frequency

1 Chronic liver disease 21%
2 Hepatosplenomegaly 17%
3 Polycystic kidneys 14%
4 Splenomegaly (without hepatomegaly) 13%
5 Transplanted kidney 9%
6 Hepatomegaly (no splenomegaly) 5%
7 Ascites 4%
8 Polycythaemia rubra vera 4%
9 Abdominal mass 2%
10 Carcinoid 2%
11 Crohn's disease 1%

12 Idiopathic haemochromatosis 1%
13 Nephrotic syndrome <1%
14 Hereditary spherocytosis <1%
15 Felty's syndrome <1%
16 Generalized lymphadenopathy <1%
17 Single palpable kidney <1%
18 Primary biliary cirrhosis <1%

Other diagnoses were: aortic aneurysm (1%), haemochromatosis (<1%), polycystic kidneys and a transplanted kidney (<1%), splenomegaly and generalized lymphadenopathy (<1%), abdominal lymphadenopathy (<1%), postsplenectomy (<1%) and normal abdomen (<1%).

Examination *routine*

Analysis of the above list reveals that in over 80% of cases, the findings in the abdomen relate to a palpable spleen, liver or kidneys. Bearing this in mind, you should approach the right-hand side of the patient and position him so that he is lying supine on one pillow (if comfortable), with the whole abdomen and chest in full view. Ideally, the genitalia should also be exposed but to avoid embarrassment to patients, who are volunteers and whose genitals are usually normal, we suggest that you ask the patient to lower his garments and ensure that these are pulled down to a level about halfway between the iliac crest and the symphysis pubis. While these preparations are being made you should be performing

1 a *visual survey* of the patient. Amongst the many relevant physical signs that you may observe in these few seconds are pallor, pigmentation, jaundice, spider naevi, xanthelasma, parotid swelling, gynaecomastia, scratch marks, tattoos, abdominal distension, distended abdominal veins, an abdominal swelling, herniae and decreased body hair. If you use the following *routine* most of these will also be noted during your subsequent examination but at this stage you should particularly note any

2 **pigmentation**. As the patient is being correctly positioned,

3 *quickly* **examine the hands*** for:
   (a) Dupuytren's contracture,
   (b) clubbing,
   (c) leuconychia,
   (d) palmar erythema, and
   (e) a flapping tremor (if relevant).

After asking you to examine the abdomen, many examiners would like, and *expect*, you to concentrate on the abdomen itself without delay, and yet they will not forgive you for missing an abnormal physical sign elsewhere. This emphasizes the importance of a good *visual survey*; a trained eye will miss nothing important on the face or in the hands while the patient is being properly positioned with the hands by his side. Thus, steps 1–3 need not occupy you for more than a few seconds; you may wish to omit steps 5 and 6 if there is no visible abnormality, and steps 7–11 can be completed as part of the *visual survey*.

*For a full list of the signs that may be visible in the hands in chronic liver disease, see Station 1, Abdominal, Case 3.

4 Pull down the lower eyelid to look for *anaemia*. At the same time check the sclerae for *icterus* and look for *xanthelasma*. The guttering between the eyeball and the lower lid is the best place to look for pallor or for any discoloration (e.g. cyanosis, jaundice, etc.).

5 Look at the lips for cyanosis (cirrhosis of the liver) and shine your pen torch into the mouth* looking for swollen lips (Crohn's), telangiectasis (Osler–Weber–Rendu), patches of pigmentation (Peutz–Jeghers) and mouth ulcers (Crohn's).

6 Palpate the neck and supraclavicular fossae for *cervical lymph nodes*.† If you do find lymph nodes you should then proceed to examine the axillae and groins for evidence of generalized lymphadenopathy (lymphoma, chronic lymphatic leukaemia). As you move from the neck to the chest, check for

7 gynaecomastia (palpate for glandular breast tissue in obese subjects),

8 spider naevi (may have been noted already on hands, arms and face and may also be present on the back), and

9 scratch marks (may have been noted on the arms, and may also be found on the back and elsewhere). Next,

10 look at the chest (in the male) and in the axillae for **paucity of hair** (if diminished, note facial hair in the male; pubic hair, if not visible, may be noted later).

11 Observe the abdomen in *three segments* (epigastric, umbilical and suprapubic) for any visible signs such as *pulsations*, generalized *distension* (ascites) or a *swelling* in one particular area. Note any scars or fistulae (previous surgery; Crohn's). Look for distended *abdominal* veins (the flow is away from the umbilicus in portal hypertension but upwards from the groin in inferior vena cava obstruction).

With practice, the examination to this point can be completed very rapidly and will provide valuable information which may be overlooked if proceeding carelessly straight to palpation of the abdomen (see Vol. 2, Section F, Experience 109). If the examiner insists that you start with abdominal palpation‡ it suggests that there is little to be found elsewhere, but you should nevertheless be prepared to use your 'wide-angled lenses' in order not to miss any of the above features.

12 Palpation of the abdomen should be performed in an orthodox manner; any temptation to go straight for a visible swelling should be resisted. Put your palm gently over the abdomen and ask the patient if he has any tenderness and to let you know if you hurt him. First systematically examine the whole of the abdomen with *light palpation*. Palpation should be done with the *pulps* of the fingers rather than the tips, the best movement being a gentle flexion at the metacarpophalangeal joints with the hand flat on the abdominal wall. Next, examine specifically for the *internal organs*. For both liver and spleen, start in the right iliac fossa (you cannot be frowned

---

*Though a brief examination of the mouth is usefully included as part of the full 'examine the abdomen' *routine*, it is worth noting that in our survey when there were the findings mentioned, the candidates were given a more specific instruction such as 'Look at this patient's mouth'.

†The supraclavicular lymph nodes, particularly on the left side, may be enlarged with carcinoma of the stomach (*Troisier's sign*; NB: *Virchow's node* behind the left sternoclavicular joint) or carcinoma of any other abdominal organ or with carcinoma of the bronchus.

‡Some examiners admit to being irritated at seeing candidates examine normal hands for a long time after being asked to examine the abdomen. They argue that the information obtainable from the face, mouth and hands can be gathered without delay during the inspection part of the examination (see Vol. 2, Section F, Anecdote 265).

upon for following this orthodox procedure*), working upwards to the right hypochondrium in the case of the *liver* and diagonally across the abdomen to the left hypochondrium in the case of the *spleen*. The organs are felt against the radial border of the index finger and the pulps of the index and middle fingers as they descend on inspiration, at which time you can gently press and move your hand upwards to meet them. The *kidneys* are then sought by bimanual palpation of each lateral region. The lower pole of the normal right kidney can sometimes be felt, especially in thin women. Palpation of the internal organs may be difficult if there is ascites. In this case, the technique is to press quickly, flexing at the wrist joint, to displace the fluid and palpate the enlarged organ ('dipping' or 'ballotting'). In a patient well chosen for the examination, a mass in the left hypochondrium may present a problem of identification (see Vol. 2, Section F, Experiences 131 and 245, and Anecdotes 268 and 270); the examiner (testing your confidence) may ask you if you are sure that it is a spleen and not a kidney or vice versa. Do not forget to establish whether you can *get above* the mass and *separate* it from the costal edge, whether you can *bimanually* palpate it and whether the percussion note over it is *resonant* (all features of an enlarged kidney; see also Station 1, Abdominal, Case 6 for the features of a spleen). Palpate *deeply* with the pulps to look for the *ascending* and *descending colons* in the flanks, and use *gentle* palpation to feel for an *aortic aneurysm* in the mid-line. Complete palpation by feeling for *inguinal lymph nodes*, noting obvious herniae and, at the same time, adding information about the distribution and thickness of pubic hair to that already gained about the rest of the body hair.

13 Percussion must be used from the nipple downwards on both sides to locate the upper edge of the liver on the right and the spleen on the left (NB: the left lower lateral chest wall may become dull to percussion before an enlarged spleen is palpable). The lower palpable edges of the spleen and liver should be defined by percussion in an orthodox manner, proceeding from the resonant to dull areas. If you suspect free fluid in the peritoneum, you must establish its presence by demonstrating

14 shifting dullness. Initially check for *stony dullness* in the flanks. There is no need to continue with the procedure of demonstrating shifting dullness if this is not present. By asking the patient with ascites to turn on his side, you can shift the dullness from the upper to the lower flank.

Before you conclude the palpation and percussion of the abdomen, ask yourself whether you have found anything abnormal. If there are no abnormal physical signs, make sure that you have not missed a polycystic kidney or a palpable splenic edge (or occasionally a mass in the epigastrium or iliac fossae). During your auscultation listen carefully for a bruit over the aorta and renal vessels. Generally speaking,

15 auscultation has very little to contribute in the examination setting, but as part of the full *routine* you should listen to the bowel sounds, check for renal artery bruits and for any other sounds such as a rub over the spleen or kidney or a venous hum (both excessively rare).

Examination of the

*Even though it is the time-honoured, orthodox procedure, many clinicians these days are opposed to this practice. They argue that a grossly enlarged spleen will be picked up on the initial light palpation which makes the approach from the right iliac fossa unnecessary. If they do not feel a mass in the left hypochondrium on initial palpation, they start deep palpation a few centimetres below the left costal edge.

16 external genitalia is not usually required in the examination for the reasons given above, and we have never heard of a case where

17 a rectal examination was required. You should, however, comment that you would like to complete your examination of the abdomen by examining the external genitalia (especially in the male with chronic liver disease – small testes; or cervical lymphadenopathy – drainage of testes to paraaortic and cervical lymph nodes) and rectum. You may of course never get this far since the examiner may interrupt you at an appropriate stage to ask for your findings. If you are allowed to conclude the examination and you have found nothing abnormal despite your careful search, on rare occasions the diagnosis of a normal abdomen will be accepted (see Station 1, Abdominal, Case 11).

See Appendix 1, Checklist 4, Abdomen.

5 | 'Examine this patient's visual fields'

Variations of instruction from our original survey
Examine this patient's visual fields and fundi*

Diagnoses from our original survey in order of frequency
1 Homonymous hemianopia 25%
2 Optic atrophy (Vol. 3, Station 5, Eyes, Case 3) 21%
3 Bitemporal hemianopia 21%
4 Unilateral hemianopia 7%
5 Partial field defect in one eye due to retinal artery branch occlusion (Vol. 3, Station 5, Eyes, Case 16) 7%
6 Bilateral homonymous quadrantic field defect 4%
7 Acromegaly (Vol. 3, Station 5, Endocrine, Case 2) 4%

Examination *routine*
Ask the patient to sit upright on the side of the bed while you position yourself in visual confrontation about a metre away. This apposition will help you to test the visual fields of his left and right eyes against those of your right and left respectively. As he is doing this, perform
1 a *visual survey* (acromegaly, hemiparesis, cerebellar signs in multiple sclerosis) of the patient. Test both temporal fields together so that you do not miss any *visual inattention*. Ask the patient to look at your eyes while you place your index fingers just inside the outer limits of your temporal fields. Then move your fingers in turn and then both at the same time, and ask him: 'Point to the finger which moves'. If there is visual inattention, the patient will only point to one finger when you move both at the same time. Next test each eye individually and ask him to cover his right eye with his right hand, and close your left eye: 'Keep looking at my eye'.

*See also Introduction.

2 Examine his **peripheral visual fields**. Test his left temporal vision against your right temporal by moving your wagging finger from the periphery towards the centre: 'Tell me when you see my finger move'.* The temporal field should be tested in the horizontal plane and by moving your finger through the upper and lower temporal quadrants. Change hands and repeat on the nasal side. By comparing his visual field with your own, any areas of field defect are thus mapped out. The visual fields of his right eye are similarly tested.

3 **A central scotoma** is tested for with a red-headed hat pin. If you have already found a field defect which does not require further examination, or if the examiner does not wish you to continue, he will soon stop you. Otherwise, comparing your right eye with the patient's left, as before, move the red-headed pin from the temporal periphery through the central field to the nasal periphery, asking the patient: 'Can you see the head of the pin? What colour is it? Tell me if it disappears or changes colour'.

Patients with optic neuropathy may report altered colour vision even if there is no absolute central loss of vision. If there is no scotoma, find his blind spot and compare it with your own. The blind spot may be enlarged in chronic papilloedema or consecutive optic atrophy.

Having found the field defect, look for

4 **additional features** (e.g. acromegaly, hemiparesis, nystagmus and cerebellar signs) if appropriate. Recall the possible causes for each type of field defect as this question, at the end of the case, is inevitable (see Station 3, CNS, Case 13).

See Appendix 1, Checklist 5, Visual fields.

6 | 'Examine this patient's cranial nerves'

Variations of instruction in initial PACES survey (resultant diagnoses in brackets)
Examine this patient's cranial nerves (right homonymous hemianopia)
Examine this patient's cranial nerves and check the reflexes in the lower limbs as this patient has had a noticeable weakness of both legs (multiple sclerosis)

Diagnoses from our MRCP surveys
1 Right homonymous hemianopia with macula sparing
2 Bulbar palsy
3 Internuclear ophthalmoplegia – multiple sclerosis
4 Cerebellopontine angle syndrome
5 Myasthenia gravis

---

*This will pick up most gross visual field defects rapidly. Moving objects are more easily detected and therefore your moving finger will be immediately noticed by the patient as it moves out of the blind area into his field of vision. Remember that his area of blindness to a stationary object may be greater than that to a moving object. In the dysphasic patient, you should ask him to point at the moving finger when he sees it rather than telling you he sees it.

6 Ocular palsy and dysarthria

7 Unilateral VIth, VIIth nerve palsies and nystagmus and possibly a XIIth nerve palsy*

8 Unilateral IXth, Xth, XIth and XIIth nerve lesions (suggesting jugular foramen syndrome†)

Examination *routine*

Perhaps surprisingly, this instruction was comparatively rare in our surveys before PACES, but seems to have experienced a slight increase in popularity in the PACES era, appearing in 4% of the PACES survey reports we have received (see Vol. 2, Section F, Experiences 26 and 30). It is one of the most feared instructions but at the same time it can provide an opportunity to score highly. More than in any other system, the well-rehearsed candidate can appear competent and professional compared with the unrehearsed. Detailed examination of the individual nerves is not usually required but rather a quick and efficient screen like that used by neurologists at the bedside or in outpatients (it is well worth attending neurology outpatients to watch quick and efficient examination techniques, if for nothing else). Not only can you look good but also the abnormalities are usually easy to detect. Although it is to be hoped that your practised *routine* will not miss out any nerves, it is preferable to perform a smooth, professional examination, which accidentally misses out a nerve, than to test your examiner's patience through a hesitant and meditative examination which takes a long time to start and may never finish! Since the examination is most easily carried out face to face with the patient, it is best, if possible, to get him to sit on the edge of the bed facing you. First

  1 take a good general and *quick* **look** at the patient, in particular his face, for any obvious abnormality. Next ask him about

  2 his sense of **smell** and **taste**: 'Do you have any difficulty with your sense of smell?' (I). Although you should have the ability to examine taste (VII, IX) and smell formally if equipment is provided, usually questioning (or possibly the judicious use of a bedside orange) is all that is required. All the examination referable to the eyes is best performed next. Unless there is a Snellen chart available, ask the patient to look at the clock on the wall or some newspaper print to give you a good idea of his

  3 **visual acuity:**

    'Do you have any difficulty with your vision?'

    'Can you see the clock on the wall?' (if he has glasses for long sight he should put them on)

    'Can you tell me what time it says?' (II).

A portable Snellen chart will enable you to perform a more formal test.

Now test the

  4 **visual fields** (see Section B, Examination *Routine* 5 above), including for *central scotoma*, with a red-headed hat pin. Follow this by examining

  5 **eye movements** (move your finger in the shape of a cross, from side to side then up and down): 'Look at my finger; follow it with your eyes' (III, IV, VI), asking the

---

*The candidate diagnosed a XIIth nerve palsy and passed (see Vol. 2, Section F, Experience 108), but see footnote * on the opposite page.

†This diagnosis was not made by the candidate.

patient at the extremes of gaze whether he sees one or two fingers. If he has diplopia, establish the extent and ask him to describe the 'false' image. As you test eye movements, note at the same time any

6 **nystagmus** (VIII, cerebellum or cerebellar connections; see Fig. C3.21, Station 3, CNS, Case 32, or

7 **ptosis** (III, sympathetic).

Remember that either extreme abduction of the eyes or gazing at a finger that is too near can cause nystagmus in normal eyes (optokinetic). Now examine

8 the **pupils** for the direct and consensual *light reflex* (II → optic tract → lateral geniculate ganglion → Edinger–Westphal nucleus of III → fibres to ciliary muscle) and for the *accommodation–convergence* reflex (cortex → III) with your finger just in front of his nose:

'Look into the distance'

'Now look at my finger' (see also Footnote, Section B, Examination *Routine* 13). Finally examine the optic discs (II) by

9 **fundoscopy** (this can be left until last if you prefer). Having finished examining the eyes, examine

10 **facial movements:**

'Raise your eyebrows'

'Screw your eyes up tight'

'Puff your cheeks out'

'Whistle'

'Show me your teeth'

$\left.\begin{array}{l} \text{} \\ \text{} \\ \text{} \\ \text{} \\ \text{} \end{array}\right\}$ VII

'Clench your teeth' – feel masseters and temporalis

'Open your mouth; stop me closing it'

$\left.\begin{array}{l} \text{} \\ \text{} \\ \text{} \end{array}\right\}$ motor V

11 then **palatal movement:**

'Keep your mouth open; say aah' (IX, X)

12 and **gag reflex*** – touch the back of the pharynx on both sides with an orange stick (IX, X). Look at

13 the **tongue** as it lies in the floor of the mouth for *wasting* or *fasciculation* (XII):

'Open your mouth again'

then get the patient to:

'Put your tongue out' – note any deviation† – 'waggle it from side to side' (XII).

14 Test the **accessory nerve:**‡

'Shrug your shoulders; keep them shrugged' – push down on the shoulders (XI).

'Turn your head to the left side, now to the right' – feel for the sternomastoid muscle on the side opposite to the turned head (XI).

Finally test

---

*This can be unpleasant, so ask the examiner's permission, explain to the patient and ask for his permission as well.

†In unilateral facial paralysis, the protruded tongue, though otherwise normal, may deviate so that unilateral hypoglossal paralysis is suspected (see Station 3, CNS, Case 35). In unilateral lower motor neurone XIIth nerve palsy there is wasting (?fasciculation) on the side of the lesion and the tongue curves to that side.

‡Painless neck weakness has only four causes: myasthenia gravis (see Station 3, CNS, Case 27), myotonic dystrophy (see Station 3, CNS, Case 2), polymyositis (see Station 3, CNS, Case 45) and motor neurone disease (see Station 3, CNS, Case 11).

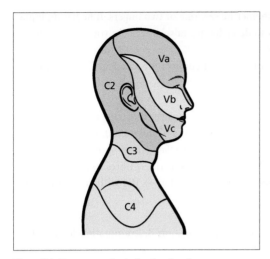

Figure B.1 Dermatomes in the head and neck.

15 **hearing:**

'Any problem with the hearing in either ear?'

'Can you hear that?' – rub finger and thumb together in front of each ear in turn (VIII – proceed to the Rinné and Weber tests* if there is any abnormality, and look in the ear if you suspect disease of the external ear, perforated drum, wax, etc.), and

16 test **facial sensation** including *corneal reflex* (sensory V; see Fig. B.1).

See Appendix 1, Checklist 6, Cranial nerves.

7 | 'Examine this patient's arms'

Variations of instruction in initial PACES survey (resultant diagnoses in brackets)

This elderly lady has had some falls and difficulty with mobility. Please examine her upper limbs (drug-induced dystonia)

This patient has a worsening tremor of his upper limbs. Please give some reasons (intention tremor and patchy peripheral sensory neuropathy)

This patient has a 20-year history of weakness in the right arm and shoulder (C5 radiculopathy)

*Weber test: sound from a vibrating tuning fork held on the centre of the forehead is conducted towards the ear if it has a conductive defect (e.g. wax or otitis media) and away from the ear if it has a nerve deafness. Rinné test: a positive test (normal) is when the sound of the tuning fork is louder by air conduction (prongs by external auditory meatus) than by bone conduction (base of fork on mastoid process). Negative is abnormal.

Examine this patient's upper limbs. There has been a weakness for about the last 5 years (motor neurone disease)

This lady has difficulty doing the housework, especially taking things out of cupboards. Look at her face and examine her hands (myotonic dystrophy)

This man had an operation which is unrelated to the case, then woke with a weak left arm. Why? (radial nerve palsy)

This 50-year-old lady has problems driving. Examine her arms to find out why (arthritis secondary to ulcerative colitis)

Diagnoses from our original survey in order of frequency

1 Wasting of the small muscles of the hand 26%
2 Motor neurone disease 19%
3 Hemiplegia 7%
4 Cerebellar syndrome 6%
5 Cervical myelopathy 6%
6 Neurofibromatosis 4%
7 Muscular dystrophy 4%
8 Psoriasis (Vol. 3, Station 5, Skin, Case 4) 4%
9 Purpura due to steroids (Vol. 3, Station 5, Skin, Case 25) 4%
10 Parkinson's disease 3%
11 Syringomyelia 3%
12 Hemiballismus 3%
13 Lichen planus (Vol. 3, Station 5, Skin, Case 11) 3%
14 Pseudoxanthoma elasticum (Vol. 3, Station 5, Skin, Case 10) 3%
15 Old polio 3%
16 Rheumatoid arthritis (Vol. 3, Station 5, Locomotor, Case 1) 3%
17 Axillary vein thrombosis 3%
18 Contracture of the elbow in a case of haemophilia 3%
19 Ulnar nerve palsy 1%
20 Pancoast's syndrome 1%
21 Herpes zoster (Vol. 3, Station 5, Skin, Case 32) 1%
22 Mycosis fungoides (Vol. 3, Station 5, Skin, Case 34) 1%
23 Polymyositis 1%

Examination *routine*

Consideration of the above list from the survey reveals that the vast majority (over 80%) of conditions behind this instruction are neurological with a handful of spot diagnoses which will usually be obvious. If the diagnosis is not an obvious 'spot' (and you should make sure that you would recognize each on the list – see individual short cases in this book and in Volume 3), your *routine* should commence in the usual way by scanning the whole patient but in particular looking at

1 the **face** for obvious abnormalities such as *asymmetry* (hemiplegia), *nystagmus* (cerebellar syndrome), *wasting* (muscular dystrophy), sad, immobile, unblinking facies (*Parkinson's* disease) or *Horner's* syndrome (syringomyelia, Pancoast's syndrome). You may return to seek a less obvious Horner's or nystagmus later, if necessary. In search of obvious abnormalities, run your eyes down to

2 the **neck** (pseudoxanthoma elasticum, lymph nodes), and then scan down the arms looking in particular at

3 the **elbows** which should be particularly inspected for *psoriasis, rheumatoid nodules* and *scars* or *deformity* underlying an ulnar nerve palsy. Before picking up the hands look for

4 a **tremor** (Parkinson's disease), then briefly inspect

5 the **hands** in the same way as you have practised under 'Examine this patient's hands' (see Section B, Examination *Routine* 15), looking at

    (a) the joints (swelling, deformity),

    (b) nail changes (pitting, onycholysis, clubbing, nail-fold infarcts), and

    (c) skin changes (colour, consistency, lesions).

If you have not already been led towards a diagnosis requiring specific action, start a full neurological examination by studying first

6 the **muscle bulk** in the upper arms, lower arms and hands, bearing in mind that in about one-quarter of cases there will be wasting of the small muscles of the hands (see Station 3, CNS, Case 52), and in one-fifth of cases there will be motor neurone disease which means wasting and

7 fasciculation.

8 Test the **tone** in the arms by passively bending the arm (with the patient relaxed) to and fro in an irregular and unexpected fashion, and in the hands by flexing and extending all the joints, including the wrist in the classic 'rolling wave' fashion used to detect cog-wheel rigidity (Parkinson's disease).

9 Ask the patient: '**Hold your arms out in front of you**' (look for *winging* of the scapulae, involuntary movements or the *myelopathy hand sign**); 'Now close your eyes' (look for *sensory wandering* – parietal drift or pseudoathetosis (see Fig. C3.17c, Station 3, CNS, Case 26).

Next test

10 power:

    (a) 'Put your arms out to the side' (demonstrate this to the patient yourself – arms at 90° to your body with elbows flexed); 'Stop me pushing them down' (deltoid – C5),

    (b) 'Bend your elbow; stop me straightening it' (biceps – C5, 6),

    (c) 'Push your arm out straight' – resist elbow extension (triceps – C7),

    (d) 'Squeeze my fingers' – offer two fingers (C8, T1),†

    (e) 'Hold your fingers out straight' (demonstrate); 'Stop me bending them' (if the patient can do this there is nothing wrong with motor C7 or the radial nerve),

    (f) 'Spread your fingers apart' (demonstrate); 'Stop me pushing them together' (dorsal interossei – ulnar nerve),

---

*With the hands outstretched and supinated, passive abduction of the little finger indicates a pyramidal lesion or ulnar nerve palsy (sensory testing should distinguish). The sign is common in, but not specific for, cervical pyramidal lesions – as the lesion becomes more severe, adjacent fingers also passively abduct.

†See Footnote, Section B, Examination *Routine* 15.

(g) 'Hold this piece of paper between your fingers; stop me pulling it out' (palmar interossei – ulnar nerve),

(h) 'Point your thumb at the ceiling; stop me pushing it down' (abductor pollicis brevis – median nerve),

(i) 'Put your thumb and little finger together; stop me pulling them apart' (opponens pollicis – median nerve).

11 Test coordination

(a) 'Can you do this?' – demonstrate by flexing your elbows at right angles and then pronating and supinating your forearms as rapidly as possible,

(b) 'Tap quickly on the back of your hand' (demonstrate),

(c) 'Touch my finger; touch your nose; backwards and forwards quickly and neatly' (demonstrate if necessary – vary the target).

12 Check the biceps (C5, 6), triceps (C7), supinator (C5, 6) and finger (C8) **reflexes**.

13 Finally perform a **sensory screen** with *light touch* and *pinprick*, bearing in mind the dermatomes shown in Fig. B.2 and the areas of sensation covered by the ulnar, median and radial nerves in the hand (see Fig. B.4, Examination *Routine* 15). Finally, check *vibration* and *joint position* sense.

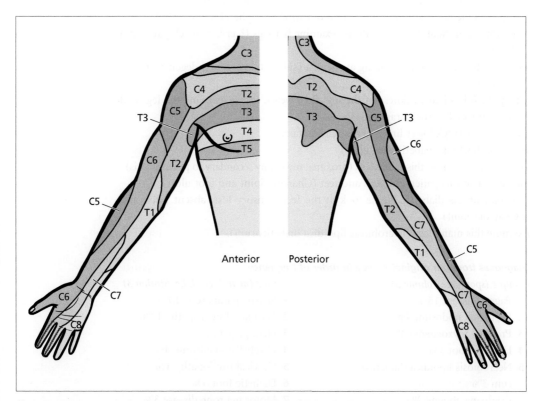

Figure B.2 Dermatomes in the upper limb. (After Foerster, 1933, Oxford University Press, *Brain* **56**: 1.) There is considerable variation and overlap between the cutaneous areas supplied by each spinal root so that an isolated root lesion results in a much smaller area of sensory impairment than the diagram indicates.

We leave you to consider where else you could look with each of the conditions given on the list in order to find additional information (see individual short cases). For example, you could look for nystagmus should you find cerebellar signs, or for Horner's syndrome should you suspect syringomyelia or Pancoast's syndrome.

See Appendix 1, Checklist 7, Arms.

8 | 'Examine this patient's legs'

Variations of instruction in initial PACES survey (resultant diagnoses in brackets)

Examine this patient's legs (subarachnoid haemorrhage; hereditary sensory and motor neuropathy; mixed upper and lower motor neurone disorders)

Examine this lady's nervous system but concentrate on the legs (Charcot–Marie–Tooth disease)

This man is unable to walk. Examine his legs (?cauda equina lesion)

This 84-year-old lady has been having difficulty walking and with her balance. Would you examine her neurologically to find out why? (peripheral neuropathy)

This lady has difficulty walking. Please examine her legs (?cervical myelopathy and diabetes)

Examine the legs but omit looking at the gait (subacute combined degeneration of the cord)

This patient has had weakness of the legs for 3 years. Please examine the legs and find out why (spastic paraparesis)

Examine this lady's lower limbs (Friedreich's ataxia)

Examine this foot (diabetic foot ulcer)

Look at, and examine, this man's legs (proximal myopathy secondary to polymyositis)

Please look at this patient's ankles and feet (Charcot's joint and foot ulcer)

This patient has diabetes. Please look at the feet (sensory loss, absent pulse and Charcot's joint)

Examine this man's legs (necrobiosis lipoidica diabeticorum).

Diagnoses from our original survey in order of frequency

Group 1 (spot – see Volume 3)	Group 2 (neurological, i.e. Station 3)
1 Paget's disease 13%	1 Spastic paraparesis 13%
2 Erythema nodosum 4%	2 Peripheral neuropathy 12%
3 Pretibial myxoedema 4%	3 Hemiplegia 5%
4 Diabetic foot 3%	4 Cerebellar syndrome 4%
5 Necrobiosis lipoidica diabetico-rum 3%	5 Cervical myelopathy 4%
6 Erythema ab igne 2%	6 Diabetic foot 3%
7 Vasculitis 2%	7 Motor neurone disease 3%
	8 Old polio 3%

8 Swollen knee 1%
9 Pemphigoid/pemphigus <1%
10 Deep venous thrombosis/ruptured Baker's cyst <1%
11 Multiple thigh abscesses <1%
12 Vasculitic leg ulcers <1%
13 Pyoderma gangrenosum <1%
14 Stigmata of sickle cell disease <1%
15 Mycosis fungoides <1%
16 Diabetic ischaemia <1%
17 Ehlers–Danlos syndrome <1%
18 Bilateral below-knee amputation <1%

9 Absent leg reflexes and extensor plantars 3%
10 Friedreich's ataxia 2%
11 Subacute combined degeneration of the cord 2%
12 Charcot–Marie–Tooth disease 1%
13 Polymyositis <1%
14 Lateral popliteal (common peroneal) nerve palsy <1%
15 Tabes <1%
16 Diabetic amyotrophy <1%

Examination *routine*

An analysis of the conditions in our survey shows that they roughly fall into the two broad groups shown above:

Group 1: a spot diagnosis (these cases are covered in Volume 3)

Group 2: a neurological diagnosis (i.e. Station 3).

Either way initial clues may be gained by first performing a brief

1 ***visual survey*** of the patient as a whole. Look at the head and face for signs such as *enlargement* (Paget's disease), *asymmetry* (hemiparesis), *exophthalmos* with or without *myxoedematous facies* (pretibial myxoedema) or obvious *nystagmus* (cerebellar syndrome). Run your eyes over the patient for other significant signs such as thyroid *acropachy* (pretibial myxoedema), *rheumatoid hands* (swollen knee), nicotine-stained fingers (leg amputations), *wasted hands* (motor neurone disease, Charcot–Marie–Tooth disease, syringomyelia) and for muscle *fasciculation* (usually motor neurone disease).

Turning to the legs, look at the skin, joints and general shape and for any

2 **obvious lesion**, especially from the list of disorders in group 1. If such a lesion is visible a further full examination of the legs will not be required in most cases. You will be able to begin your description and/or diagnosis immediately (see individual short cases). If there is no obvious lesion look again specifically for

3 **bowing** of the tibia (see Vol. 2, Section F, Experience 182), with or without enlargement of the skull. Though the changes of vascular insufficiency (absence of hair, shiny skin, cold pulseless feet, peripheral cyanosis, digital gangrene, painful ulcers) barely occurred in our survey, these should be *briefly* looked for (because they will direct you to examine the pulses, etc. rather than the neurological system).

Observing the legs from the neurological point of view, note whether there is

4 **pes cavus** (Friedreich's ataxia, Charcot–Marie–Tooth disease) or

5 **one leg smaller** than the other (old polio, infantile hemiplegia). Next note

6 **muscle bulk**. Bear in mind that some generalized disuse atrophy may occur even in a limb with upper motor neurone weakness (e.g. severe spastic paraparesis; see Vol. 2, Section F, Experience 109). There may be unilateral loss of muscle bulk (old

polio), muscle wasting that stops part of the way up the leg (Charcot–Marie–Tooth disease), isolated anterior thigh wasting (e.g. diabetic amyotrophy) or generalized proximal muscle wasting (polymyositis) or muscle wasting confined to one peroneal region (lateral popliteal nerve palsy). Look specifically for

7 fasciculation (nearly always motor neurone disease).

8 Examine the **muscle tone** in each leg by passively moving it at the hip and knee joints (with the patient relaxed, roll the leg sideways, backwards and forwards on the bed; lift the knee and let it drop, or bend the knee and partially straighten in an irregular and unexpected rhythm).

9 Test **power:***

    (a) 'Lift your leg up; stop me pushing it down' (L1,2),

    (b) 'Bend your knee; don't let me straighten it' (L5, S1,2),

    (c) (Knee still bent) 'Push out straight against my hand' (L3,4),

    (d) 'Bend your foot down; push my hand away' (S1),

    (e) 'Cock up your foot; point your toes at the ceiling. Stop me pushing your foot down' (L4,5).

Moving smoothly into testing

10 coordination, take your hand off the foot and run your finger down the patient's shin below the knee, saying

    (f) 'Put your heel just below your knee then run it smoothly down your shin; now up your shin, now down . . .' etc.†

11 Check the knee (L3,4) and ankle (S1,2) **jerks‡** and by forced dorsiflexion with the leg held in slight knee flexion. Check for *ankle clonus* (and patellar clonus if there may be pyramidal disease).

12 Test the **plantar response,** remembering that in slight pyramidal lesions an extensor plantar is more easily elicited on the outer part of the sole than the inner.§

13 Turning to **sensation,** dermatomes L2 to S1 on the leg (see Fig. B.3) are tested if you examine *light touch* (dab cotton wool lightly) and *pinprick* once each on the outer thigh (L2), inner thigh (L3), inner calf (L4), outer calf (L5), medial foot (L5) and lateral foot (S1). The most common sensory defect is a peripheral neuropathy with stocking distribution loss. Demonstrate this with light touch (usually the most sensitive indicator) and pinprick.

Test somewhere above the suspected sensory level:

    'Does the pin feel sharp and prickly?' – 'Yes'.

Test on the feet:

---

*The screen of instructions from (a) to (e) will identify most legs in which there are abnormalities of motor function. You may wish to embellish these, where necessary, with instructions to test hip extension, hip adduction, hip abduction and hip rotation.

†If there is possible or definite cerebellar disease, you may wish to demonstrate dysdiadochokinesis in the foot by asking the patient to tap his foot quickly on your hand.

‡One study has suggested that the plantar strike technique for examining ankle jerks may be more reliable than the better-known tendon strike technique, especially in the elderly (*Lancet* 1994. **344**: 1619–20).

§In slight pyramidal disease the extensor plantar is first elicited on the dorsilateral part of the foot (*Chaddock's manoeuvre*). As the degree of pyramidal involvement increases, the area in which a *Babinski's sign* may be elicited first increases to cover the whole sole and then spreads beyond the foot until *Oppenheim's sign* (extensor response when the inner border of the tibia is pressed heavily; see Fig. C3.17b, Station 3, CNS, Case 26) or *Gordon's reflex* (extensor response on pinching the Achilles tendon) can be elicited. In such cases the big toe may be seen to go up as the patient takes his socks off.

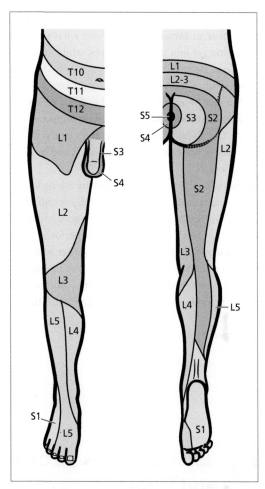

Figure B.3 Dermatomes in the lower limb. (After Foerster, 1933, Oxford University Press, *Brain* **56**: 1.) There is considerable variation and overlap between the cutaneous areas supplied by each spinal root so that an isolated root lesion results in a much smaller area of sensory impairment than the diagram indicates.

'Does the pin feel sharp and prickly?' – 'No'.

'Tell me when it changes'.

Work up the leg to the sensory level and confirm afterwards by demonstrating the same level medially and laterally.* The level of the peripheral neuropathy may be different on the two legs. *Vibration* should be tested on the medial malleoli (and

*The same method can be used for rapid demonstration of a higher sensory level: normal sensation is demonstrated above the lesion, e.g. on the shoulder or chest. The pin is then rapidly moved up the whole body from the foot until the patient announces that the sensation is changing to normal. That area is then worked over rapidly to detect the actual sensory level.

knee, iliac crest, etc., if it is impaired), and *joint position* sense in the great toes (remember to explain to the patient what you mean by 'up' and 'down' in his toes before you get him to close his eyes; whilst testing the position sense hold the toe by the lateral aspects).

Sometimes the examiner will stop you before you get this far. If the lesion is predominantly motor, he may break in before you have tested sensation, and if predominantly sensory, he may lead you to test sensation earlier or stop you at this point. You should, however, be sufficiently deft to perform the full examination described above quickly and efficiently, and be prepared to complete it by examining the patient's

14 gait (check the patient can walk by asking for either his or the examiner's permission to examine the gait). First, watch his *ordinary walk* to a defined point and back (see Station 3, CNS, Case 5) and then watch him walk *heel-to-toe* (ataxia), on his *toes* and on his *heels* (foot-drop). Finally perform

15 Romberg's test with the feet together and the arms outstretched. You must be ready to catch the patient if there is any possibility of ataxia. Romberg's test is only positive (sensory ataxia, e.g. subacute combined degeneration, tabes dorsalis) if the patient is more unsteady (tends to fall) with the eyes closed than open.

See Appendix 1, Checklist 8, Legs.

9 | 'Examine this patient's legs and arms'

Variations of instruction in initial PACES survey (resultant diagnoses in brackets)
This man has had a collapse – can you examine his limbs (left hemiplegia and atrial fibrillation)?

Diagnoses from our original survey in order of frequency
1 Motor neurone disease 29%
2 Cervical myelopathy 14%
3 Syringomyelia 14%
4 Friedreich's ataxia 14%
5 Parkinson's disease 7%

Examination *routine*
As appropriate from 'Examine this patient's arms' (see Section B, Examination *Routine* 7) and 'Examine this patient's legs' (see Section B, Examination *Routine* 8).

10 | 'Examine this patient's gait'

Variations of instruction in initial PACES survey (resultant diagnoses in brackets)
Examine this patient's gait (ankylosing spondylitis)
This man has difficulty walking and falls especially at night. Examine his gait and
then his legs (cerebellar signs and sensory neuropathy)
This patient has difficulty in walking. Please examine him (cerebellar signs)
Examine the gait and anything else which is relevant (no diagnosis reached)

Diagnoses from our surveys in order of frequency
1 Ataxia 50%
2 Spastic paraparesis 20%
3 Parkinson's disease 10%
4 Charcot–Marie–Tooth disease 5%
5 Ankylosing spondylitis 5%
6 A nightmare (see Vol. 2, Section F, Experience 42) 5%

Examination *routine*
As you approach the patient, perform
  1 a *quick **visual survey***, noting any *cerebellar signs* (nystagmus, intention tremor)
or obvious signs of conditions such as *Parkinson's* disease (facies, tremor), *Charcot–
Marie–Tooth* disease (peroneal wasting, pes cavus, etc.) or *ankylosing spondylitis*.
Introduce yourself to the patient and ask him
  2 whether he can walk without help (*cerebellar dysarthria* heard during his reply
may be a useful clue). If he reports difficulty, reassure him that you will stay with
him in case of any problems.
  3 Ask him to walk to a defined point and back whilst you look for any of the classic
abnormal gaits (see Station 3, CNS, Case 5), particularly ataxic (cerebellar or sensory),
spastic, steppage (Charcot–Marie–Tooth) or parkinsonian (?pill-rolling tremor). As
the patient walks, make sure you note specifically
  4 the **arm swing** (Parkinson's) and
  5 any *clumsiness* on **the turns** (ataxia, Parkinson's) or 'sticky feet' with gait apraxia
(slow, shuffling, short steps) or marche à petit pas (small, quick steps – also known
as senile gait). Next test
  6 heel-to-toe gait (demonstrate as you ask the patient to do this) which will
exacerbate ataxia (note the side to which the patient tends to fall). Ask the patient to
walk
  7 on his toes (S1) and then
  8 on his heels (L5; foot-drop – lateral popliteal nerve palsy, Charcot–Marie–Tooth
disease). If he has a spastic gait or a hemiparesis he may find both these tests difficult
to perform.
  9 Now ask him to stand with his *feet together*, *arms out* in front; when you are satis-
fied with the degree of steadiness with the eyes open, ask him to *close his eyes* (you
should be standing nearby to catch him if he shows a tendency to fall). **Romberg's**

test is only positive (*sensory ataxia*) if the patient is more unsteady (tends to fall) with the eyes closed than with them open (dorsal column disease, e.g. subacute combined degeneration, tabes dorsalis, etc.).

10 If you suspect sensory ataxia, a further test is to ask the patient to **close his eyes while walking** (he will become *more* ataxic). Again you should be ready to catch the patient should he fall. As always, be ready to look for

11 additional features of the conditions on the list if appropriate (see individual short cases, and consider what you would do with each).

See Appendix 1, Checklist 10, Gait.

11 | 'Ask this patient some questions'

Variations of instruction from our original survey
Talk to this patient
Examine this patient's speech
Converse with this patient

Diagnoses from our original survey in order of frequency
1 Dysphasia 24%
2 Cerebellar dysarthria 16%
3 Raynaud's 11%
4 Systemic sclerosis/CREST (Vol. 3, Station 5, Locomotor, Case 3) 8%
5 Pseudobulbar palsy 8%
6 Myxoedema (Vol. 3, Station 5, Endocrine, Case 9) 5%
7 Graves' disease (Vol. 3, Station 5, Endocrine, Case 3) 5%
8 Crohn's disease 5%
9 Ankle oedema due to nephrotic syndrome 5%
10 Senile dementia 5%
11 Parkinson's disease 3%

Examination *routine*
Inspection of the list of cases in our survey which provoked this instruction reveals that they fall into four groups, each with a very different reason for the instruction:
Group 1: to spot the diagnosis and confirm it by eliciting *revealing answers* 39%
Group 2: to demonstrate and diagnose the type of a dysarthria 32%
Group 3: to diagnose a dysphasia 24%
Group 4: to assess higher mental function 5%.
With the group 1 patients you may have been given a lead such as 'Look at the hands' (Raynaud's) or 'Look at the face' (systemic sclerosis, myxoedema, etc.) before the instruction 'Ask this patient some questions'. At any rate you should start your examination as usual with

1 a **visual survey** of the patient from head to foot, particularly looking for evidence of: (i) the spot diagnosis in group 1 patients (Raynaud's, systemic sclerosis/CREST, hypo- or hyperthyroidism, Crohn's, nephrotic syndrome – see Volume 3); (ii) a *hemiplegia* which may be associated with dysphasia; or (iii) any of the conditions associated with dysarthria (see Station 3, CNS, Case 36), especially *nystagmus* or *intention tremor* (which may be revealed by even minor movements) in cerebellar disease, *pes cavus* in Friedreich's ataxia and the *facies/tremor* of Parkinson's disease. In the group 1 patients, once you are on to the diagnosis, the sort of

2 **specific questions** the examiners are looking for (see also the individual short cases in Volume 3) are:

Raynaud's (see also Vol. 2, Section F, Anecdote 262):

'Do your fingers change colour in the cold?'

'What colour do they go?' ('Is there a particular sequence of colours?')

'How long have you had the trouble?'

'What is your job?' (vibrating tools, etc.)

and if there is any possibility of connective tissue disease:

'Do you have any difficulty with swallowing?' etc.

Systemic sclerosis:

'Do you have any difficulty with swallowing?'

'Do your fingers change colour in the cold?'

'Do you get short of breath?' (on hills? on flat? etc.)

We leave you to work out the straightforward questions you would ask the slow, croaking patient with *myxoedematous facies*, the patient with *exophthalmos*, or the one who has *lid retraction* and is *fidgety*, or the patient who has *multiple scars* and *sinuses* on his abdomen. In the young patient who may have nephrotic syndrome, you would be looking for the history of a sore throat.

If there are no features suggesting a group 1 patient, it is likely that the problem is either a dysarthria or dysphasia and, as already mentioned, there may be clues pointing to one of these. You need to ask the patient

3 some **general questions** to get him *talking*:

'My name is . . . Please could you tell me your name?'

'What is your address?'

If you still need to hear a patient speak further ask

4 **more questions** which require *long answers* such as: 'Please could you tell me all the things you ate for breakfast/lunch'.

To test

5 **articulation,** ask the patient to repeat traditional words and phrases such as 'British Constitution', 'West Register Street', 'biblical criticism' and 'artillery'. As well as testing articulation, such

6 **repetition** is useful for assessing speech when the patient only gives one-word answers to questions. If necessary ask the patient to repeat long sentences after you. Information gained from repetition may also be useful in your assessment of dysphasia (see below).

If the problem is *dysarthria*, it is really a spot diagnosis to test your ability to recognize and demonstrate the features of the different types (see Station 3, CNS, Case 36). It is recommended that you find as many patients as possible with the conditions causing the various types of dysarthria and listen to them speak so that, as with murmurs, the diagnosis is a question of instant recognition. This is particularly true of the ataxic dysarthria of cerebellar disease. When you have heard enough to make the diagnosis, you should either describe the speech (see Station 3, CNS, Case 36) and, with supporting signs seen on inspection, give the diagnosis, or proceed to look for

7 additional signs (in the same way as you might do after the 'What is the diagnosis?' instruction).

If the patient has a *dysphasia* (see Station 3, CNS, Case 40), you may wish to demonstrate that

8 comprehension is good (expressive dysphasia) or impaired (receptive dysphasia). Perform a few simple commands *without gesturing*, e.g.

> 'Please put your tongue out'
> 'Shut your eyes'
> 'Touch your nose', etc.

Assuming these are performed adequately, proceed to look for expressive dysphasia by asking the patient to name some everyday items, e.g. a comb, pen, coins. If the patient is unable to name the objects, test for

9 nominal dysphasia. Hold up your keys:

> 'What is this?' – patient does not answer.
> 'Is this a spoon?' – 'No'.
> 'Is it a pen?' – 'No'.
> 'Is it keys?' – 'Yes'.

If the patient is able to name objects, test the ability to form sentences by asking the patient to describe something in more detail, e.g.

> 'Could you tell me where you live and how you would get home from here?'
> 'Could you tell me the name of as many objects in this room as possible?'

If there are expressive problems you should check to see if the problem is true expressive dysphasia or whether there is

10 orofacial dyspraxia.* Ask the patient to perform various orofacial movements (assuming there is no receptive dysphasia). These should be tested first by command *without gesture*, e.g.

> 'Please show me your teeth'
> 'Move your tongue from side to side'.

Subsequently ask the patient to obey the same commands but *with gesture*, i.e. so the patient can mimic. This should give some idea as to whether the patient has either ideational or ideomotor dyspraxia.†

Our survey showed that it is extremely rare for candidates to be asked to assess

---

*It is important to make this distinction so that the type of speech therapy is appropriate. In orofacial dyspraxia the therapist needs to work on mouth movements rather than concentrating only on linguistic problems. It has recently been established that the lesion which leads to orofacial dyspraxia is in the operculum.

†Again it is relevant to therapy to establish if the patient can make movements when aided by gesture.

11 higher mental functions.* This is, however, an assessment which every Membership candidate should be equipped to make. The following is the 'abbreviated mental test' – more than four of the questions wrong suggests a well-established dementia:

    1 Age

    2 Time (to nearest hour)

    3 Address for recall at end of test – this should be repeated by the patient to ensure it has been heard correctly: 42 West Street

    4 Year

    5 Name of this place

    6 Recognition of two persons (doctor, nurse, etc.)

    7 Date of birth (day and month sufficient)

    8 Year of First World War

    9 Name of present monarch

    10 Count backwards from 20 to 1.

Agnosia, apraxia, dyslexia, dysgraphia and dyscalculia are considered in Station 3, CNS, Case 8.

See Appendix 1, Checklist 11, Ask some questions.

12 | 'Examine this patient's fundi'

Variations of instruction in initial PACES survey (resultant diagnoses in brackets)

Examine this patient's fundi (diabetic retinopathy – many cases, all stages; unilateral optic atrophy and angioid streaks)

Look at the fundi (diabetic retinopathy – many cases, all stages)

Examine the eyes of this patient with diabetes (panretinal photocoagulation and exudates near macula)

This patient feels as if he is walking on cotton wool and has had recurrent Bell's palsies. Please examine his eyes (it turned out to be preproliferative diabetic retinopathy)

This patient is blind. Examine his fundi (retinitis pigmentosa and cataracts)

This man had sudden-onset blindness. Please look at the fundi and suggest why (glaucoma and retinal artery occlusion)

*Rare at the time of writing (see Vol. 2, Section F, Anecdote 286), though it is conceivable that any examiners who see this book will be given ideas as to the areas they are neglecting!

This patient has visual loss. Please examine the fundi (diabetic maculopathy)

Your house officer has examined this lady's fundi. She is a 23-year-old nurse. He is worried and has asked for your opinion (myelinated nerve fibres)

Examine this man's fundus – just the right one (diabetic retinopathy)

Look at the fundi and describe what you find (cataracts and diabetic retinopathy)

This man has trouble with his vision. Examine the fundi (retinitis pigmentosa)

Examine the fundi. The patient has a central scotoma (retinitis pigmentosa and diabetic maculopathy)

This elderly man has had sudden onset of blindness in the right eye. Please examine him and tell me why (optic atrophy)

Diagnoses from our survey in order of frequency

1 Diabetic retinopathy (Vol. 3, Station 5, Eyes, Case 1) 41%
2 Retinitis pigmentosa (Vol. 3, Station 5, Eyes, Case 2) 16%
3 Optic atrophy (Vol. 3, Station 5, Eyes, Case 3) 6%
4 Papilloedema (Vol. 3, Station 5, Eyes, Case 8) 4%
5 Retinal vein thrombosis (Vol. 3, Station 5, Eyes, Case 6) 2%
6 Old choroiditis (Vol. 3, Station 5, Eyes, Case 7) 2%
7 Cataracts (Vol. 3, Station 5, Eyes, Case 9) 2%
8 Albinism (Vol. 3, Station 5, Eyes, Case 11) 2%
9 Myelinated nerve fibres (Vol. 3, Station 5, Eyes, Case 13) 1%
10 Hypertensive retinopathy (Vol.3, Station 5, Eyes, Case 14) 1%
11 Glaucoma (Vol. 3, Station 5, Eyes, Case 15) 1%
12 Laurence–Moon–Bardet–Biedl (Vol. 3, Station 5, Eyes, Case 19) <1%
13 Asteroid hyalosis (Vol. 3, Station 5, Eyes, Case 17) <1%
14 Retinal artery occlusion (Vol. 3, Station 5, Eyes, Case 16) <1%
15 Drusen (Vol. 3, Station 5, Eyes, Case 18) <1%
16 Cytomegalovirus choroidoretinitis (AIDS) (Vol. 3, Station 5, Eyes, Case 20) <1%
17 Normal (Vol. 3, Station 5, Eyes, Case 21) <1%

Special note

Although, with the new Station 5, a fundus case is no longer mandatory, the College has made it clear that fundoscopy continues to be a skill that all MRCP candidates should be competent in. Though there are only a limited number of possibilities, it is clear from our surveys that a lot of candidates experience more difficulty with a fundus than with any other short case. On our questionnaire, a considerable number of candidates reported 'I said optic atrophy . . .' or 'I said diabetic retinopathy . . . but I hadn't got a clue what it was' (see Vol. 2, Section F, Experiences 158–160). Clearly, there is not a lot that a book like this can do to help other than to warn you in advance of the problem, to provide you with a list of the likely conditions and to describe them (see individual short cases). Other than this, the art of fundoscopy and fundal diagnoses can only be acquired with practice. With a moderate degree of clinical expertise and common sense, most candidates ought to be able to overcome this hurdle.

Examination *routine*

Almost invariably, if you are asked to look at the fundus the diagnosis must be in the fundus. However, it is good practice to precede fundoscopy with

1 a **quick general look** at the patient (this will rarely help but the occasional person with diabetes in the examination may also have *foot ulcers* or *necrobiosis lipoidica* or may be wearing a *Medic-Alert* bracelet or neck chain), at his eyes (*arcus lipidus* at an inappropriately young age may suggest diabetes), and at his pupils (usually, but not always, dilated for the examination).

Turning to ophthalmoscopy, it may be your practice to focus immediately on the fundus and, in the vast majority of cases, this will provide the diagnosis. However, it would be preferable to cultivate the habit (if you can gain sufficient expertise to do it quickly and efficiently) of looking first at

2 the structures in front of the fundus, particularly the **lens** (people with diabetes will often reward you with early *cataract* formation; your examiner will sometimes not have noticed it, but as long as you are right when he checks, you may increase your score). Adjust the lenses of the ophthalmoscope so that you move down through

3 the **vitreous,** noting any *opacities* (e.g. asteroid hyalinosis; see Vol. 3, Station 5, Eyes, Case 17), *haemorrhages, fibrous tissue* or *new vessel formation* (diabetes) until you get to

4 the **fundus**. Localize the disc and examine it and its margins for *optic atrophy,** *papillitis* (see Vol. 3, Station 5, Eyes, Case 3) or *papilloedema* (see Vol. 3, Station 5, Eyes, Case 8) and for *myelinated nerve fibres* (see Vol. 3, Station 5, Eyes, Case 13). Trace the

5 arterioles and **venules** out from the disc, noting particularly their calibre, light reflex (*silver wiring*) and AV crossing points (*AV nipping*; see Vol. 3, Station 5, Eyes, Case 14).

6 Examine **each quadrant** of the fundus and especially the **macular area** and its temporal aspect.† You are looking particularly for *haemorrhages* (dot, blot, flame-shaped), *microaneurysms, exudates* both hard (well-defined edges; increased light reflex) and soft (fluffy with ill-defined edges; *cotton-wool spots*). If hard exudates are present see if these form a ring (*circinates* in diabetes).

If you see haemorrhages you must look specifically for

(a) dot haemorrhages/microaneurysms,

(b) new vessel formation, and

(c) photocoagulation scars.

If you diagnose diabetic retinopathy, your examiner will expect you to be able to comment on the presence or absence of all of these (see Vol. 2, Section F, Experience 160). If you cannot find these diagnostic clues, you may have noted the features that suggest hypertensive rather than diabetic retinopathy (silver wiring, AV nipping,

---

*There are normal variations in disc colour; in both infancy and old age it is naturally pale, as is the enlarged disc of a myopic eye. The advice of a well-known neurologist and experienced MRCP teacher to his MRCP candidates was: 'Don't diagnose optic atrophy unless it is a "barn door" optic atrophy'. It is well worth bearing this advice in mind (see Vol. 2, Section F, Experience 159). Temporal pallor of the disc due to a lesion in

the papillomacular bundle is often seen in multiple sclerosis. However, temporal pallor is not always pathological.
†The macula will come into view if you ask the patient with a dilated pupil to look at the ophthalmoscopic light. Ideally, you should use the dot light for this, if it is available in your ophthalmoscope.

more soft exudates than hard, haemorrhages which are mainly flame-shaped, early disc swelling with loss of venous pulsation* or frank papilloedema).

In the patient with diabetic retinopathy, it is of particular clinical significance to assess whether lesions (especially hard exudates) involve or threaten (i.e. are near to) the centre of the fovea.†

It would be useful if you knew that the patient has diabetes (see Vol. 2, Section F, Experience 204 and Quotation 379) but if you remain in doubt, remember that diabetes and hypertension often coexist in a patient, and that it is more important that you have checked comprehensively for the above features, and report your findings honestly (mentioning the features in favour of one diagnosis or the other), than to guess or make up findings. In PACES, the College is keen that the instruction tells you the patient has diabetes if he/she does. In general, this does not help as many of the patients with different types of retinal pathologies in the exam have diabetes, because patients with diabetes are the one group having regular fundal checks which may turn up pathologies other than diabetic retinopathy, e.g. drusen, old choroiditis, myelinated nerve fibres, etc. However, in the patient with haemorrhages and exudates it is of great value to know if the patient has diabetes.

We leave you to master the findings of the other fundal short cases and to ensure that you would recognize each (see individual short cases in this book and in Volume 3). The final point in this important *routine* is to

7 **keep examining until** you have finished and are **ready** to present your findings. Do not be put off by the impatient words or mumblings of your examiner; these will be forgotten when you present accurate findings and get the diagnosis right. Conversely, it is too late to go back and check if the examiner asks whether you saw a ... and you are not sure (Vol. 2, Section F, Experience 160). You need to be able to give a clear and unequivocal 'yes' or 'no'. Thus, the best tip we can offer as you look around the fundus is to stop at the disc, the macula and in each quadrant of each eye and ask yourself the question: 'Are there any abnormalities? What are they?' before moving on to the next area.

See Appendix 1, Checklist 12, Fundi.

---

*Observation of venous pulsation is an expertise which comes with much practice of looking at normal as well as abnormal fundi. Though it could be useful if you have acquired this expertise before the examination, do not get bogged down studying the venous pulsation for too long if you are not used to it. See also Vol. 3, Station 5, Eyes, Case 8.

†The UK National Screening Committee diabetic retinopathy screening guidelines suggest that patients with hard exudates within one disc diameter of the centre of the fovea should be referred to an ophthalmologist (see Vol. 3, Station 5, Eyes, Case1).

13 | 'Examine this patient's eyes'

Variations of instruction in initial PACES survey (resultant diagnoses in brackets)

Examine this patient's eyes (retinitis pigmentosa; Graves' disease; complete IIIrd nerve palsy; IIIrd, IVth, VIth nerve palsy)

Examine the eyes and anything else appropriate (Graves' eye disease and signs of hyperthyroidism)

Look at this patient's eyes (exophthalmos; IIIrd nerve palsy)

This woman presents with painful eyes. Please examine her (chemosis and goitre)

Examine this lady's eye movements (partial IIIrd nerve palsy)

This lady has had neurosurgery. Please examine her eyes (right upper homonymous hemianopia)

This man is followed up in the eye clinic. Have a look at him and tell me why (exophthalmos and lid lag)

Diagnoses from our original survey in order of frequency

1 Exophthalmos (Vol. 3, Station 5, Eyes, Case 12) 27%
2 Ocular palsy (Vol. 3, Station 5, Eyes, Case 4) 23%
3 Nystagmus 11%
4 Diabetic retinopathy (Vol. 3, Station 5, Eyes, Case 1) 8%
5 Optic atrophy (Vol. 3, Station 5, Eyes, Case 3) 7%
6 Myasthenia gravis 4%
7 Visual field defects 3%
8 Ptosis 3%
9 Retinitis pigmentosa (Vol. 3, Station 5, Eyes, Case 2) 2%
10 Horner's syndrome 2%
11 Holmes–Adie pupil 1%
12 Argyll Robertson pupils 1%
13 Cataracts (Vol. 3, Station 5, Eyes, Case 9) 1%
14 Papilloedema (Vol. 3, Station 5, Eyes, Case 8) 1%

Other diagnoses were: buphthalmos in a patient with Sturge–Weber syndrome (1%), normal eyes in a patient who was supposed to have internuclear ophthalmoplegia (1%) and retinal detachment (<1%).

Examination *routine*

A study of the above list maps out your examination steps when you hear this instruction. It is basically going to be a part of your cranial nerves *routine* (see Section B, Examination *Routine* 6) but carried out in slightly more detail. It should be your habit to commence all examination *routines* by *scanning* the whole patient. The patient with nystagmus due to cerebellar disease (see Station 3, CNS, Case 7) may have an *intention tremor* which will occasionally be noticeable even with minor movements. The patient with exophthalmos may have *pretibial myxoedema* or *thyroid acropachy*. A number of other conditions with stigmata elsewhere on the body may cause eye signs. Though these conditions were not prominent in our survey, they should be borne in mind as you complete this *visual survey*: face and hands of acromegaly, foot ulcers in diabetes, pes cavus in Friedreich's ataxia, the long, lean look of myotonic dystrophy, etc. As you finish your *visual survey* briefly look again at

1 the **face** (e.g. myasthenic facies, tabetic facies, facial asymmetry in hemiparesis), and then concentrate on

2 the **eyes**. Ask yourself if there is

(a) exophthalmos,

(b) strabismus,

(c) ptosis, or

(d) other abnormalities such as xanthelasma or arcus senilis.

Look at

3 the **pupils** for inequality of size and shape; whether one or both are small (Argyll Robertson, Horner's) or large (Holmes–Adie, IIIrd nerve palsy). Remember it may be necessary to use subdued light to elicit anisocuria, particularly due to unilateral Horner's syndrome. Also check for iris abnormalities such as Lisch nodules in neurofibromatosis. Next, it is traditional to check

4 the **visual acuity** by asking the patient to read a newspaper or other print which you hold up, and by asking him to look at the clock on the wall (see Section B, Examination *Routine* 6); alternatively it would be preferable to pull out a pocket-sized Snellen chart.* In the traditional *routine* you should next test

5 **visual fields** (see Section B, Examination *Routine* 5). However, in the majority of cases the important findings are on testing

6 **eye movements** (see Section B, Examination *Routine* 6). We leave you to decide if you wish to follow the traditional *routine* or check eye movements before acuity and visual fields (see Vol. 2, Section F, Experience 145 and Quotation 388). You are looking for

(a) ocular palsy (see Station 3, CNS, Case 16),

(b) diplopia,

(c) nystagmus, or

(d) lid lag.

In order to test

7 the **pupillary light reflex**, take out your pen torch and shine the light twice (*direct* and *consensual*) in each eye. Then test

8 the **accommodation–convergence reflex** – hold your finger close to the patient's nose:

'Look into the distance',

then suddenly

'Now look at my finger'.†

Finally, examine

9 the **fundi** (see Section B, Examination *Routine* 12).

---

*We advise you to take a pocket-sized Snellen chart. It will enable you to put an approximate value on the patient's visual acuity while taking no extra time.

†Some neurologists believe that as this traditional method of examining the accommodation–convergence reflex may involve a change in optical axis and luminance, it is better to get the patient to follow a target down the optical axis over 2 m.

As usual, when you have the diagnosis, think what else you could look for (e.g. cerebellar signs in a patient with nystagmus; sympathectomy scar over the clavicle in a patient with Horner's syndrome; absent limb reflexes in Holmes–Adie pupil) before shouting out the diagnosis even if it is obvious (e.g. exophthalmos).

See Appendix 1, Checklist 13, Eyes.

14 | 'Examine this patient's face'

Variations of instruction in initial PACES survey (resultant diagnoses in brackets)
Look at the face (hereditary haemorrhagic telangiectasia)
Look at this patient's face (lupus pernio)
Look at this man's face and examine whatever else you think is necessary

Diagnoses from our original survey in order of frequency
  1 Lower motor neurone VIIth nerve lesion 12%
  2 Lupus pernio (Vol. 3, Station 5, Skin, Case 19) 8%
  3 Ptosis 7%
  4 Sturge–Weber syndrome (Vol. 3, Station 5, Skin, Case 24) 7%
  5 Hypothyroidism (Vol. 3, Station 5, Endocrine, Case 5) 7%
  6 Osler–Weber–Rendu syndrome (Vol. 3, Station 5, Skin, Case 3) 7%
  7 Myotonic dystrophy 4%
  8 Jaundice 4%
  9 Horner's syndrome 4%
 10 Systemic sclerosis/CREST (Vol. 3, Station 5, Locomotor, Case 3) 3%
 11 Peutz–Jeghers syndrome (Vol. 3, Station 5, Skin, Case 26) 3%
 12 Upper motor neurone facial weakness 3%
 13 Systemic lupus erythematosus (Vol. 3, Station 5, Locomotor, Case 16) 3%
 14 Parkinson's disease 3%
 15 Cushing's syndrome (Vol. 3, Station 5, Endocrine, Case 6) 2%
 16 Neurofibromatosis (Vol. 3, Station 5, Skin, Case 2) 2%
 17 Superior vena cava obstruction 2%
 18 Plethora (polycythaemia rubra vera) 2%
 19 Hypopituitarism (Vol. 3, Station 5, Endocrine, Case 8) 2%
 20 Vitiligo and a goitre (Vol. 3, Station 5, Skin, Case 8 and Endocrine, Case 4) 2%
 21 Cyanosis 2%
 22 Paget's disease (Vol. 3, Station 5, Locomotor, Case 7) 1%
 23 Bilateral parotid enlargement (Vol. 3, Station 5, Other, Case 1) 1%
 24 Exophthalmos (Vol. 3, Station 5, Eyes, Case 12) 1%
 25 Acromegaly (Vol. 3, Station 5, Endocrine, Case 2) 1%
 26 Dermatomyositis (hands and face) (Vol. 3, Station 5, Skin, Case 6) 1%
 27 Xanthelasma and arcus senilis (Vol. 3, Station 5, Skin, Case 7) 1%

28 Acne rosacea 1%

29 Dermatitis herpetiformis (Vol. 3, Station 5, Skin, Case 39) 1%

30 Malar flush 1%

Examination *routine*

This instruction is really just a variation on the 'spot diagnosis' theme (see Section B, Examination *Routine* 22), only easier because you are told where the abnormalities lie. In a way similar to that described in the 'What is the diagnosis?' *routine*,

1 *survey* the patient from head to foot and then

2 scan the face and skull. The abnormality will usually be obvious (see above list) but if you find none then proceed to

3 break down the parts of the face into their constituents and scrutinize each, asking yourself the question: 'Is it normal?'. Thus, if you have scanned the eyes and have not been struck by any obvious abnormality (e.g. ptosis or an abnormal pupil), you should look at all the structures such as the *eyelids* (mild degree of ptosis, heliotrope rash on the upper lid in dermatomyositis), *eyelashes* (sparse in alopecia*), *cornea* (arcus senilis, ground-glass appearance in congenital syphilis), *sclerae* (icteric, congested in superior vena cava obstruction and polycythaemia), *pupils* (small, large, irregular, dislocated lens in Marfan's, cataract in myotonic dystrophy) and *iris* ('muddy iris' in iritis)† on both sides. Look at the *face* for any erythema or infiltrates (lupus pernio, SLE, dermatomyositis, malar flush), around the *mouth* for tight, shiny, adherent skin (systemic sclerosis) or pigmented macules (Peutz–Jeghers) and, if indicated, in the mouth for telangiectases (Osler–Weber–Rendu), cyanosis or pigmentation (Addison's). The whole face can be rapidly covered in this manner. Having spotted the abnormality and, you hope, made the diagnosis, you should, if appropriate, try to score extra points by demonstrating

4 additional features in the same way as described under 'What is the diagnosis?'. Go through each diagnosis on the list and work out what additional features you would see elsewhere. Thus, if you find a lower motor neurone VIIth nerve lesion, demonstrate the weakness in the upper as well as the lower part of the face (see Station 3, CNS, Case 35), then be seen to examine the ears for evidence of herpes zoster (Ramsay Hunt syndrome).

If despite carrying out the above routine there is still no apparent abnormality then examine the facial musculature (see 'Examine this patient's cranial nerves') for evidence of a VIIth nerve lesion which is not obvious.

See Appendix 1, Checklist 14, Face.

---

*May be associated with the organ-specific autoimmune diseases (see Vol. 3, Station 5, Skin, Cases 8 and 14).

†Another uncommon but important sign which may occur in the iris is neovascularization in diabetes (rubeosis iridis).

However, it is unlikely that this would occur in the context of 'Examine this patient's face' at the examination.

15 | 'Examine this patient's hands'

Variations of instruction in initial PACES survey (resultant diagnoses in brackets)

Examine this patient's hands (rheumatoid hands and nodules; rheumatoid hands and cervical collar; osteoarthritis; psoriasis; rheumatoid arthritis)

Examine these hands (psoriasis; scleroderma; neurofibromatosis; deforming arthropathy, ?type)

Please examine this patient's hands. He is a 15-year-old boy who presented with carpopedal spasm as a child (pseudohypoparathyroidism?)

This man has a painful knee. Please examine his hands and suggest why (gout)

This man has had painful hands. Please examine him (rheumatoid hands)

Look at this patient's hands (rheumatoid arthritis)

This is a lady of about 80 years. Please look at her hands (osteoarthritis and gout)

Examine the hands and any other relevant joints (CREST)

Examine these hands (chronic tophaceous gout)

This patient has rheumatoid arthritis. Please check the functional status (rheumatoid arthritis)

Have a look at this lady's hand and talk me through your examination (rheumatoid hands)

Diagnoses from our original survey in order of frequency

 1 Rheumatoid hands (Vol. 3, Station 5, Locomotor, Case 1) 22%
 2 Systemic sclerosis/CREST (Vol. 3, Station 5, Locomotor, Case 3) 13%
 3 Wasting of the small muscles of the hand 12%
 4 Psoriatic arthropathy/psoriasis (Vol. 3, Station 5, Locomotor, Case 2) 11%
 5 Ulnar nerve palsy 9%
 6 Clubbing (Vol. 3, Station 5, Skin, Case 17) 7%
 7 Raynaud's (Vol. 3, Station 5, Skin, Case 22) 3%
 8 Vasculitis (Vol. 3, Station 5, Locomotor, Case 10) 3%
 9 Steroid changes (especially purpura) (Vol. 3, Station 5, Skin, Case 25) 3%
10 Acromegaly (Vol. 3, Station 5, Endocrine, Case 2) 2%
11 Motor neurone disease 2%
12 Xanthomata (Vol. 3, Station 5, Skin, Case 7) 2%
13 Cyanosis 2%
14 Chronic liver disease 2%
15 Thyroid acropachy (Vol. 3, Station 5, Endocrine, Case 12) 2%
16 Carpal tunnel syndrome 2%
17 Osteoarthrosis (Vol. 3, Station 5, Locomotor, Case 8) 2%
18 Osler–Weber–Rendu syndrome (Vol. 3, Station 5, Skin, Case 3) 1%
19 Tophaceous gout (Vol. 3, Station 5, Locomotor, Case 5) 1%

Other diagnoses were: neurofibromatosis (<1%), systemic lupus erythematosus (<1%), cervical myelopathy (<1%), dermatomyositis ('examine hands and face', <1%), nail–patella syndrome ('examine hands and knees', <1%), Charcot–Marie–Tooth disease

(<1%), superior vena cava obstruction (<1%), facioscapulohumeral muscular dystrophy (<1%), Addison's disease (<1%) and Marfan's syndrome (<1%).

Examination *routine*

Analysis of the list given above suggests that when you hear this instruction, rheumatoid arthritis is likely to be present in about a quarter of the cases, and scleroderma, wasting of the small muscles of the hand, psoriasis, ulnar nerve palsy or clubbing in about a further half. As you approach the patient you should bear this in mind and look specifically at

1 the **face** for typical expressionless facies, with adherent shiny skin, sometimes with telangiectasia (*systemic sclerosis*). It is clear from the survey list that a variety of other conditions may show signs in either the face or in the general appearance, particularly *cushingoid* facies (steroid changes in a patient with rheumatoid arthritis), *acromegalic* facies, *arcus senilis* or *xanthelasma* (xanthomata), *icterus* and *spider naevi* (chronic liver disease) or *exophthalmos* (thyroid acropathy). We leave you to consider the changes you may note as you approach the patient with any of the other conditions on the list (see individual short cases in this book and in Volume 3). Even if the diagnosis is not immediately clear on looking at the face, it is likely that in many cases it will become rapidly apparent as you

2 **inspect the hands**. Run quickly through the six main conditions that make up 75% of cases

   (a) *rheumatoid arthritis* (proximal joint swelling, spindling of the fingers, ulnar deviation, nodules),

   (b) *systemic sclerosis* (sclerodactyly with tapering of the fingers, sometimes with gangrene of the fingertips, tight, shiny, adherent skin, calcified nodules, etc.),

   (c) generalized *wasting* of the small muscles of the hand, perhaps with dorsal guttering,

   (d) *psoriasis* (pitting of the nails, terminal interphalangeal arthropathy, scaly rash),

   (e) *ulnar nerve palsy* (may be a typical claw hand or may be muscle wasting which spares the thenar eminence; often this diagnosis will only become apparent when you have made a sensory examination), and

   (f) *clubbing*.

The changes that you may see in the other conditions in the list are dealt with under the individual short cases in this book and in Volume 3, but if in these first few seconds you have not made a rapid spot diagnosis, study first the dorsal and then the palmar aspects of the hands, looking specifically at

3 the **joints** for swelling, deformity or Heberden's nodes,

4 the **nails** for pitting, onycholysis, clubbing, nail-fold infarcts (vasculitis – usually rheumatoid) or splinter haemorrhages (unlikely),

5 the **skin** for *colour* (pigmentation, icterus, palmar erythema), for *consistency* (tight and shiny in scleroderma; papery thin, perhaps with purpuric patches in steroid therapy; thick in acromegaly), and for *lesions* (psoriasis, vasculitis, purpura, xanthomata, spider naevi, telangiectasis in Osler–Weber–Rendu and systemic sclerosis, tophi, neurofibromata, other rashes),

6 the **muscles** for isolated *wasting* of the thenar eminence (median nerve lesion), for generalized wasting especially of the first dorsal interosseous but sparing the

thenar eminence (ulnar nerve lesion), for generalized wasting from a T1 lesion or other cause (see Station 3, CNS, Case 52) or for *fasciculation* which usually indicates motor neurone disease, though occasionally it can occur in other conditions such as syringomyelia, old polio or Charcot–Marie–Tooth disease.

Before leaving the inspection it is worth looking specifically for *skin crease pigmentation* (see Vol. 2, Section F, Experience 186) before moving to

7 palpation of the hands for Dupuytren's contracture, nodules (may be palpable in the palms in rheumatoid arthritis), calcinosis (scleroderma/CREST), xanthomata, Heberden's nodes or tophi. In the vast majority of cases you will have, by now, some findings demanding either specific further action (see below) or a report with a diagnosis. Nonetheless, you should be prepared to continue with a full neurological examination of the hands to confirm a suspected neurological lesion, or if you have still made no diagnosis. If the hands appear normal it may be that there is a sensory defect. In these cases, it is more efficient, therefore, to commence the examination by testing

8 sensation. Ask the patient if there has been any numbness or tingling in his hands and if so, when (?worse at night – carpal tunnel syndrome) and where. Bearing in mind the classic patterns of sensory defect in ulnar and median nerve lesions (see Fig. B.4) and the dermatomes (see Fig. B.2), seek and define an area of deficit to *pinprick* and *light touch* (dab cotton wool lightly), and check the *vibration* and *joint position* sense. With incomplete sensory loss due to either an ulnar or a median nerve defect, if you stroke the medial border of the little finger and the lateral border of the index finger with your fingers simultaneously, the patient may sense that the one side feels different from the other.

9 Check the **tone** of the muscles in the hand by flexing and extending all the joints including the wrist in a 'rolling wave' fashion.

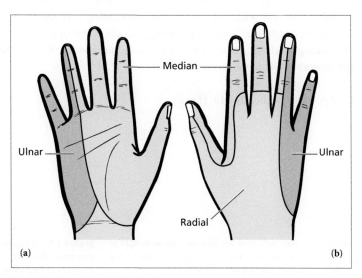

(a)   **(b)**

Figure B.4 Dermatomes in the hand.

10 The **motor** system of the hands can be tested with the instructions

(a) 'Open your hands; now close them; now open and close them quickly' (myotonic dystrophy)*

(b) 'Squeeze my fingers' – offer two fingers (C8, T1)†

(c) 'Hold your fingers out straight' (demonstrate); 'stop me bending them' (C7)

(d) 'Spread your fingers apart' (demonstrate); 'stop me pushing them together' (dorsal‡ interossei – ulnar nerve)

(e) 'Hold this piece of paper between your fingers; stop me pulling it out' (palmar‡ interossei – ulnar nerve)

(f) 'Point your thumb at the ceiling; stop me pushing it down' (abductor pollicis brevis – median nerve)

(g) 'Put your thumb and little finger together; stop me pulling them apart' (opponens pollicis – median nerve).

Finally, for the sake of completeness, check the

11 **radial pulses.**

The action you take after finding an abnormality at any stage during the above *routine* will depend on what you find. Most commonly, an abnormality found during the inspection will lead to most of the above being skipped in favour of a search for other evidence of the condition you suspect. It is worth emphasizing that there may be clues at

12 **the elbows** in several of the common conditions: rheumatoid arthritis (nodules), psoriatic arthropathy (psoriatic plaques), ulnar nerve palsy (scar, filling of the ulnar groove, restriction of range of movement at the elbow or evidence of fracture) and xanthomata. On the evidence of our survey, you will need to examine the elbows in over 40% of cases (do not be put off by rolled-down sleeves). It is worth considering where else you would look, what for and what other tests you would do with the other conditions on the list (see individual short cases in this book and in Volume 3), but in particular remember to look for *tophi* on the ears if you suspect gout, and if you have diagnosed acromegaly seek an associated *carpal tunnel syndrome* (see Vol. 2, Section F, Experience 116). If on inspection you suspect a neurological deficit in the hand, you may wish to confirm it by performing only that part of the above *routine* relevant to that lesion, e.g. testing abduction and opposition of the thumb and seeking the classic sensory pattern if you see lone wasting of the thenar eminence and suspect carpal tunnel syndrome.

See Appendix 1, Checklist 15, Hands.

---

*Alternatively, you could miss this step out and go straight to step (b), but then issue the instruction 'Let go' and if there is any suspicion of myotonic dystrophy move to step (a).

†Some neurologists prefer to test the deep finger flexors by trying to extend flexed fingers, whilst steadying the wrist (flexor digitorum profundus, C8).

‡Remember DAB and PAD: DAB = dorsal abduct, PAD = palmar adduct.

16 | 'Examine this patient's skin'

Variations of instruction in initial PACES survey (resultant diagnoses in brackets)
Examine this patient's skin (psoriasis; neurofibromatosis)
Look at this patient's skin (psoriasis)
Examine this lady's skin (neurofibromatosis)
This man has itchy skin. Please examine (eczema)

Diagnoses from our original survey in order of frequency*
1 Psoriasis (Vol. 3, Station 5, Skin, Case 4) 15%
2 Vitiligo (Vol. 3, Station 5, Skin, Case 8) 10%
3 Systemic sclerosis/CREST (Vol. 3, Station 5, Locomotor, Case 3) 10%
4 Radiation burn on the chest (Vol. 3, Station 5, Skin, Case 31) 10%
5 Epidermolysis bullosa dystrophica 10%
6 Purpura (Vol. 3, Station 5, Skin, Case 25) 5%
7 Pseudoxanthoma elasticum (Vol. 3, Station 5, Skin, Case 10) 5%
8 Localized scleroderma (Vol. 3, Station 5, Skin, Case 35) 5%

Examination *routine*

This instruction is a rather more specific variation of the 'spot diagnosis' *routine* (see Section B, Examination *Routine* 22). You should
1 perform a *visual survey* of the patient, from scalp to sole, with regard to the fact that most dermatological lesions have a predilection for certain areas. It is as well to remember some of the regional associations as you *survey* the patient.

Scalp Psoriasis (look especially at the hairline for redness, scaling, etc.), alopecia,† ringworm (very uncommon)

Face Systemic sclerosis (tight, shiny skin, pseudorhagades, beaked nose, telangiectasis), discoid lupus erythematosus (raised, red, scaly lesions with telangiectasis, scarring and altered pigmentation), xanthelasma, dermatomyositis (heliotrope colour to eyelids), Sturge–Weber, rodent ulcer (usually below the eye or on the side of the nose, raised lesion with central ulcer, the edges being rolled and having telangiectatic blood vessels)

Mouth Osler–Weber–Rendu, Peutz–Jeghers, lichen planus (white lace-like network on mucosal surface), pemphigus, candidiasis (white exudate inside the mouth usually associated with a disease requiring multiple antimicrobial therapy or an immunosuppressive disorder, e.g. leukaemia, AIDS, etc.), herpes simplex, Behçet's

---

*You may be asked to 'Examine this patient's skin'. However, it may be 'Examine this patient's hands, face or rash' or just 'Look at this patient'. The figures here apply only to when the instruction was to examine the skin.

†Some causes of alopecia:
1 Diffuse – male pattern baldness, cytotoxic drugs, hypothyroidism, hyperthyroidism, iron deficiency
2 Patchy – alopecia areata, ringworm; with scarring – discoid lupus erythematosus, lichen planus.

Neck	Pseudoxanthoma elasticum, tuberculous adenitis with sinus formation (?ethnic origin)
Trunk	Radiotherapy stigmata, morphoea, neurofibromatosis, dermatitis herpetiformis (itching blisters over scapulae, buttocks, elbows, knees), herpes zoster along the intercostal nerves, pityriasis rosea, Addison's (areolar and scar pigmentation), pemphigus (trunk and limbs)
Axillae	Vitiligo, acanthosis nigricans (pigmentation and velvety thickening of axillary skin, perianal, areolar and lateral abdominal skin, 'tripe palms', mucous membranes involved, may be underlying insulin resistance or malignancy)
Elbows	Psoriasis (extensor), pseudoxanthoma elasticum (flexor), xanthomata (extensor), rheumatoid nodules (extensor), atopic dermatitis (flexor), olecranon bursitis, gouty tophi
Hands	Systemic sclerosis (sclerodactyly, infarcts of finger pulps, prominent capillaries at nail-folds), lichen planus (wrists), dermatomyositis (heliotrope lesions – Gottron's papules – on the joints of the dorsum of the fingers/hands, nail-fold capillary dilation and infarction), Addison's (skin crease pigmentation), granuloma annulare, erythema multiforme (polymorphic eruption, 'target' lesions, mucous membrane involvement, macules, vesicles, bullae, etc.), SLE (erythematous patches over the dorsal surface of the phalanges), scabies (not in MRCP PACES!)
Nails	Psoriasis (pitting, onycholysis), iron deficiency (koilonychia), fungal dystrophy, tuberous sclerosis (periungal fibromata)
Genitalia	Behçet's (iridocyclitis, uveitis, pyodermas, ulcers, etc.), lichen sclerosus (white plaques), candidiasis
Legs	Leg ulcer (diabetic, venous, ischaemic, pyoderma gangrenosum), necrobiosis lipoidica diabeticorum, pretibial myxoedema, erythema nodosum, Henoch–Schönlein purpura, tendon xanthomata in Achilles, erythema ab igne, pemphigoid (legs and arms), lipoatrophy
Feet	Pustular psoriasis, eczema, verrucae, keratoderma blenorrhagica (?eyes, joints, etc.)

During this *survey* you should consider

2 the **distribution** of the lesions (psoriasis on extensor areas, lichen planus in flexor areas, candidiasis on mucous membranes, tuberous sclerosis on nails and face, necrobiosis lipoidica diabeticorum usually bilateral, gouty tophi in the joints of hands, elbows and on the ears, etc.). Then after the *survey* (which should take a few seconds)

3 examine the **lesions** (see Section B, Examination *Routine* 17, 'Examine this patient's rash'), looking in particular for the *characteristic* features, e.g. scaling in psoriasis, shiny purple polygonal papules with Wickham's striae in lichen planus, etc. If you have made a diagnosis, consider whether you need to look for any

4 **associated lesions** (arthropathy and nail changes with psoriasis, evidence of associated autoimmune disease with vitiligo, etc.). Go through the skin conditions which our survey has suggested occur in the exam and make sure that you would recognize each, would know what else to look for, and what to say in your presentation.

See Appendix 1, Checklist 16, Skin.

17 | 'Examine this patient's rash'

Variations of instruction in initial PACES survey (resultant diagnoses in brackets)

Take a look at this lady's rash (?examiners didn't know either – rash of uncertain cause)

This lady has a rash. Examine it (mixed connective tissue disease)

Diagnoses from our original survey in order of frequency*

1 Psoriasis (Vol. 3, Station 5, Skin, Case 4) 20%
2 Purpura (Vol. 3, Station 5, Skin, Case 25) 10%
3 Vasculitis (Vol. 3, Station 5, Locomotor, Case 10) 10%
4 Neurofibromatosis (Vol. 3, Station 5, Skin, Case 2) 10%
5 Juvenile chronic arthritis (Still's disease) (Vol. 3, Station 5, Locomotor, Case 18) 10%
6 Xanthomata (Vol. 3, Station 5, Skin, Case 7) 5%
7 Necrobiosis lipoidica diabeticorum (Vol. 3, Station 5, Skin, Case 18) 5%
8 Radiation burn on the chest (Vol. 3, Station 5, Skin, Case 31) 5%

Examination *routine*

This *routine* is generally the same as that discussed under 'Examine this patient's skin (see Section B, Examination *Routine* 16)'

1 You should quickly conduct a *visual survey* as described under 'skin' and note if there are any similar or related lesions elsewhere. Look at the

2 **distribution** of the lesions, whether confined to a single area (morphoea, erythema nodosum, rodent ulcer, melanoma, alopecia areata, etc.) or present in other areas such as psoriasis, neurofibromatosis, acanthosis nigricans, dermatomyositis, etc. While concentrating on the lesion in question, it is important to look at the

3 **surrounding skin** for any helpful clues such as *scratch marks* as evidence of itching,† *radiotherapy field markings* on the skin in the vicinity of a radiation burn, or *paper-thin skin* with purpura (corticosteroid therapy), etc. You should now

4 **examine the lesion** in detail. To determine the *extent* of the lesion, you may have to ask the patient to undress, a procedure which will provide you with a little more time to survey other areas. Decide if the rash is *pleomorphic* or *monomorphic* (all the lesions are similar). If so, examine one typical lesion carefully in terms of:

   (a) *colour*, e.g. erythematous or pigmented,
   (b) *size*,
   (c) *shape*, e.g. oval, circular, annular, etc.,
   (d) *surface*, e.g. scaling or eroded,
   (e) *character*, e.g. macule, papule, vesicle, pustule, ulcer, etc.,
   (f) *secondary features*, e.g. crusting, lichenification, etc.

---

*See Footnote, Section B, Examination *Routine* 16. The same sentiment applies here.
†Some causes of itching:
1 Dermatological – scabies, dermatitis herpetiformis, lichen planus, eczema

2 Medical – cholestasis, chronic renal failure, lymphoma, polycythaemia rubra vera.

It is advisable to be familiar with the correct use of the terms to describe rashes (especially if you do not recognize the lesion!). To say 'skin lesion' or 'skin rash' conveys no diagnostic meaning. In your presentation, you should be able to describe the lesion with respect to the above six features, especially if you do not know the diagnosis. The following are some of the useful terms employed in describing skin lesions:

Macules: flat, circumscribed lesions, not raised above the skin – size and shape vary

Papules: raised, circumscribed, firm lesions up to 1 cm in size

Nodules: like papules but larger; usually lie deeper in skin

Tumours: larger than nodules, elevated or very deeply placed in the skin

Weals: circumscribed elevations associated with itching and tingling

Vesicles: small well-defined collections of fluid

Bullae: large vesicles

Pustules: circumscribed elevations containing purulent fluid which may, in some cases, be sterile (e.g. Behçet's)

Scales: dead tissue from the horny layer which may be dry (e.g. psoriasis) or greasy (e.g. seborrhoeic dermatitis)

Crusts: these consist of dried exudate

Ulcers: excavations in the skin of irregular shape; remember that every ulcer has a shape, an edge, a floor, a base and a secretion, and it forms a scar on healing

Scars: the result of healing of a damaged dermis.

5 Finally, if indicated, look for **additional features** (arthropathy in psoriasis or Still's disease, cushingoid facies if purpura is due to steroids, clubbing with radiation burns on the chest, etc.).

See Appendix 1, Checklist 17, Rash.

18 | 'Examine this patient's neck'

Variations of instruction in initial PACES survey (resultant diagnoses in brackets)

Examine this patient's neck (goitre; pseudoxanthoma elasticum; multinodular goitre)

This patient has noticed a swelling in his neck – please examine (goitre)

This patient has a goitre. Please examine her (exophthalmos and non-nodular goitre)

Diagnoses from our original survey in order of frequency

1 Goitre (Vol. 3, Station 5, Endocrine, Case 4) 46%

2 Generalized lymphadenopathy 17%

3 Graves' disease (Vol. 3, Station 5, Endocrine, Case 3) 12%

4 Jugular vein pulse abnormality 6%

5 Bilateral parotid enlargement/Mikulicz's syndrome (Vol. 3, Station 5, Other, Case 1) 4%

6 Supraclavicular mass with Horner's syndrome 4%

7 Facioscapulohumeral muscular dystrophy 4%

8 Ankylosing spondylitis (Vol. 3, Station 5, Locomotor, Case 6) 2%

9 Hypothyroidism (Vol. 3, Station 5, Locomotor, Case 5) 2%

10 Acanthosis nigricans (Vol. 3, Station 5, Skin, Case 48) <1%

Examination *routine*

As usual, the first step is to

1 *survey* the patient quickly from head to foot (exophthalmos, myxoedematous facies, ankle oedema, etc.) and then to

2 **look at the neck.** According to the survey, the reason for the instruction in half of the cases will be a *goitre*. If another abnormality is visible, your further action will be dictated by what you see and we suggest you go through the list and establish a sequence of actions for each abnormality (e.g. if you see giant *v* waves you would wish to examine the heart and liver; see Station 3, Cardiovascular, Case 11). If you do see a goitre, offer a drink to the patient:

'Take a sip of water and hold it in your mouth';

look at the neck:

'Now swallow'.

Watch the movement of the goitre, or the *appearance* of a *nodule* not visible before swallowing (behind sternomastoid; see Fig. C5.64c2, Vol. 3, Station 5, Endocrine, Case 4). Next ask the patient's permission to feel the neck, and then approach him from behind. If there has been no evidence of a goitre so far you may wish to palpate the neck for lymph nodes *before* feeling for a goitre. Otherwise

3 **palpate** the thyroid. With the right index and middle fingers, feel below the thyroid cartilage where the isthmus of the thyroid gland lies over the trachea. Then palpate the two lobes of the thyroid gland which extend laterally behind the sternomastoid muscle. Ask the patient to swallow again while you continue to palpate the thyroid, ensuring that the neck is slightly flexed to ease palpation. Remember that if there is a goitre, when you give your presentation you are going to want to comment on its *size*, whether it is *soft* or *firm*, whether it is *nodular* or *diffusely enlarged*, whether it *moves* readily on swallowing, whether there are *lymph nodes* (see below) and whether there is a vascular *murmur* (see below). Extend palpation upwards along the medial edge of the sternomastoid muscle on either side to look for a *pyramidal lobe* which may be present. Apologize for any discomfort you may cause because the deep palpation necessary to feel the thyroid gland causes pain,* particularly in patients with Graves' disease. *Percussion* over the upper sternum is used to assess any retrosternal extension of goitre. Next palpate laterally to examine for

4 **lymph nodes.** If you find lymph node enlargement, check not only in the *supraclavicular fossae* and right up the neck but also in the *submandibular, postauricular* and *suboccipital* areas, ensuring that the head is slightly flexed on the side

*In viral thyroiditis (rare) the patient may complain of a painful thyroid and the thyroid may be overtly tender on light palpation.

under palpation to allow access and scrutiny of slightly enlarged lymph nodes. Ascertain whether the lymph nodes are *separate* (reactive hyperplasia, infectious mononucleosis, lymphoma, etc.) or *matted* together (neoplastic, tuberculous), *mobile* or *fixed* to the skin or deep tissues (neoplastic), or whether they are *soft, fleshy, rubbery* (Hodgkin's disease) or *hard* (neoplastic). Particularly if you find lymph nodes without a goitre, examine for lymph nodes in the axillae and groins (lymphoma, chronic lymphatic leukaemia, etc.) and, if allowed, feel for the spleen.

5 **Auscultate** over the thyroid for evidence of increased vascularity. You may need to occlude venous return to rule out a venous hum, and listen over the aortic area to ensure that the thyroid bruit you hear is not, in fact, an outflow obstruction murmur conducted to the root of the neck.

6 If there is any evidence of thyroid disease, consider beginning an assessment of **thyroid status** (see Section B, Examination *Routine* 19, 'Assess this patient's thyroid status') by feeling and counting the pulse (NB: do not miss *atrial fibrillation*, whether slow or fast). The examiner will soon stop you if he wishes to hear your description of a multinodular goitre in a euthyroid patient.

See Appendix 1, Checklist 18, Neck.

19 | 'Assess this patient's thyroid status'

Variations of instruction in initial PACES survey (resultant diagnoses in brackets)
Examine this lady's thyroid status (euthyroid)
This lady has had previous problems with her thyroid. Examine her to determine her thyroid status (euthyroid)

Diagnoses from original survey in order of frequency
1 Euthyroid Graves' disease (Vol. 3, Station 5, Endocrine, Case 3) 42%
2 Hyperthyroidism (Vol. 3, Station 5, Endocrine, Case 3) 17%
3 Euthyroid simple goitre (Vol. 3, Station 5, Endocrine, Case 4) 8%

Examination *routine*
Although the patient usually has signs of thyroid disease (exophthalmos, goitre), you are not being asked to examine these but rather to assess whether the patient is clinically hypo-, eu- or hyperthyroid. Perform a speedy
1 *visual survey*, looking specifically for *signs of thyroid disease* (exophthalmos, goitre, thyroid acropachy, pretibial myxoedema – all can occur in association with *any* thyroid status), and ask yourself if the facies are in any way myxoedematous. Observe the patient's

2 composure, whether *hyperactive, fidgety* and *restless* (hyperthyroid); normal, composed demeanour (euthyroid); or if she is somewhat *immobile* and *uninterested* in the people around her (hypothyroid).

3 Take the pulse and *count* it for 15 seconds, noting the presence or absence of *atrial fibrillation* (slow, normal rate or fast). If the pulse is slow (less than 60) or if you suspect hypothyroidism, proceed immediately to test for

4 slow relaxation of the ankle,* supinator or other jerks. To test the reflexes, you will require the patient's cooperation and the ensuing conversation may provide you with helpful clues (slow hesitant speech, slow movements, etc.). Otherwise,

5 feel the **palms**, whether *warm* and *sweaty* or cold and sweaty (anxiety) and then

6 ask the patient to stretch out his hands to full extension of the wrist and elbow. If the **tremor** is not obvious, place your palm against his outstretched fingers to feel for it. Alternatively, you can place a piece of paper on the dorsum of his outstretched hands – it will oscillate if a fine tremor is present.

7 Look at the **eyes**, noting exophthalmos (sclera visible above the lower lid, a sign not related to thyroid status) but looking specifically for *lid retraction* (sclera visible above the cornea). Test for lid lag (lid lag and retraction may diminish as the hyperthyroid patient becomes euthyroid).

8 Examine the **thyroid** as described under 'Examine this patient's neck (see Examination *Routine* 18), remembering the steps are (i) look, (ii) palpate and (iii) auscultate.†

Putting the above findings together, it should be possible to provide a definite conclusion about thyroid status; this is considered a very basic skill and it will not be taken lightly if, in your state of nerves, you make fundamental errors. Though the examiner may put you under pressure to test your confidence, keep calm and be particularly wary of being led to diagnose hypo- or hyperthyroidism in the presence of a normal pulse rate (see Vol. 2, Section F, Experience 191).

9 Be prepared with the **standard questions** for assessment of thyroid status (temperature preference, weight change, appetite, bowel habits, palpitations, change of temper, etc; see Vol. 3, Station 5, Endocrine, Case 5) if there is any doubt about the thyroid status after the above examination.

See Appendix 1, Checklist 19, Thyroid status.

---

*The slow relaxing ankle jerk in hypothyroidism is best demonstrated with the patient kneeling on a chair or bed with the feet hanging over the edge, and the examiner standing behind the patient. This manoeuvre is useful for the dressed patient in the outpatient department and may be useful in the PACES exam if the patient is dressed and sitting on a chair.

†A thyroid bruit is good evidence of thyroid overactivity; if present, it can be heard over the isthmus and lateral lobe of the thyroid; it will not be obliterated by occluding the internal jugular vein (venous hum) or by rotation of the head and it will not be influenced by pressure of the stethoscope (use light pressure to avoid causing non-thyroid bruits).

20 | 'Examine this patient's knee'

Possible diagnoses
Rheumatoid arthritis
Seronegative spondyloarthropathy
   Psoriatic arthritis
   Ankylosing spondylitis
   Inflammatory bowel disease
   Reactive arthritis
Gout
Pseudogout
Septic arthritis
Osteoarthritis
Haemarthrosis
Prepatellar bursitis
Baker's cyst
Charcot's joint

Examination *routine*

If asked to examine a patient's knees, you should bear the following in mind:
   (a) is it an *inflammatory* or *non-inflammatory* problem?
   (b) is it a *monoarthritis* or part of a more widespread arthropathy (*oligo-* or *polyarthropathy* or *spondyloarthropathy*)?
   (c) is the pain (if any) referred from elsewhere (i.e. hip)?
   (d) are there any extraarticular features?
   (e) what is the functional impairment?

1 On approaching the patient, **observe** for any other obvious features of joint disease (e.g. symmetrical deforming polyarthritis in the hands of *rheumatoid arthritis*, an asymmetrical arthritis and skin plaques of *psoriatic arthritis*, or podagra of the first MTP joint as seen in gout).

2 Ask the patient if he has any pain and expose the leg from the upper thigh to the foot.

3 Inspect the leg. Is there any obvious deformity (*valgus* or *varus* deformity or *flexion* deformity)? Are there any scars or wounds to suggest entry for infection? Is there any muscle wasting (*quadriceps*)? Is the knee swollen or erythematous? Look for loss of the medial and lateral dimples around the knees to suggest the presence of an effusion. Compare one side with the other as you progress through the examination.

4 Palpate the joint. Is it warm? Place your whole hand gently over the patient's knee and rest it there for a few seconds. Compare the temperature of this knee with the mid calf and mid thigh on the same side as well as the opposite knee. Do not be too quick to move your hands as you may miss subtle differences in temperature. Watch the patient's face for any sign that you are causing him discomfort. Ask if the knee is tender on palpation.

By this stage you should have an idea of whether this is an inflammatory or non-inflammatory problem and how active it is.

5 Examine for an **effusion**. For a small effusion look for the *bulge sign*. With your index finger, firmly wipe any fluid from the medial joint recess (moving from distal to proximal) into the lateral joint recess. Now apply a similar wiping motion from distal to proximal in the lateral joint recess. A distinct bulge will be seen to appear back in the medial compartment as the fluid moves back to this side of the joint. For larger effusions the bulge sign is absent and the presence of fluid needs to be assessed by the *patellar tap*. Firm pressure is applied over the suprapatellar pouch with the flat of one hand, using the thumb and index finger to push any fluid from the medial and lateral joint compartments into the retropatellar space. With the index finger or thumb of the other hand, apply a short jerky movement to the patella. The presence of significant fluid is indicated by a spongy feel followed by a 'tap' as the patella hits the anterior aspect of the lower end of the femur.

6 Assess **movement**. Ask the patient to flex the knee as far as possible. Observe the degree of flexion (and any discomfort). Normal flexion is 135°.

7 Palpate for any **crepitus** over the joint as flexion occurs and feel behind the knee for a

8 Baker's cyst.

9 Assess for joint **instability**. Examine for *cruciate* instability (anterior and posterior draw test*) and medial and lateral ligament instability. *McMurray's sign* can be used to examine for cartilage tears. The knee is fully flexed and then internally rotated before being straightened by the examiner. Pain, or a clunking feeling, over the knee joint suggests a cartilage tear. The test is repeated with external rotation of the knee.

10 Ask to examine the **other joints**. Do not forget to ask about examining the other knee and spine (for associated inflammatory spondylitis). Are there any features of *psoriasis, inflammatory bowel disease, reactive arthritis* (enthesitis, keratoderma blenorrhagica, conjunctivitis, balanitis) or tophi to suggest *gout*?

Finally, think of relevant *investigations* such as X-rays for changes of rheumatoid arthritis, osteoarthrosis or pseudogout; synovial fluid analysis for crystals (negative or positive birefringence on polarized microscopy, gram stain and culture for infection).

See Appendix 1, Checklist 20, Knee.

---

*With the patient supine, flex the knee to 90 degrees, place your hands around the upper calf and gently pull forward or push backward looking for significant anterior or posterior movement of the tibia plateau. Compare with the other side.

21 | 'Examine this patient's hip'

Possible diagnoses
Osteoarthrosis
Rheumatoid arthritis
Seronegative spondyloarthritis
   Ankylosing spondylitis
   Psoriatic arthritis
   Inflammatory bowel disease
   Reactive arthritis (chronic)
Septic arthritis
Avascular necrosis
Paget's
Iliopsoas bursitis
Sciatica

Examination *routine*

1 Inspect the leg. Is the hip held in a flexed position? Is there any shortening of the leg? Is the leg externally rotated? Look for any scars. Are there any other obvious stigmata of rheumatic disease (e.g. rheumatoid arthritis, psoriatic arthropathy, ankylosing spondylitis, osteoarthritis)? Look for any walking aids.

2 Ask the patient if they have any pain. Ask them to show the location of the pain. Pain in the groin is more suggestive of hip disease.

3 Assess **movement**. With the patient lying flat and with his knee bent, ask him to flex his hip to the chest. Then, assess the degree of internal and external rotation. With both the knee and hip flexed to 90°, rotate the hip joint internally and externally using the foot as a pointer and the knee as a pivot. Estimate the degree of rotation. Next, assess hip abduction and adduction by placing one hand on the opposite iliac crest (to keep the pelvis stationary); then, place your other hand under the ankle of the leg being examined and abduct and adduct the hip. The normal range of movement is flexion 120°, internal rotation 30°, external rotation 45°, abduction 60°, adduction 30°. A hip flexion deformity may be masked by an increased spinal lordosis. Flex the opposite hip (with knee bent) to flatten out the lumbar lordosis (feel with your hand under the patient's spine). Any fixed flexion deformity of the opposite hip will be brought out by the flattening of the lumbar spine (*Thomas's test*).

4 If no abnormality is detected then consider whether the pain may be coming from the patient's spine. Carry out a **straight leg raise**. Slowly raise the patient's leg by taking hold of his heel and lifting the leg slowly. Stop if pain occurs. Pain in the leg to the foot is indicative of pain originating in the *spine* – nerve root entrapment. You may need to undertake a *neurological assessment* to test for abnormalities in muscle strength (particularly of ankle plantarflexion), sensation or reflexes (be prepared to differentiate a nerve root from a peripheral nerve lesion).

5 Check for **tenderness** over the greater trochanter (trochanteric bursitis).

6 You may need to check for **leg length** inequality* (measure from the anterior superior iliac crest to the medial malleolus on the same side, compare with other leg).

7 Ask the patient to **walk**. An antalgic gait occurs when there is pain in one hip and the patient leans to the other side to avoid putting weight on the affected side. A waddling gait is indicative of hip muscle weakness (e.g. osteomalacia, myositis).

You would be interested to see X-rays of the pelvis. Consider what other investigations you would request for the conditions on the list above.

See Appendix 1, Checklist 21, Hip.

22 | 'What is the diagnosis?'

Variations of instruction in initial PACES survey (resultant diagnoses in brackets)
What is the diagnosis? (psoriasis)
This lady has had multiple fractures. What is your diagnosis? (?Turner's syndrome)
Examine this gentleman. What do you notice? (cushingoid due to steroids)
Examine this patient (peripheral and central cyanosis)
Look at this patient (acromegaly; scleroderma; drug eruption)
This woman has glycosuria. Look at her and examine anything that is relevant (acromegaly and xanthelasma)
This patient is tired all the time. Why is that? (koilonychia)
Examine this patient's spine (ankylosing spondylitis and aortic incompetence)
This lady has been having headaches. Please examine the appropriate systems (acromegaly)
Describe this lady's abnormalities (systemic sclerosis)
Look at this man and examine the patient as you feel appropriate (acromegaly)
This lady has had headaches. Please examine her (acromegaly)
You must know the diagnosis of this patient (neurofibromatosis)
This lady complains of some abnormalities in her gums. Please examine her (lichen planus)
This lady has uncontrolled hypertension. Please examine her (pituitary tumour)

*The reasons to examine for a shorter leg are: (i) for protrusio acetabulum, which occurs mainly in rheumatoid arthritis when the femoral head migrates through the acetabulum because of regional osteoporosis. (ii) Where there has been a fracture which has gone undetected at the neck of femur. (iii) When a patient has had a joint replacement (mainly hip, but knee also) where there has been a need to shorten the bone a bit more than the prosthesis allows. (iv) Where a Girdlestone procedure is carried out – when no hip joint prosthesis is placed (or removed) because of sepsis or patient's general health does not allow a major operation and, basically, the neck of the femur and femoral head are excised and the femur is held in place by the joint capsule, but migrates upwards. (v) Where there is apparent leg shortening which occurs due to pelvic tilt secondary to spinal disease – in this case the leg is not actually shortened, hence the need to measure both leg lengths.

This middle-aged man complains of headaches. Would you like to assess him and tell me why? (acromegaly)

Have a look at this lady who presented to the A & E department with acute shortness of breath and tell me why (spontaneous pneumothorax due to tuberous sclerosis)

Look at the hands, look at the face and give the diagnosis (hypertrophic pulmonary osteoarthropathy)

What do you think of this lady? (cushingoid due to steroids)

Diagnoses from our original survey in order of frequency

1 Acromegaly (Vol. 3, Station 5, Endocrine, Case 2) 11%
2 Parkinson's disease 5%
3 Hemiplegia 5%
4 Goitre (Vol. 3, Station 5, Endocrine, Case 4) 5%
5 Jaundice 5%
6 Myotonic dystrophy 4%
7 Pigmentation (Vol. 3, Station 5, Endocrine, Case 7) 4%
8 Graves' disease (Vol. 3, Station 5, Endocrine, Case 3) 4%
9 Exophthalmos (Vol. 3, Station 5, Endocrine, Case 1) 4%
10 Paget's disease (Vol. 3, Station 5, Locomotor, Case 7) 3%
11 Ptosis 3%
12 Choreoathetosis 3%
13 Drug-induced parkinsonism 3%
14 Breathlessness 2%
15 Purpura (Vol. 3, Station 5, Skin, Case 25) 2%
16 Hypopituitarism (Vol. 3, Station 5, Endocrine, Case 8) 2%
17 Addison's/Nelson's (Vol. 3, Station 5, Endocrine, Case 7) 2%
18 Cushing's syndrome (Vol. 3, Station 5, Endocrine, Case 6) 2%
19 Psoriasis (Vol. 3, Station 5, Skin, Case 4) 2%
20 Hypothyroidism (Vol. 3, Station 5, Endocrine, Case 5) 2%
21 Systemic sclerosis/CREST (Vol. 3, Station 5, Locomotor, Case 3) 2%
22 Sturge–Weber syndrome (Vol. 3, Station 5, Skin, Case 24) 2%
23 Spider naevi and ascites 1%
24 Marfan's syndrome (Vol. 3, Station 5, Locomotor, Case 9) 1%
25 Neurofibromatosis 1%
26 Cyanotic congenital heart disease 1%
27 Pretibial myxoedema (Vol. 3, Station 5, Endocrine, Case 9) 1%
28 Uraemia and dialysis scars 1%
29 Horner's syndrome 1%
30 Cachexia 1%
31 Osler–Weber–Rendu syndrome (Vol. 3, Station 5, Skin, Case 3) 1%
32 Ankylosing spondylitis (Vol. 3, Station 5, Locomotor, Case 6) 1%
33 Ulnar nerve palsy 1%
34 Turner's syndrome (Vol. 3, Station 5, Endocrine, Case 11) 1%
35 Down's syndrome (Vol. 3, Station 5, Other, Case 5) 1%
36 Bilateral parotid enlargement/Mikulicz's syndrome (Vol. 3, Station 5, Other, Case 1) 1%

37 Old rickets (Vol. 3, Station 5, Locomotor, Case 17) 1%
38 Torticollis 1%
39 Congenital syphilis 1%
40 Syringomyelia <1%
41 Herpes zoster (Vol. 3, Station 5, Skin, Case 32) <1%
42 Pemphigoid/pemphigus (Vol. 3, Station 5, Skin, Case 30) <1%
43 Bell's palsy <1%
44 Necrobiosis lipoidica diabeticorum (Vol. 3, Station 5, Skin, Case 18) <1%
45 Primary biliary cirrhosis <1%

Examination *routine*

Advice commonly given by the candidates in our survey as a result of their Membership experiences was to 'keep calm'. When you stand before a patient with a condition from the above list and hear the instruction under consideration, you are being asked to do what you do every day of your medical life. There are two differences, however, between everyday medical life and the examination: (i) the patients in the examination usually have classic, often florid, signs and should be easier to diagnose than most patients seen in the clinic; and (ii) in the examination, you may be overwhelmed by nerves and, as a result, make the most fundamental errors. You must indeed try to keep calm and remind yourself that this is likely to be an easy case, and that you will not only make a diagnosis (as you would with ease in the clinic), but will also find a way of scoring some extra marks. Unlike some of the instructions requiring long examination *routines*, the 'spot diagnosis' may be solved in seconds leaving time for something extra which you may be able to dictate, rather than leaving it to the examiner to lead. You should start with

1 *a visual survey* of the patient, running your eyes from the head via the neck, trunk, arms and legs to the feet, seeking the areas of abnormality, and thereby the diagnosis. We would suggest that you rehearse presenting the *records* for the various possibilities on the list (see individual short cases in this book and in Volume 3). If you are well prepared with the features of these short cases, then in the majority of instances you should be able to make a diagnosis, or likely diagnosis, which you can confirm or highlight by demonstrating additional features (see below). If you have scanned the patient briefly and not found any obvious abnormality, then

2 retrace the same ground, scrutinizing each part more thoroughly and asking yourself at each stage, 'Is the head normal?', 'Is the face normal?', etc. If it is not normal, describe the abnormality to yourself in the mind, trying to match it up with one of the short case *records*. In this way, cover the

(a) head (think especially of *Paget's* and *myotonic dystrophy* with frontal balding),
(b) face (think especially of *acromegaly*, *Parkinson's*, the facial asymmetry of *hemiplegia*, the long lean look of myotonic dystrophy, tardive dyskinesia, hypopituitarism, Cushing's, hypothyroidism, systemic sclerosis),
(c) eyes (*jaundice, exophthalmos*, ptosis, Horner's, xanthelasma),
(d) neck (*goitre*, Turner's, ankylosing spondylitis, torticollis),
(e) trunk (pigmentation, ascites, purpuric spots, spider naevi, wasting, pemphigus, etc.),
(f) arms (choreoathetosis, psoriasis, Addison's, spider naevi, syringomyelia),

(g) hands (acromegaly, *tremor*, clubbing, sclerodactyly, arachnodactyly, claw hand, etc.),

(h) legs (bowing, purpura, pretibial myxoedema, necrobiosis lipoidica diabeticorum), and

(i) feet (pes cavus).

If you still do not have the diagnosis

3 specifically consider **abnormal colouring** such as *pigmentation, icterus* or pallor, and then cover the same ground again but in even more detail,

4 breaking down each part into its constituents, scrutinizing them, and continually asking yourself the question: 'Is it normal?'. This procedure is most profitable on the face (Section B, Examination *Routine* 14).

Once you have the diagnosis, the natural impulse for most people is to give it in one word, and then stand back and wait for the applause. However, it is worth remembering that the majority of the candidates, who have all worked hard and prepared for the examination, are likely to 'spot' the diagnosis and yet only a few end up with the diploma. Do not let this opportunity pass you by; try to make more of the case yourself by proceeding to

5 look for **additional** and **associated features**, and then by making your presentation more elaborate. Describe the findings in detail (see individual short cases in this book and in Volume 3) and highlight the key features to support your diagnosis (lenticular abnormalities in myotonic dystrophy and Marfan's; thyroid bruit in Graves' disease; webbed neck in Turner's syndrome, and so on). It is worth going through the diagnoses on the list yourself, and considering what additional features you would look for, and how you could really go to town on an easy case. For example, if you diagnose acromegaly you could demonstrate the massive sweaty palms, commenting on the increased skin thickening and on the presence or absence of thenar wasting (carpal tunnel syndrome; see Vol. 2, Section F, Experience 116), and then proceed to test the visual fields. If you suspect Parkinson's disease, take the hands and test for cog-wheel rigidity at the wrist, demonstrate the glabellar tap sign (despite its unreliability) and then ask the patient to walk. If you diagnose hemiplegia, confirm that any facial weakness is upper motor neurone (see Station 3, CNS, Case 8), and then check for atrial fibrillation. If you see a goitre, examine it and then assess the thyroid status.

See Appendix 1, Checklist 22, 'Spot' diagnosis.

Section C
Short Case *Records*

*'Be professional in presentation. I agree it's an easy exam – it's easy to fail'.**

*Vol. 2, Section F, Quotation 346.

These books exist as they are because of many previous candidates who, over the years, have completed our surveys and given us invaluable insight into the candidate experience. Please give something back by doing the same for the candidates of the future. For all of your sittings, whether it be a triumphant pass or a disastrous fail . . .

Remember to fill in the survey at www.ryder-mrcp.org.uk

THANK YOU

In this section and in Section I in Volume 3, we present aides-mémoire (clinical descriptions for presentation to the examiner) for over 226 short cases. We have called these aides-mémoire *records*. They are divided into the eight station subsections of the three clinical stations of PACES. The order in each subsection has been determined by the frequency with which, according to our surveys, these short cases have appeared in the PACES examination for that station. Thus, short case no. 1 in a particular station subsection occurred most commonly, followed by short case no. 2 and so on. The percentages given represent our best estimate of your chance of meeting a particular short case in that station subsection in any one attempt at the MRCP PACES examination.

It cannot be overstressed that the first short cases we have dealt with in each station subsection occurred very commonly and the last very rarely, with all grades in between. The implications for your priorities are obvious. There are those who are tempted to ignore the less common cases and, indeed a good case can be made for this approach, but it is a risky business (see Footnote, Station 3, CNS, Case 44).

In this section, the style of each *record* imagines you to be in the examination situation with the patient displaying the typical features of a particular condition; you are 'churning out' these to the examiner along with the answers to various anticipated questions. Thus, you play the *record* of the condition to the examiner. Of course, the cases in the actual examination will only have some of the features (the *record* tends to describe the 'full house' case) and it is hoped that by becoming familiar with the whole *record*, you will be well equipped:

1 to pick up all the features present in the cases you meet on the day by scanning through the *records* in your mind; and

2 to adapt the *record* for the purpose of presenting those features which are present. To facilitate quick revision, the main points of each short case are highlighted in italics. The small print is a mixed bag of additional features and facts, lists of differential diagnoses and answers to some of the questions that might be asked. With the lists of differential diagnoses, we have tended to put the most important ones (which you should consider first) in large print with longer lists in the smaller print. The lists are not necessarily meant to be comprehensive. Next to the diagnoses on these lists we have used brackets to give some of the features of the conditions concerned, or perhaps one or two features you could look for (indicated by ?). The question mark is put there as a cue for you to look for important diagnostic features. We make no apology for repeating some of the features often, in the hope that by constant reinforcement they will become more firmly embedded in your memory. When unilateral signs could affect either side, we have not usually specified the side in the *record* but have indicated this by R/L. In these cases, however, each R/L in the *record* refers to the same side. Also, . . . is occasionally used for a sign in the lung fields or retina which could occur in any zone or to indicate the size of an organ or sign where the size is unspecified.

Presentation to the examiner

Becoming familiar with the short case *records* will arm you for the examination, though obviously it will not always be necessary, or desirable, for you to use them. Sometimes it may be appropriate just to give the diagnosis; even so, it may still be possible to enrich it with some of the well-known features from the *record*. If the examiner's question is: '*What is the diagnosis?*' you could answer 'Mitral stenosis' and await his reaction. On the other hand, if you are certain of your diagnosis, it would be better to say: 'The diagnosis is mitral stenosis because there is a rough, rumbling mid-diastolic murmur localized to the apex of the heart, there is a sharp opening snap and a loud first heart sound, a tapping impulse, an impalpable left ventricular apex, a left parasternal heave and a small volume pulse. Furthermore, the chaotic rhythm suggests atrial fibrillation and the patient has a malar flush'.

If you enlarge your response to 'What is the diagnosis?' by giving the features in this way, it is best to give the evidence in order of its importance to the diagnosis (as shown in the example). However, if the question is: '*What are your findings?*' it is best to give them in the order they are elicited: 'The patient has a malar flush and is slightly breathless at rest. The pulse is irregular in rate and volume. The jugular venous pressure is not elevated and the cardiac apex is not palpable but there is a tapping impulse parasternally on the left side and there is a left parasternal heave. The first heart sound is loud and there is an opening snap followed closely by a mid-diastolic rumble which is localized to the apex. These signs suggest that the patient has mitral stenosis'. Either way you score all the points under the heading 'Identifying physical signs'. If there is a differential diagnosis (and there usually is) then you should obviously give it to score the points under that heading. However, if there is no differential diagnosis don't make one up just because of this heading! – simply state you do not believe there is a differential diagnosis in the case concerned. There is also a need to score points under the heading 'Clinical judgement'. Depending on the circumstances, there may be cases where you can take the initiative and continue your dialogue to discuss investigation and management of the case concerned. The advantage of this is that you control the subject under discussion and can show knowledge by talking in areas that you know. The disadvantage of constantly stopping to make the examiner ask questions is that (a) this makes the examiner work and it is nice for the examiner to rest while you do all the talking, and (b) you are not in control of the subject matter. If the examiner asks all the questions he is in control and may ask in areas where your knowledge is weaker!

Remember, if you are talking in front of the patient, to avoid using words like 'cancer', 'motor neurone disease' and 'multiple sclerosis'. Use euphemisms such as 'neoplastic disease', 'anterior horn cell disease' and 'demyelinating disease'.

Remember that you can influence any discussion that follows by what you say. For example, the words 'The diagnosis is aortic incompetence' may produce an interrogation by the examiner about anything he would like to ask you. However, if you say: 'He has aortic incompetence for which there are several causes', this invites the examiner to ask you the causes. It is, therefore, a good answer – as long as you know them!

Station 1
Respiratory

Short case	Checked and updated as necessary for this edition by
1 Interstitial lung disease (fibrosing alveolitis)	Dr Omer Khair*
2 Pneumonectomy/lobectomy	Dr Omer Khair*
3 Chronic bronchitis and emphysema	Dr Omer Khair*
4 Bronchiectasis	Dr Omer Khair*
5 Dullness at the lung bases	Dr Omer Khair*
6 Rheumatoid lung	Dr Omer Khair*
7 Old tuberculosis	Dr Omer Khair*
8 Chest infection/consolidation/pneumonia	Dr Omer Khair*
9 Yellow nail syndrome	Dr Shireen Velangi*
10 Kyphoscoliosis	New short case for this edition by Dr Dev Banerjee*
11 Stridor	Dr Omer Khair*
12 Marfan's syndrome	Dr David Carruthers*
13 Carcinoma of the bronchus	Dr Omer Khair*
14 Klippel–Feil syndrome	Dr David Carruthers*
15 Kartagener's syndrome	Dr Omer Khair*
16 Lung transplant	Dr Omer Khair*
17 Cystic fibrosis	Dr Omer Khair*
18 Obesity/Pickwickian syndrome	Dr Omer Khair*
19 Pneumothorax	Dr Omer Khair*
20 Cor pulmonale	Dr Omer Khair*
21 Collapsed lung/atelectasis	New short case for this edition by Dr Rahul Mukherjee*
22 Superior vena cava obstruction	Dr Omer Khair*
23 Tuberculosis/apical consolidation	Dr Omer Khair*
24 Normal chest	Dr Bob Ryder

*All suggested changes by these specialty advisors were considered by Dr Bob Ryder and were accepted, edited, added to or rejected with Dr Ryder making the final editorial decision in every case.

Dr Omer Khair, Consultant Chest Physician, City Hospital, Birmingham, UK
Dr Shireen Velangi, Consultant Dermatologist, City Hospital, Birmingham, UK
Dr Dev Banerjee, Consultant Chest Physician, Heartlands Hospital, Birmingham, UK
Dr David Carruthers, Consultant Rheumatologist, City Hospital, Birmingham, UK
Dr Rahul Mukherjee, Consultant Chest Physician, Heartlands Hospital, Birmingham, UK

Case 1 | Interstitial lung disease (fibrosing alveolitis)

Frequency in survey: main focus of a short case or additional feature in 34% of attempts at PACES Station 1, Respiratory.

Record

The patient is breathless on minimal exertion (and may be on long-term oxygen therapy). There is bilateral *clubbing* of the fingers. There is evidence of steroid purpura peripherally, (may be) *cyanosis*, reduced but symmetrical expansion of the chest (there may be dullness to percussion at the bases) and *fine inspiratory crackles* at the bases.

The likely diagnosis is diffuse interstitial lung fibrosis.

Causes of diffuse interstitial lung disease*

Acute (less likely in the exam)

Vasculitis/haemorrhage (haemoptysis, falling haemoglobin)

Eosinophilic lung disease (drugs, fungi/parasites/allergic bronchopulmonary aspergillosis (ABPA))

Infection (immunosuppression)

Acute respiratory distress syndrome (ARDS) (complicating acute severe illness often with septicaemia)

Chronic (more likely in the exam)

Cryptogenic fibrosing alveolitis† (most common cause is usual interstitial pneumonia (UIP) (histological diagnosis) with insidious onset, dyspnoea and cough)

Rheumatoid lung disease (?hands, nodules)

Systemic sclerosis (?mask-like facies, telangiectasia, sclerodactyly; see Vol. 3, Station 5, Locomotor, Case 3)

---

*Over 200 separate entities falling within the spectrum of diffuse parenchymal lung disease have been described.

†The umbrella term of cryptogenic fibrosing alveolitis encompasses the most common group of interstitial lung diseases – the *idiopathic interstitial pneumonias* (IIPs) that present with progressive breathlessness, diffuse interstitial infiltrates on chest X-ray and fine end-inspiratory crepitations on auscultation. The separate IIPs have widely differing prognoses and have distinct radiological and pathological patterns. Consequently, in 2002 they were reclassified by a consensus committee of the American Thoracic Society (ATS) and European Respiratory Society. *Idiopathic pulmonary fibrosis* (IPF) is the most common IIP with histological lesions of UIP and poor prognosis (median survival 2.8–4 years).

Non-specific interstitial pneumonia (NSIP) is clinically indistinguishable from IPF except that it has a better prognosis (median

survival 6–7 years). *Cryptogenic organizing pneumonia* (COP), previously also known as bronchiolitis obliterans organizing pneumonia, typically presents with rapidly progressive breathlessness coming on over a 3–4-week period, with lethargy, loss of appetite, low-grade fever and cough productive of clear sputum. Plain chest X-ray reveals consolidation that is impossible to distinguish from infection or malignancy and diagnosis is made by biopsy. COP is important because, unlike many of the other interstitial lung diseases, the majority of patients achieve full resolution of their disease with corticosteroids. *Acute interstitial pneumonia* (AIP) is an idiopathic form of acute respiratory distress syndrome (ARDS). It tends to affect individuals in the fourth or fifth decade of life. There is rapidly progressive breathlessness, usually proceeding to respiratory failure within a period of a few weeks. Prognosis is poor.

Systemic lupus erythematosus (?typical rash; see Vol. 3, Station 5, Locomotor, Case 16)

Polymyositis (?proximal muscle weakness and tenderness; see Vol. 3, Station 5, Locomotor, Case 15)

Dermatomyositis (?heliotrope rash on eyes/hands and polymyositis; see Vol. 3, Station 5, Skin, Case 6)

Sjögren's syndrome (?dry eyes and mouth)

Mixed connective tissue disease

Ankylosing spondylitis (?male with fixed kyphosis and stooped 'question mark' posture; see Vol. 3, Station 5, Locomotor, Case 6)

Sarcoidosis (?extrapulmonary features, e.g. lupus pernio; see Vol. 3, Station 5, Skin, Case 19)

Extrinsic allergic alveolitis also known as hypersensitivity pneumonitis (HP) (acute pulmonary and systemic symptoms occur 6 h following inhaled allergen – ?farmer, pigeon racer, etc.)

Asbestosis (?occupational history – lagger, etc.)

Silicosis (?occupational history – slate worker or granite quarrier, etc.)

Drug induced (e.g. bleomycin, busulphan, nitrofurantoin, amiodarone)

Radiation fibrosis

Chemical inhalation (e.g. beryllium, mercury)

Poison ingestion (e.g. paraquat)

ARDS (also called acute interstitial pneumonia)

Investigations include

Chest X-ray (bilateral interstitial shadowing, reticulonodular, loss of lung volumes)*

High-resolution CT (subpleural reticulation, traction bronchiectasis, basal honey-combing, ground-glass attenuation)†

Pulmonary function tests (restrictive defect, reduced lung volumes, impaired gas transfer)

Serology:

Eosinophilia – Churg–Strauss syndrome, eosinophilic pneumonia

Serum calcium – raised in 5–15% of cases of sarcoidosis

Serum angiotensin converting enzyme (ACE) – may be raised in sarcoidosis

Antineutrophil cytoplasmic antibody (ANCA) – raised in a cytoplasmic pattern in Wegener's granulomatosis and in a perinuclear pattern in Churg–Strauss syndrome

Rheumatoid factor, and an autoimmune profile – connective tissue disease

Serum precipitins – may be raised in hypersensitivity pneumonitis (HP). Inflammatory markers – frequently raised in interstitial lung disease

---

*The distribution of changes on chest X-ray may provide diagnostic clues:

upper zone – hypersensitivity pneumonitis, ankylosing spondylitis, radiation fibrosis, sarcoidosis
lower zone – idiopathic pulmonary fibrosis, NSIP, drug-induced, connective tissue, asbestosis

†A number of interstitial lung diseases have a characteristic HRCT appearance such that biopsy is not needed to make the diagnosis in the fourth or fifth decade of life. Rapidly progressive breathlessness usually proceeding to respiratory failure within a period of a few weeks. Prognosis is poor.

Histology – gold standard for diagnosis; depending on the suspected diagnosis, tissue samples can be obtained:

Endobronchially, e.g. sarcoidosis

Transbronchially, e.g. sarcoidosis, amyloid, cryptogenic organizing pneumonia (COP)

Surgically, either by open biopsy or as is more usual by video-assisted thoracoscopic surgery (VATS)

Bronchoscopy with bronchoalveolar lavage (BAL) (characteristic patterns of macrophages, lympohocytes, eosinophils and neutrophils in different diseases)

Echocardiogram (to exclude coexistent pulmonary hypertension)

Six-minute walk (patients with IPF desaturating below 88% or who manage less than 200 metres fall into a poorer prognostic group)

Gallium scanning (sarcoidosis)

24-hour urine collection for hypercalciuria in sarcoidosis – may lead to the development of calculi

Case 2 | Pneumonectomy/lobectomy

Frequency in survey: main focus of a short case or additional feature in 13% of attempts at PACES Station 1, Respiratory. Additional feature in a further 1%.

Survey note: some candidates had to discuss the chest X-ray of their pneumonectomy short case. It would usually show a 'white out' on one side, deviated trachea and compensatory hyperinflation on the other side.

Record 1

There is a deformity of the chest with *flattening* on the R/L and a *thoracotomy scar* on that side. The trachea is *deviated* to the R/L and the apex beat is *displaced* in the same direction. On the R/L *expansion* is reduced, the percussion note is *dull* and the *breath sounds* are *diminished*. There is an area of bronchial breathing in the R/L upper zone (over the grossly deviated trachea).

These findings suggest a R/L pneumonectomy.

In the patient with lobectomy, as opposed to total pneumonectomy, the signs will be more confined. For example see *Record 2*.

Record 2

There is a *deformity** of the chest with the left lower ribs *pulled in** and a left-sided *thoracotomy scar*. The *trachea* is central (may be displaced) but the *apex beat* is displaced* to the left. The *percussion note is dull* over the left lower zone and *breath sounds* are *diminished* in this area.

These signs suggest a left lower lobectomy.*

Surgical resection and the lung

Surgery has little role in the management of *small cell carcinoma*. In others, after a full assessment which includes clinical examination, lung function tests, bone and liver biochemistry, isotope bone scan, ultrasound or CT scan of the liver, mediastinal CT scan and, if necessary, mediastinoscopy, 25% of *non-small cell* lung cancers will be suitable for attempted surgical resection. The operative mortality for lobectomy is about 2–4% and this rises to about 6% for total pneumonectomy, which may be required if the tumour involves both divisions of a main bronchus or more than one lobe.

Surgical resection is often required for *solitary pulmonary nodules* of uncertain cause. The possibility of

undiagnosed small cell cancer in this instance is not necessarily a reason for avoiding thoracotomy; resection of small cell lung cancer presenting as a solitary pulmonary nodule may have a 5-year survival comparable to that of other forms of nodular bronchogenic carcinoma treated surgically (approximately 25%).

Surgical resection is indicated in the treatment of *bronchiectasis* (see Station 1, Respiratory, Case 4) when other forms of treatment have failed to control symptoms, particularly if it is localized and if recurrent haemoptysis is present.

In the days before antituberculous chemotherapy, tuberculosis was sometimes treated surgically (see Station 1, Respiratory, Case 7).

---

*In lower lobectomy there may not be deformity (or it may be subtle) and the ribs may not be pulled in and apex beat not displaced because the remaining lung may expand to occupy the space.

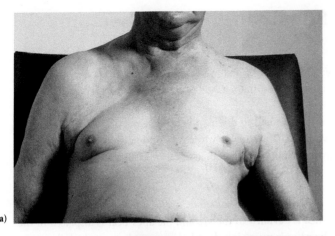

(a)

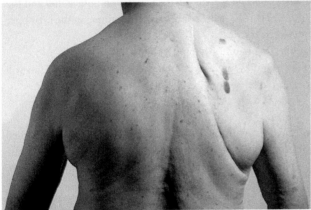

(b)

Figure C1.1 (a) Deformity of the right chest with flattening. (b) Right-sided thoracotomy scar on the back.

Case 3 | Chronic bronchitis and emphysema*

Frequency in survey: main focus of a short case or additional feature in 11% of attempts at PACES Station 1, Respiratory.

Survey note: usually the patients in the examination fall between the extremes of the classic *Records* below.

Record 1

This thin man (with an anxious, drawn expression) presents the classic 'pink puffer' appearance. He has *nicotine staining* of the fingers. He is tachypnoeic at rest with *lip pursing* during expiration, which is *prolonged*. The suprasternal notch to cricoid distance is reduced (a sign of hyperinflation; normally >3 finger breadths). His chest is *hyperinflated, expansion* is mainly *vertical* and there is a *tracheal tug*. He uses his *accessory muscles* of respiration at rest and there is *indrawing* of the *lower ribs* on inspiration (due to a flattened diaphragm). The percussion note is hyperresonant, obliterating cardiac and hepatic dullness, and the breath sounds are quiet (this is so in classic pure emphysema – frequently, though, wheezes are heard due to associated bronchial disease).

These are the physical findings of a patient with emphysema (inspiratory drive often intact).†

Record 2

This (male) patient (who smokes, lives in a foggy city, works amid dust and fumes, and has probably had frequent respiratory infections) presents the classic 'blue bloater' appearance. He has *nicotine staining* on the fingers. He is stocky and *centrally cyanosed* with suffused conjunctivae. His chest is *hyperinflated*, he uses his *accessory muscles* of respiration; there is *indrawing* of the *intercostal muscles* on inspiration and there is a *tracheal tug* (both signs of hyperinflation). His pulse is 80/min, the venous pressure is not elevated (may be raised with ankle oedema and hepatomegaly if cor pulmonale is present), the trachea is central, but the suprasternal notch to cricoid distance is reduced. *Expansion* is equal but *reduced* to 2 cm and the percussion note is resonant; on auscultation, the expiratory phase is prolonged and he has widespread *expiratory rhonchi* and (may be) coarse inspiratory crepitations. (His forced expiratory time (see Section B, Examination *Routine* 3) is 8 sec.) There is no flapping tremor of the hands (unless he is in severe hypercapnoeic respiratory failure in which case ask to examine the fundi – ?papilloedema).

These are the physical findings of advanced chronic bronchitis‡ (inspiratory drive often reduced) producing chronic small airways obstruction (and, if ankle oedema, etc., right heart failure due to cor pulmonale).

---

*Chronic obstructive pulmonary disease (COPD), which encompasses both chronic bronchitis and emphysema, includes the criteria of an obstructive spirometry (i.e. one can have chronic bronchitis only without an obstructive spirometry and hence such a person technically does not have COPD but only chronic bronchitis).

†Emphysema is, however, a histological or CT diagnosis.
‡Chronic bronchitis, though, is defined as sputum production (not due to specific disease such as bronchiectasis or TB) on most days for 3 months of the year for 2 consecutive years.

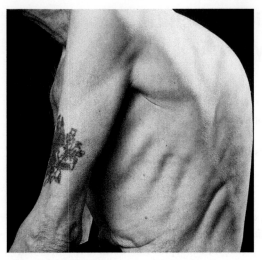

Figure C1.2 Hyperinflated rib cage. Note indrawing of intercostal muscles.

Causes of emphysema

Smoking (usually associated with chronic bronchitis; mixed centrilobular and panacinar)

α1-antitrypsin deficiency (?young patient; lower zone emphysema, panacinar in type; ?icterus, hepatomegaly, etc. of hepatitis or cirrhosis)

Coal dust (centrilobular emphysema – simple coal worker's pneumoconiosis – only minor abnormalities of gas exchange)

Macleod's (Swyer–James) syndrome – rare (unilateral emphysema following childhood bronchitis and bronchiolitis with subsequent impairment of alveolar growth; breath sounds diminished on affected side – more likely to meet this in the 'pictures' section of MRCP Part 2 written examination)

Record 1 (continuation)

The decreased breath sounds over the . . . zone of the R/L lung of this patient with emphysema raises the possibility of an emphysematous bulla.

Investigations include:

Pulmonary function tests:

FEV_1 <80% predicted value for height, age and sex (diagnostic)

FEV_1/FVC ratio <0.7 (diagnostic)

TLC elevated

RV elevated

TLCO or KCO (transfer factor) reduced

Reversibility testing may be helpful in distinguishing COPD from asthma

Chest X ray:

Hyperinflation (>7 posterior ribs visible)

Flattened diaphragm

Irregular distribution of lung vasculature

Bullae

FBC – ?polycythaemia

Arterial blood gases

Pulse oximetry

α1-antitrypsin – young age or family history

High-resolution CT thorax:

Bullae

Destruction of normal lung parenchyma and architecture

ECG and echocardiography if possible cor pulmonale

Functional assessement – 6-min walking test with oximetry during exercise

Case 4 | Bronchiectasis

Frequency in survey: main focus of a short case or additional feature in 9% of attempts at PACES Station 1, Respiratory.

Record

This patient (who may be rather *underweight, breathless* and *cyanosed*) has *clubbing* of the fingers (not always present) and a frequent *productive cough* (the patient may cough in your presence;* there may be a *sputum pot* by the bed). There are (may be) *inspiratory clicks* heard with the unaided ear. There are *crepitations* over the . . . zone(s) (the area(s) where the bronchiectasis is) and (may be) widespread *rhonchi*.

The diagnosis could well be bronchiectasis. The frequent productive cough and inspiratory clicks are in favour of this. Other possibilities (clubbing and crepitations) are:

1 Fibrosing alveolitis* (marked sputum production and clicks are against this)
2 Sarcoidosis
3 Post TB
4 Lung abscess
5 Carcinoma of the lung (?heavy nicotine staining, lymph nodes, etc.).

Possible causes of bronchiectasis

Respiratory infection in childhood (especially whooping cough, measles, TB)

Cystic fibrosis (young, thin patient, may have malabsorption and steatorrhoea; see Station 1, Respiratory, Case 17)

Bronchial obstruction due to foreign body, carcinoma, granuloma (tuberculosis, sarcoidosis) or lymph nodes (e.g. tuberculosis)

Fibrosis (complicating tuberculosis, unresolved or suppurative pneumonia with lung abscess, mycotic infections or sarcoidosis)

Hypogammaglobulinaemia (congenital and acquired)

Allergic bronchopulmonary aspergillosis (proximal airway bronchiectasis)

Marfan's syndrome (?tall, long extremities, high-arched palate; see Station 3, Cardiovascular, Case 13)

Yellow nail syndrome (?excessively curled yellow nails with bulbous fingertips; lymphoedema of extremities; see Vol. 3, Station 5, Skin, Case 12)

Congenital disorders such as sequestrated lung segments, bronchial atresia and Kartagener's syndrome†

Associated with smoking-related chronic obstructive pulmonary disease (COPD)‡

Investigations include

Chest X-ray ('tramlines', indicating thickened airways, 'ring shadows', and segmental or lobar collapse)

High-resolution thin-section CT thorax (tramlines (non-tapering of bronchi), the 'signet ring' sign (end-on dilated bronchi larger than accompanying pulmonary artery), crowding of the bronchi with associated lobar volume loss, mucous plugging of

---

*It is worth asking the patient to 'give a cough' as it may help you differentiate bronchiectasis from fibrosing alveolitis.
†The features of Kartagener's syndrome are dextrocardia, situs inversus, infertility, dysplasia of frontal sinuses, sinusitis and otitis media. Patients have ciliary immotility.

‡The majority of bronchiectasis patients seen in chest clinics nowadays have no obvious cause but also have COPD from smoking. One study showed that a distinct proportion of COPD patients (up to 30%) also have bronchiectasis (as confirmed by CT).

dilated bronchi (flame and blob sign), thickening and plugging of small airways resulting in numerous nodular and V- or Y-shaped opacities)

Arterial blood gas

Exercise capacity

Pulmonary function tests (combined restrictive/obstructive features)

Sputum culture (NB: *Pseudomonas* colonization) including AFB

Total immunoglobulin levels of IgG, IgM, IgA, IgE

Specific antibodies to pneumococcus and tetanus antigens

Aspergillus radioallergosorbent test (IgE) and precipitins (IgG)

Rheumatoid factor

Protein electrophoretic strip

α1-antitrypsin

Sweat test, nasal potentials, cystic fibrosis genotyping

Cilia studies (if nasal mucociliary clearance is prolonged or nasal nitric oxide low, proceed to light microscopy of ciliary beat frequency and then electron microscopy)

Case 5 | Dullness at the lung base

Frequency in survey: main focus of a short case or additional feature in 7% of attempts at PACES Station 1, Respiratory.

Record

The pulse is regular and the venous pressure is not elevated. The trachea is central,* the expansion is normal, but the percussion note is *stony dull* at the R/L base(s), with *diminished* tactile *fremitus* and vocal *resonance*, and *diminished breath sounds*. There is (may be) an area of bronchial breathing above the area of dullness.

The diagnosis is R/L pleural effusion.†

Causes of pleural effusion

Exudate (protein content $>30\,\mathrm{g\,L^{-1}}$)‡

Bronchial carcinoma (?nicotine staining, clubbing, radiation burns on chest, lymph nodes)

Secondary malignancy (?evidence of primary especially breast, lymph nodes, radiation burns)

Pulmonary embolus and infarction (?DVT; blood-stained fluid will be found at aspiration)

Pneumonia (bronchial breathing/crepitations, fever, etc.)§

Tuberculosis

Mesothelioma (asbestos worker, ?clubbing)

Rheumatoid arthritis (?hands and nodules)

Systemic lupus erythematosus (?typical rash)

Lymphoma (?nodes and spleen)

Transudate (protein content $<30\,\mathrm{g\,L^{-1}}$)

Cardiac failure (?JVP ↑, ankle and sacral oedema, large heart, tachycardia, S_3 or signs of a valvular lesion)

Nephrotic syndrome (?generalized oedema, patient may be young; see Station 1, Abdominal, Case 20)

Cirrhosis (?ascites, generalized oedema, signs of chronic liver disease; see Station 1, Abdominal, Case 3)

---

*The trachea may be deviated if the effusion is very large. A large effusion without any mediastinal shift (clinically and on chest X-ray) raises the possibility of collapse as well as effusion.

†On your initial inspection there may be biopsy or aspiration needle marks, or the marks of a sticking plaster removed by the invigilator at the beginning of the day, as a clue that you are going to find a pleural effusion.

‡Although the protein content $>30\,\mathrm{g\,L^{-1}}$ is not necessarily 100% sensitive and specific, it is still the most simple way of dividing exudate from transudate. Also, in exudates, the fluid to serum protein ratio is usually greater than 0.5, with an LDH of $>200\,\mathrm{IU}$ and a fluid to serum LDH ratio of >0.6.

§Up to 57% of patients with pneumonia develop a pleural effusion and, of these, over 4% develop frank pleural infection. The associated mortality is about 20%. Diagnostic thoracentesis should be performed in all suspected cases, using image guidance if the effusion is small or heavily loculated. Aspiration of overt pus confirms empyema. About 40% of infected pleural effusions are culture negative and, in this situation, biochemical pleural fluid markers (pH, LDH, white blood cell count and glucose) are central in establishing a diagnosis. Pleural fluid pH <7.2 suggests pleural infection. Pleural fluid glucose concentration can be used if pH measurement is unavailable. The amplification of bacterial DNA from culture-negative fluid improves diagnostic sensitivity.

Other causes of pleural effusion

Meigs' syndrome (ovarian fibroma)

Subphrenic abscess (?recent abdominal disease or surgery)

Peritoneal dialysis

Hypothyroidism (?facies, pulse, ankle jerks)

Pancreatitis (more common on the left; fluid has high amylase)

Dressler's syndrome (recent myocardial infarction, ?pericardial friction rub)

Trauma

Asbestos exposure

Yellow nail syndrome (yellowish-brown beaked nails usually associated with lymphatic hypoplasia; see Vol. 3, Station 5, Skin, Case 12)

Chylothorax (trauma or blockage of a major intrathoracic lymphatic, usually by a neoplastic process)

Other causes of dullness at a lung base

Raised hemidiaphragm (e.g. hepatomegaly, phrenic nerve palsy)

Basal collapse

Collapse/consolidation (if the airway is blocked by, for example, a carcinoma there may be no bronchial breathing)

Pleural thickening (e.g. old TB or old empyema or asbestos-induced with or without mesothelioma)

Pleural biopsy

Biopsy is carried out using an 'Abram's biopsy needle'. The specificity for detecting TB and malignancy is better with a pleural biopsy than with a pleural aspiration on its own. Remember that any biopsies for TB cultures should be placed in normal saline and not formalin.

Thoracoscopy

This is a technique involving visual inspection of the pleural cavity for diagnostic and therapeutic purposes (e.g. pleurodesis).

Case 6 | Rheumatoid lung

Frequency in survey: main focus of a short case or additional feature in 4% of attempts at PACES Station 1, Respiratory.

Record

There is (may be) cyanosis (there may also be dyspnoea) and the principal finding in the chest is of *fine inspiratory crackles* (or crepitations – whichever term you prefer) on auscultation at both bases.

In view of the *rheumatoid* changes (see Vol. 3, Station 5, Locomotor, Case 1) in the *hands* (there may also be clubbing), the likely diagnosis is pulmonary fibrosis associated with rheumatoid disease (rheumatoid lung).

Classic fibrosing alveolitis develops in 2%* of patients with rheumatoid arthritis and has a poor prognosis. It may progress to a honeycomb appearance on chest X-ray, bronchiectasis, chronic cough and progressive dyspnoea. Pulmonary function tests show reduced diffusion capacity, diminished compliance and a restrictive ventilatory pattern.

Gold, used in the therapy of rheumatoid arthritis, can also induce interstitial lung disease; it is indistinguishable from rheumatoid pulmonary fibrosis except that the gold-induced disease may reverse when the drug is discontinued.

Other pulmonary manifestations of rheumatoid disease

Pleural disease.† Though frequently found at autopsy, rheumatoid pleural disease is usually asymptomatic. The rheumatoid patient may have a pleural rub or pleural effusion but only occasionally would the latter be of sufficient size to cause respiratory limitation. The pleural fluid at diagnostic aspiration is never blood-stained and often contains immune complexes and rheumatoid factor; it is high in protein (exudate) and

LDH and low in glucose, C3 and C4. The white count in the pleural fluid is variable but usually <5000/μL.

Intrapulmonary nodules. Single or multiple radiological nodules may be seen in the lung parenchyma before or after the onset of arthritis. They are usually asymptomatic but may become infected and cavitate. As they have a predilection for the upper lobes and can cause haemoptysis, they can resemble tuberculosis or even carcinoma. They can rupture into the pleural space, causing a pneumothorax. Massive confluent pulmonary nodules may be seen in rheumatoid lungs in association with pneumoconiosis (*Caplan's syndrome*).

Obliterative bronchiolitis. Rarely, small airways obstruction may develop into a necrotizing bronchiolitis, classically associated with dyspnoea, hyperinflation and a high-pitched expiratory wheeze or 'squawk' on auscultation. This complication may also result from therapy with gold or penicillamine.

Two other manifestations are *pulmonary arteritis* (reminiscent of polyarteritis nodosa) and *apical fibrobullous disease.*

---

*Though fibrosing alveolitis becomes overt in only 2% of patients, 25% of patients with rheumatoid arthritis show interstitial changes on chest X-ray and 50% have reduced diffusion capacity, suggesting that subclinical fibrosing alveolitis is common. There is no relationship between the extent of lung disease and the titre of rheumatoid factor.

†Though our surveys have not thrown up a case of pleural effusion and rheumatoid hands, it would nevertheless be worth a glance at the hands of a patient with a pleural effusion for possible rheumatoid changes as well as for clubbing.

Case 7 | **Old tuberculosis**

Frequency in survey: main focus of a short case or additional feature in 3% of attempts at PACES Station 1, Respiratory.

Record 1

The trachea is *deviated* to the R/L. The R/L upper chest shows *deformity* with *decreased expansion, dull percussion* note, *bronchial breathing* and *crepitations*. The apex beat is (may be) *displaced* to the R/L. There is a *thoracotomy scar* posteriorly with evidence of rib resections.

The patient has had a R/L thoracoplasty for treatment of tuberculosis before the days of chemotherapy.

Record 2

The tracheal deviation to the R/L and the diminished expansion and crackles at the R/L apex suggest R/L apical fibrosis.

Old tuberculosis is the likely cause.

Record 3

Expansion is diminished on the R/L with dullness and reduced/absent breath sounds at the R/L lung base. There is a R/L supraclavicular scar (there may also be crepitations).

The patient has had a phrenic nerve crush for TB before the days of chemotherapy.

Treatment of pulmonary tuberculosis*

First 2 months (intensive phase†):
  isoniazid
  rifampicin
  pyrazinamide
  ethambutol
Four-month continuation phase:
  rifampicin
  isoniazid

---

*Treatment does not have to be initiated in hospital and patients do not need to be kept in hospital if their treatment is initiated there. Treating patients at home does not put their co-habitants at increased risk.

†The aim of the intensive phase is to render the patient non-infectious. Ninety percent of the mycobacteria are killed within the first week. With fewer organisms, the risk of secondary drug resistance falls until after 2 months it is safe to reduce to two bactericidal drugs.

Case 8 | Chest infection/consolidation/pneumonia

Frequency in survey: main focus of a short case or additional feature in 3% of attempts at PACES Station 1, Respiratory.

Record

There is reduced movement of the R/L side of the chest. There is *dullness* to percussion over ... (describe where) with *bronchial breathing, coarse crepitations, whispering pectoriloquy* and a *pleural friction rub.*

These features suggest consolidation (say where).

Most common causes of consolidation

Bacterial pneumonia (pyrexia, purulent sputum, haemoptysis, breathlessness)

Carcinoma (with infection behind the tumour; ?clubbing, wasting, etc; see Station 1, Respiratory, Case 13)

Pulmonary infarction (fever less prominent, sputum mucoid, occasionally haemoptysis and blood-stained pleural effusion)

Causes of community-acquired pneumonia in hospital studies*

Microbe	Percentage
Streptococcus pneumoniae	39
Chlamydia pneumoniae	13.1
Mycoplasma pneumoniae	10.8
Haemophilus influenzae	5.2

Microbe	Percentage
Legionella spp	3.6
Chlamydia psittaci	2.6
Staphylococcus aureus	1.9
Moraxella catarrhalis	1.9
All viruses	12.8

Investigations may include

Chest X-ray (consolidation, air bronchograms, cavitation, parapneumonic effusions)

Full blood count and inflammatory markers

Renal and hepatic indices (derangement may indicate increased severity or a multisystem involvement of atypical pneumonias – *Mycoplasma, Chlamydia, Legionella*)

Oximetry

Arterial blood gases

Sputum and blood cultures

*Recommended antimicrobial therapy if microbe identified

Streptococcus pneumoniae	Amoxicillin
Chlamydia pneumoniae	Clarithromycin
Mycoplasma pneumoniae	Erythromycin
Haemophilus influenzae	Co-amoxiclav
Legionella	Clarithromycin +/– rifampicin
Chlamydia psittaci	Tetracycline
Staphylococcus aureus	Flucloxacillin +/– rifampicin
Methicillin-resistant *Staph. aureus*	Vancomycin
Pseudomonas aeruginosa	Ceftazidime + aminoglycoside

Urinary antigen tests for pneumococcus and *Legionella* infections

Paired serological tests for other atypical pneumonias

Diagnostic pleural tap

The CURB-65 score

Confusion

Urea >7 mmol/L

Respiratory rate >30/min

Blood pressure (BP); systolic BP <90 mmHg or diastolic BP <60 mmHg

65 years and above

One or fewer of the above is associated with a low mortality (1.5%) and perhaps suitability for home treatment, whereas three or more features are suggestive of a severe pneumonia with a higher mortality (22%) and the advisability of consideration of ICU support.

Case 9 | Yellow nail syndrome

Frequency in survey: main focus of a short case or additional feature in 2% of attempts at PACES Station 1, Respiratory.

Survey note: see Vol. 2, Section F, Anecdotes 89 and 90.

Yellow nail syndrome is dealt with in Vol. 3, Station 5, Skin, Case 12.

Case 10 | Kyphoscoliosis

Frequency in survey: main focus of a short case or additional feature in 2% of attempts at PACES Station 1, Respiratory.

Survey note: see Vol. 2, Section F, Anecdotes 91 and 92.

Record

On inspection of the chest from the side (of this patient whom you have been told has been referred for investigation of *breathlessness*), I note an *increase in thoracic curvature*. There is no suggestion of any prominent angular features indicative of a gibbus and no evidence of any reversal of the normal lumbar lordosis. Further inspection of the patient when bending forwards shows restriction in the mobility of the spine. Inspection of the back shows no evidence of neurofibromatosis, spina bifida (hairy patch), thoracotomy scars, or spinal surgery scars. Whilst sitting down and *bending forwards*, the *curvature remains*, suggesting that the scoliosis is fixed. There is a *rib hump*. Palpation of the spine reveals no tenderness. Sliding the fingers down the spine reveals no evidence of a palpable step at the lumbo-sacral junction (feature of spondylolisthesis). Whilst the patient is standing, he demonstrates that he cannot touch his toes on flexion, and there is reduced extension when asked to bend back, whilst keeping the pelvis steady. There is evidence of reduced lateral flexion and rotation. There are no other features suggestive of old poliomyelitis or any obvious muscle atrophy in any of the limbs. The patient is (may be) *cyanosed*. *Chest expansion* is *reduced* but percussion and breath sounds are normal.

The patient demonstrates a scoliosis, most likely idiopathic in origin. The breathlessness is likely to be due to hypoventilation secondary to the deformity.

Scoliosis is a lateral curvature of the spine. Deformity of the spine will suggest a structural scoliosis rather than a non-structural scoliosis where the vertebrae are normal and the curvature can be due to compensatory reasons, e.g. tilting of the pelvis, sciatic due to unilateral muscle spasm or postural. In structural scoliosis, the deformity cannot be altered by a change in posture.

Kyphosis is the term used to describe the increased forward curvature. Therefore kyphoscoliosis describes an abnormal curvature of the spine in both coronal and sagittal planes. There may be varying degrees of kyphosis and scoliosis in an individual patient.

Causes of kyphoscoliosis include

1 Congenital, e.g. hemivertebra, fused verterbrae or absent/fused ribs

2 Paralytic secondary to the loss of supportive action of the trunk and spinal muscles, e.g. anterior poliomyelitis

3 Neuropathic as a complication of neurofibromatosis, spina bifida, cerebral palsy, syringomyelia, Friedreich's ataxia

4 Myopathic, e.g. muscular dystrophy (Duchenne's muscular dystrophy, arthrogryposis)

5 Metabolic, e.g. cystine storage disease, Marfan's syndrome
6 Idiopathic, the most common (approximately 65% of all cases of scoliosis)

Prognosis depends on age of onset, the level of the spine affected (the higher the level, the worse the prognosis), the number of primary curves, the type of structural scoliosis (congenital versus idiopathic).

Causes of kyphosis *only* include
1 Postural
2 Degenerative spine (e.g. osteoporosis)
3 Scheuermann's disease
4 Congenital
5 Nutritional (vitamin D deficiency)
6 Post tuberculosis of the spine (gibbus)
7 Post traumatic (vertebral fractures)

Investigations include
X-ray of spine and chest – concavity, with displacement of the spine and narrowing of the pedicles. On convexity there will be widening of the rib spaces. Angular deformity can be measured more accurately using the Cobb method*

MRI of the spine may be considered to look at the spinal cord

Spirometry – restrictive picture with a reduced FEV_1 and FVC. FVC of under 1 L will increase the risk of hypercapnic respiratory failure secondary to hypoventilation

Non-invasive ventilation
The need for domiciliary NIV should be assessed in the presence of breathlessness, poor sleep quality, and type II respiratory failure from blood gas analysis. Long-term follow-up by NIV specialists is necessary. Pulmonary hypertension is common in untreated respiratory failure.

*The Cobb angle, named after the American orthopaedic surgeon John Robert Cobb (1903–1967), was originally used to measure coronal plane deformity on anteroposterior plain radiographs in the classification of scoliosis and has subsequently been adapted to classify sagittal plane deformity. It is defined as the angle formed between a line drawn parallel to the superior endplate of one vertebra above the deformity and a line drawn parallel to the inferior endplate of the vertebra one level below the deformity.

Case 11 | Stridor

Frequency in survey: main focus of a short case or additional feature in 1% of attempts at PACES Station 1, Respiratory.

Record

The patient is comfortable at rest. From the *bedside* I can hear a noisy, *high-pitched sound* with each inspiration. Her respiratory rate is 12/min. Chest expansion is normal, resonance is normal and auscultation reveals *normal vesicular breath sounds* and no added sounds. There is (may be) a *healed tracheostomy scar* present.

In view of the tracheostomy scar, it is likely that the inspiratory stridor is due to tracheal stenosis following prolonged ventilatory support via a tracheostomy.

Inspiratory stridor usually implies upper airways obstruction and tracheal narrowing (extrathoracic).

Causes of inspiratory stridor

1 Acute (infective epiglottitis, croup)
2 Trauma (foreign body, smoke inhalation)
3 Chronic (neoplastic, tracheal stenosis)

Expiratory stridor is usually found with lower intrathoracic obstruction.

Causes of expiratory stridor

1 Foreign body
2 Intraluminal mass/neoplasm
3 Lower tracheal stenosis
4 Bronchial stenosis

Causes of tracheal stenosis

1 Congenital (webs, tracheomalacia), *or*
2 Acquired (tracheostomy or intubation)
3 Post trauma, *or*
4 Post infections (e.g. TB)
5 Neoplasia

Management would include referral to thoracic surgeon who would consider rigid bronchoscopy with possible dilation and/or stent insertion. Primary reconstruction may be considered as definitive treatment.

Case 12 | Marfan's syndrome

Frequency in survey: main focus of a short case or additional feature in 1% of attempts at PACES Station 1, Respiratory.

Survey note: see Vol. 2, Section F, Experience 27 and Anecdote 88.

Marfan's syndrome is dealt with in Vol. 3, Station 5, Locomotor, Case 9.

Case 13 | Carcinoma of the bronchus

Frequency in survey: main focus of a short case or additional feature in 0.8% of attempts at PACES Station 1, Respiratory.

Survey note: candidates reported a variety of signs. The three *records* given are typical.

Record 1

There is *clubbing* of the fingers which are *nicotine-stained*. There is a hard *lymph node* in the R/L supraclavicular fossa. The pulse is 80/min and regular, and the venous pressure is not raised. The trachea is central, chest expansion normal, but the percussion note is *stony dull* at the R/L base and *tactile fremitus, vocal resonance* and *breath sounds* are all *diminished* over the area of dullness.

The likely diagnosis is carcinoma of the bronchus causing a *pleural effusion*.

Record 2

The patient is *cachectic*. There is a *radiation burn* on the R/L upper chest wall. There is *clubbing* of the fingers which are *nicotine-stained*. The pulse is 80/min, venous pressure is not elevated and there are no lymph nodes. The *trachea* is *deviated* to the R/L and *expansion* of the R/L upper chest is *diminished*. *Tactile vocal fremitus* and *resonance* are *increased* over the upper chest where the *percussion note* is *dull* and there is an area of *bronchial breathing*.

It is likely that this patient has had radiotherapy for carcinoma of the bronchus which is causing *collapse* and *consolidation of the R/L upper lung*.

Record 3

There is a *radiation burn* on the chest. There are *lymph nodes* palpable in the R/L axilla. The trachea is central. I did not detect any abnormality in expansion, vocal fremitus, vocal resonance or breath sounds, but there is *wasting* of the *small muscles* of the R/L *hand*, and *sensory loss* (plus pain) over the *T1** dermatome. There is a R/L *Horner's syndrome* (see Station 3, CNS, Case 41).

The diagnosis is *Pancoast's syndrome* (due to an apical carcinoma of the lung involving the lower brachial plexus and the cervical sympathetic nerves).

Other complications of carcinoma of the bronchus

1 Other local effects such as:
   Superior vena cava obstruction (?oedema of the face and upper extremities, suffusion of eyes, fixed engorgement of neck veins and dilation of superficial veins, etc; see Station 1, Respiratory, Case 22)
   Stridor (often associated with superior vena cava obstruction; dysphagia may occur)

2 Metastases and their effects (pain, ?hepatomegaly, neurological signs, etc.)

*The weakness, sensory loss and especially pain may be more widespread (C8, T1, 2).

3 Non-metastatic effects such as:

Hypertrophic pulmonary osteoarthropathy (?clubbing plus pain and swelling of wrists and/or ankles – subperiosteal new bone formation on X-ray)

Neuropathy (peripheral neuropathy – sensory, motor or mixed; cerebellar degeneration and encephalopathy; proximal myopathy, polymyositis, dermatomyositis, reversed myasthenia – Eaton–Lambert syndrome)

Endocrine (inappropriate antidiuretic hormone, ectopic ACTH, ectopic parathormone or parathormone-related peptide,* carcinoid)

Gynaecomastia (if rapidly progressive and painful may be due to a HCG-secreting tumour)

Thrombophlebitis migrans (?DVT)

Non-bacterial thrombotic endocarditis

Anaemia (usually normoblastic; occasionally leucoerythroblastic from bone marrow involvement)

Pruritus

Herpes zoster (see Vol. 3, Station 5, Skin, Case 32)

Acanthosis nigricans (grey-brown/dark brown areas in the axillae and limb flexures, in which skin becomes thickened, rugose and velvety with warts; see Vol. 3, Station 5, Skin, Case 48)

Erythema gyratum repens (irregular wavy bands with a serpiginous outline and marginal desquamation on the trunk, neck and extremities)

Record 4 (lobectomy)

There is a R/L *thoracotomy scar*. The *trachea* is *deviated* to the R/L. On the R/L side *chest expansion* is *diminished*, percussion note more resonant and breath sounds are harsher. The patient has had a R/L lobectomy to remove a tumour, resistant lung abscess or localized area of bronchiectasis.

Treatment for lung cancer

1 Surgical resection for limited disease
2 Chemotherapy/radiotherapy or combination
3 Radiofrequency ablation (alternative to surgery in early stages)
4 Palliative care

---

*Hypercalcaemia may also be due to bone secondaries.

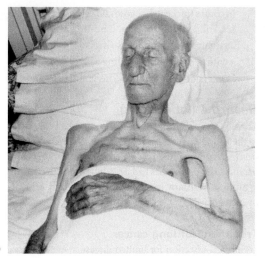

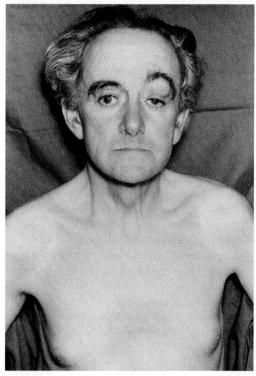

Figure C1.3 (a) Cachexia due to carcinoma of the bronchus (note radiotherapy ink marks). (b) Pancoast's tumour (note gynaecomastia and left Horner's syndrome).

Case 14 | Klippel–Feil syndrome

Frequency in survey: main focus of a short case or additional feature in 0.8% of attempts at PACES Station 1, Respiratory.

Survey note: see Vol. 2, Section F, Anecdote 91.

Klippel–Feil syndrome is dealt with in Vol. 3, Station 5, Other, Case 7.

Case 15 | Kartagener's syndrome

Frequency in survey: main focus of a short case or additional feature in 0.7% of attempts at PACES Station 1, Respiratory.

Record

This patient (who may be rather *underweight, breathless* and *cyanosed*) has *clubbing* of the fingers (not always present) and a frequent *productive cough* (the patient may cough in your presence;* there may be a *sputum pot* by the bed). There are (may be) *inspiratory clicks* heard with the unaided ear. There are *crepitations* over the . . . zone(s) (the area(s) where the bronchiectasis is) and (may be) widespread *rhonchi*.

The apex beat is *not palpable on the left side,* and the heart sounds can barely be heard there but can be heard instead on the *right* side. The patient has dextrocardia.†

The findings in the chest are in keeping with bronchiectasis and this in association with dextrocardia suggests that the diagnosis is Kartagener's syndrome.

Features of Kartagener's syndrome

1 Dextrocardia
2 Bronchiectasis
3 Situs inversus
4 Infertility
5 Dysplasia of frontal sinuses
6 Sinusitis
7 Otitis media

Patients with Kartagener's syndrome have ciliary immotility.

---

*It is worth asking the patient to 'give a cough' as it may help you differentiate bronchiectasis from fibrosing alveolitis.

†Consider the possibility of this diagnosis if you cannot feel the apex beat and then have difficulty hearing the heart sounds. As you gradually move the stethoscope towards the right side of the chest, they get louder.

Case 16 | Lung transplant

Frequency in survey: main focus of a short case or additional feature in 0.7% of attempts at PACES Station 1, Respiratory.

Record 1

This *young* man (who has had a *major operative procedure* for a *severe chronic respiratory problem*) is not breathless at rest. His respiratory rate is 12/min. He is bilaterally clubbed. He has a *mid-sternotomy scar*. Expansion is equal and normal both sides. Percussion is normal and *breath sounds* are *vesicular* with no added sounds in both lungs.

In view of his age I suspect that the chronic respiratory problem requiring a surgical procedure was cystic fibrosis and I suspect that he has had a double lung transplantation that has been successful.

Record 2

This middle-aged man (who had a right lung transplant and has been increasingly breathless in recent months) has an *increased respiratory rate* of 18/min. He is taking *oxygen* $2\,\mathrm{L\,min^{-1}}$ via nasal cannulae. He is bilaterally clubbed. He has features of *Cushing's* syndrome. There is a *right thoracotomy scar*. He has reduced expansion in both lungs. The left base is dull to percussion. There are fine inspiratory crackles to the mid-zones in the left lung and a few scattered *inspiratory squeaks* in the right lung.

The findings in the left lung suggest that the lung transplant was for pulmonary fibrosis. It may be that he has had recurrent episodes of acute rejection during recent months and has now developed bronchiolitis obliterans syndrome (BOS) for which he takes large doses of steroids and is on continuous oxygen therapy. (He will have a spirometry recording book to demonstrate the fall in FEV_1 and FVC over the last 12 months and may be on the active retransplant list – look for the bleeper.)

Indications for lung transplantation

1 Pulmonary vascular: primary pulmonary hypertension, pulmonary hypertension secondary to systemic disease and Eisenmenger's syndrome
2 Restrictive pulmonary diseases: idiopathic pulmonary fibrosis, fibrosis secondary to connective tissue disease, sarcoidosis and chronic allergic alveolitis
3 Obstructive diseases: emphysema with or without α1-antitrypsin deficiency, Langerhans cell granulomatosis and lymphangioleiomyomatosis
4 Suppurative disease including cystic fibrosis and bronchiectasis

Complications of lung transplantation

1 Perioperative, e.g. dehiscence of graft
2 Infection: viral, especially cytomegalovirus, but also herpes simplex; bacterial; fungal – *Candida, Aspergillus*; other opportunistic infections, e.g. pneumocystis
3 Rejection: may be hyperacute (within hours) or acute; most patients experience one or two episodes during the first 6 months. *Bronchiolitis obliterans syndrome* is progressive airways obstruction with rapid progression and poor survival. Acute

rejection is a major prognostic factor. It is characterized by non-productive cough, dyspnoea and malaise. Pulmonary function shows irreversible airflow obstruction, reduced total lung capacity and gas transfer. No effective treatment is available. A regimen of immunosuppressives is commonly employed. Retransplantation may be considered.

4 Side-effects of drugs, e.g. azathioprine, cyclosporin, corticosteroids

Case 17 | Cystic fibrosis

Frequency in survey: main focus of a short case or additional feature in 0.7% of attempts at PACES Station 1, Respiratory.

Record

This young patient (who is usually *underweight*, of *short stature* and rather pale, but may also be *breathless* and *cyanosed*) has *clubbing* of the fingers (often present) and a *productive cough* (there may be a *sputum pot* by the bed). There are (may be) *inspiratory clicks* and *expiratory wheeze* (heard with the unaided ear). There are *crepitations* over . . . (the area of bronchiectasis – state where). There is (may be) widespread *polyphonic expiratory wheeze*.

These features suggest *bronchiectasis* (see Station 1, Respiratory, Case 4) and as this is a young patient, this suggests that the underlying disorder is cystic fibrosis. If so, the patient is also likely to have *pancreatic insufficiency* and *malabsorption*.* The diagnosis can be confirmed by the *sweat sodium test*.†

Some patients have well-developed *cor pulmonale* with *cyanosis, ankle oedema* and *right heart failure*.

Cystic fibrosis is a genetic disorder (autosomal recessive) and a child born to two heterozygote carriers has a 25% chance of having the disease. The disorder usually occurs in Caucasians; Africans and Asians are seldom affected.

---

*In most cases there is a history of frequent large foul stools which are difficult to flush down. These patients are under-achievers in weight and height for their age; they have a good appetite, steatorrhoea and a protuberant abdomen. Hepatic symptoms are relatively uncommon but there may be *jaundice*. Sometimes there may be *portal hypertension*, glycosuria, biliary cirrhosis, cholelithiasis, intussusception and aspermia.

†A history of recurrent respiratory infections and of gastrointestinal symptoms, especially recurrent abdominal pain and faecal impaction, is highly suggestive of cystic fibrosis. The sodium and chloride levels are in excess of $70\,mmol\,L^{-1}$ in the sweat, and these levels do not fall after the administration of aldosterone $(0.1\,mg\,kg^{-1})$ for a week.

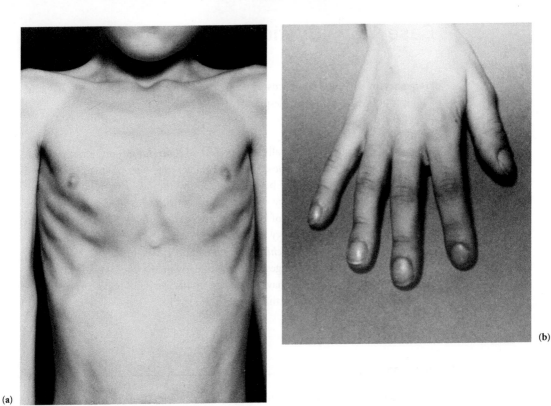

Figure C1.4 (a) Hyperinflated rib cage with rib recession in an undernourished patient. (b) Clubbing of cyanosed fingers.

Case 18 | Obesity/Pickwickian syndrome

Frequency in survey: main focus of a short case or additional feature in 0.5% of attempts at PACES Station 1, Respiratory.

Survey note: most cases revolved around features of the Pickwickian syndrome, though there was one case with an apronectomy scar and small testes in which Klinefelter's was suggested.

Record

The patient is *massively obese* and *cyanosed*. He has (may have) rapid and shallow breathing (or hypoventilating), his *venous pressure is elevated* and there is *ankle oedema*.

These features suggest *cor pulmonale* secondary to the extreme obesity – the Pickwickian syndrome.*

Respiratory problems associated with obesity

Severe obesity leads to increased demand for ventilation, increased breathing workload, respiratory muscle inefficiency, decreased functional reserve capacity and expiratory reserve volume. There is alveolar hypoventilation and reduced ventilatory sensitivity to CO_2. Peripheral lung units can close, resulting in a ventilation–perfusion mismatch. The overall result is chronic hypoxaemia with cyanosis and hypercapnia; the end-stage is the *Pickwickian syndrome* in which nocturnal obstructive apnoea† and hypoventilation are so marked that the patient can only have undisturbed sleep when upright (more usually sitting than standing as in the original description!*), often in the daytime.

Pulmonary hypertension occurs, there are usually morning headaches and impotence and there

may be polycythaemia. Eventually cardiac failure supervenes.

Sleep apnoea is very common in the severely obese. The most obese are not necessarily the most severely affected. It may be obstructive or central.† Daytime somnolence is common and is partly due to the hypoxia and partly from the continual disturbance of sleep at night – the patient tends to wake after each episode of sleep apnoea (cessation of breathing for 10 sec or longer).

Body Mass Index (BMI) = weight (kg)/height (m)². As a rule of thumb, health risks increase as BMI increases above 25; however, BMI normally increases with age and one study found that the BMI associated with the lowest mortality was approximately: 19.5 at age 20, 21 at age 30, 22.5 at age 40, 24.5 at age 50, nearly 26 at age 60 and 27.5 at age 70.

---

*The term is derived from the character in Charles Dickens' *Pickwick Papers* and was first applied by Osler. The character, Joe, kept beating the door even after hearing a response from inside the room, because if he stopped, he would fall asleep standing on his feet! (See *American Journal of Medicine* 1956, **21**: 811–18 to read Dickens' wonderful description.)

†*Obstructive sleep apnoea* – the upper pharyngeal cavity collapses due to the negative intrathoracic pressure and the process is aided by a short neck and large accumulations of fat often in combination with micrognathia and enlarged tonsils. There are

vigorous thoracoabdominal movements but no air entry into the lungs. The obstruction leads to hypoventilation and hypoxia which somehow trigger apnoeic episodes, making the hypoxia and hypercapnia worse. Weight loss and sometimes surgical removal of the obstructive tissues may help. *Central sleep apnoea* – cessation of ventilatory drive from the brain centres so that diaphragmatic excursions stop for periods of 10–30 sec. There are no thoracoabdominal movements and there is no activity. It is not known why the obese are prone to this.

Body fat can be estimated by measuring skinfold thickness with callipers at the biceps, triceps, subscapular and suprailiac regions.

Adipocytes increase in size and then number as necessary to accommodate excess nutrient calories; but once formed, though they can decrease in size with weight loss, their total number does not decrease (the 'ratchet effect'). *Lipoprotein lipase* (LPL) generates free fatty acids (FFA) from circulating chylomicrons and VLDL, and the FFA can then enter adipocytes. LPL activity is high in obese people and rises with initial weight loss and this may be a factor in the accelerated weight regain of many patients. Maintained weight loss, however, is associated with a decrease in LPL activity. Fat cells from the upper body are probably different in responsiveness to testosterone and oestrogens than lower body fat cells leading to:

Android fatness: fat distributed in upper body above the waist,

Gynaecoid fatness: fat predominantly in lower body – lower abdomen, buttocks, hips, thighs.

Android fatness carries a greater risk for hypertension, cardiovascular disease, hyperinsulinaemia, diabetes, gallbladder disease, stroke and a higher mortality than does gynaecoid fatness. A waist:hip (circumference) ratio greater than 0.85 for women and 1.0 for men is abnormal.

Other clinical manifestations of obesity

Insulin resistance (enlarged adipocytes less sensitive to the antilipolytic and lipogenic actions of insulin; decreased number of insulin receptors as well as postreceptor defects; liver and muscle also less sensitive to insulin; basal and stimulated hyperinsulinaemia results*)

Diabetes mellitus (type 2 diabetes approximately three times higher in the overweight; 85% of type 2 patients in the USA are obese; though the development of type 2 diabetes requires the appropriate genetic legacy, obesity by enhancing insulin resistance tends to unmask and exacerbate the underlying propensity)

Hypertension* (prevalence three times higher in the obese; mechanism is uncertain – hyperinsulinaemia*

leading to increased tubular reabsorption of sodium may be a factor; weight loss by dieting lowers blood pressure even without dietary salt restriction)

Cardiovascular disease (in obesity increased blood volume, stroke volume, left ventricular end-diastolic volume and filling pressure result in high cardiac output; this leads to left ventricular hypertrophy and dilation, the former being exacerbated by hypertension; the result is greater risk of congestive heart failure and sudden death)

Lipid abnormalities (obesity is associated with low HDL cholesterol;* LDL may be elevated; hypertriglyceridaemia* is more prevalent, possibly because the insulin resistance and hyperinsulinaemia* cause increased hepatic production of triglycerides; the hypertriglyceridaemia tends to improve with weight loss; if a true genetic lipoprotein disorder coexists, more intensive therapy may be required)

Venous circulatory disease (severe obesity is often associated with varicose veins and venous stasis; congestive cardiac failure adds to the dependent oedema; increased propensity for thrombophlebitis and thromboembolism)

Cancer (obese women have a higher incidence of endometrial cancer, postmenopausal breast cancer, and cancer of the gallbladder and the biliary system; obese men have a higher mortality from cancer of the colon, rectum and prostate, for unknown reasons)

Gastrointestinal disease (cholesterol gallstones leading to cholecystitis; obesity may be associated with fatty liver with modest abnormalities of liver function tests)

Arthritis (osteoarthritis due to excess stress placed on the joints of the lower extremities and back; multifactorial elevation in uric acid levels in the obese)

Skin (intertrigo in redundant folds of skin; fungal and yeast infections; *acanthosis nigricans*, which should always be looked for in obese patients, may be associated with severe insulin resistance; see Vol. 3, Station 5, Skin, Case 48)

Increased mortality (obesity itself may make an independent contribution to mortality, though the effect generally occurs through linkage with factors such as hypertension, diabetes and hyperlipidaemia.*

*NB: the metabolic syndrome. This refers to the clustering of insulin insensitivity, hyperinsulinaemia, varying degrees of glucose intolerance, hypertension, increased triglycerides and

decreased HDL, a clustering which may predispose to vascular disease, in particular coronary artery disease. It is postulated that insulin insensitivity is the underlying factor.

Endocrine causes of obesity

(<1% of obese patients)

Hypothyroidism (thickened and coarse facial features, dry skin, non-pitting swelling of subcutaneous tissues, hoarse voice, thinning hair, slow pulse, slow relaxing ankle jerks; see Vol. 3, Station 5, Endocrine, Case 5)

Polycystic ovarian syndrome (hirsutism, oligo- or amenorrhoea, excess androgen production of ovarian origin, ultrasound scan may show polycystic ovaries; patients with polycystic ovaries are often obese and insulin resistant)

Hypothalamic disease (damage to hypothalamic appetite systems and tracts by surgery, trauma, inflammation, craniopharyngioma or other tumours may lead to hyperphagic obesity)

Cushing's (truncal obesity, moon face, purple striae, proximal muscle weakness; see Vol. 3, Station 5, Endocrine, Case 6).

Rare genetic diseases associated with obesity include

Prader–Willi syndrome (obesity may be massive, almond-shaped eyes, acromicria, mental retardation, diabetes, hypogonadism; see Vol. 3, Station 5, Endocrine, Case 12)

Laurence–Moon–Bardet–Biedl syndrome (?retinitis pigmentosa, hypogonadism, dwarfism, mental retardation, polydactyly; see Vol. 3, Station 5, Eyes, Case 19)

Alström syndrome (see Vol. 3, Station 5, Eyes, Case 19)

Cohen's syndrome (microcephaly, mental retardation, short stature, facial abnormalities and obesity)

Carpenter's syndrome (see Vol. 3, Station 5, Eyes, Case 19)

Blount's disease (bowed legs, tibial torsion, obesity).

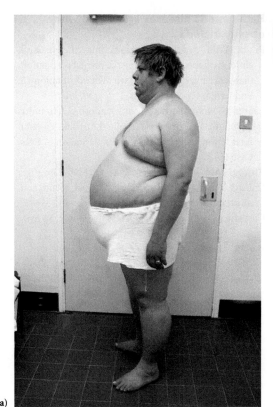

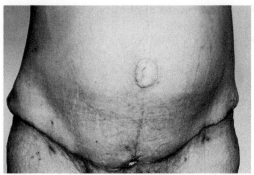

Figure C1.5 (a) Pickwickian syndrome. (b) Apronectomy scar.

Case 19 | Pneumothorax

Frequency in survey: main focus of a short case or additional feature in 0.5% of attempts at PACES Station 1, Respiratory.

Record

The R/L *side* of the chest (of this tall, thin, young adult male – old patients are usually bronchitic) *expands poorly* compared with the other side. Though the *percussion note* on the R/L side is *hyperresonant*, the tactile fremitus, vocal resonance and *breath sounds* are all *diminished* (large pneumothorax of one side may push the *trachea* and apex beat to the opposite side).

These findings suggest a pneumothorax of the R/L side.

Male-to-female ratio is 6/1.

A 'crunching' sound in keeping with the heart beat may be heard when the pneumothorax is small.

Treatment is not required in a healthy individual with a small pneumothorax (i.e. if only a quarter of one side is affected). Drainage is indicated for:

Larger pneumothorax associated with dyspnoea, increasing in size or not resolving after 1 week

Tension pneumothorax

Pneumothorax complicating underlying severe chronic bronchitis with emphysema

Pneumothorax exacerbating acute severe asthma (hence a chest X-ray is mandatory in acute severe asthma).

When drainage is indicated, simple aspiration (with a plastic cannula, syringe and three-way tap so that aspirated air can be removed) should usually be attempted before resorting to intercostal drainage via a tube attached to an underwater seal. Tension pneumothorax should be released urgently by stabbing an intravenous cannula through the chest wall at the second intercostal space, mid-clavicular line, pending the insertion of an intercostal drain.

Recurrent spontaneous pneumothorax is treated by obliteration of the pleural space (pleurectomy; inser-tion of irritating substances into the pleural cavity; scarification of the pleura followed by intrapleural suction).

Causes of pneumothorax

Traumatic

Penetrating chest wounds

Iatrogenic (chest aspiration, intercostal nerve block, subclavian cannulation, transbronchial biopsy, needle aspiration lung biopsy, positive pressure ventilation)

Chest compression injury (including external cardiac massage)

Spontaneous

Primary (a common cause in young men*)

Secondary

  chronic obstructive pulmonary disease

  asthma

  congenital cysts and bullae

  pleural malignancy

  rheumatoid lung disease (see Station 1, Respiratory, Case 6)

  bacterial pneumonia (see Station 1, Respiratory, Case 5)

  tuberculosis

---

*The risk of a second pneumothorax in a young adult following the first episode is of the order of 25%. After a second episode, the risk increases to the order of 50%.

cystic fibrosis (see Station 1, Respiratory, Case 17)
tuberous sclerosis (see Vol. 3, Station 5, Skin, Case 9)
endometriosis of the pleura
Marfan's syndrome (see Station 3, Cardiovascular, Case 13)

sarcoidosis
histiocytosis X
whooping cough
oesophageal rupture
Pneumocystis carinii pneumonia

Case 20 | Cor pulmonale

Frequency in survey: main focus of a short case or additional feature in 0.3% of attempts at PACES Station 1, Respiratory.

Record

The patient's fingers are *nicotine-stained* and there is *central cyanosis*. There is (may be) *finger clubbing* (if associated with pulmonary fibrosis). The pulse is regular, the *venous pressure is raised* (give height) with prominent small *a* waves and giant *v* waves (if there is secondary tricuspid incompetence), and there is *ankle* and *sacral oedema*. *Expiration is prolonged and noisy*. The *accessory muscles* of respiration are in use at rest, and there is a *tracheal tug*. The trachea is central, expansion is equal, the percussion note is resonant, and tactile fremitus and vocal resonance are normal. There is a *left parasternal heave* and a palpable second heart sound* (?pansystolic murmur of tricuspid incompetence (rare)). The heart sounds are often difficult to hear due to hyperexpansion of the lungs. There are (may be) widespread *expiratory rhonchi* and coarse inspiratory crepitations and the forced expiratory time (see Section B, Examination *Routine* 3) is 8 sec. (There is no *flapping tremor* of the hands – if there were, you would want to examine the fundi for papilloedema.)

These findings suggest cor pulmonale due to chronic bronchitis and emphysema. (Right heart failure is often precipitated by acute infection.)

The auscultatory cardiac signs of pulmonary hypertension, some of which may be audible,* are:

Loud pulmonary second sound

Pulmonary early systolic ejection click

Right ventricular fourth heart sound

Pansystolic murmur of functional tricuspid incompetence (giant *v* waves)

Early diastolic murmur of functional pulmonary incompetence (Graham Steell murmur).

Causes of pulmonary hypertension

COPD (with or without emphysema; by far the most common cause; see Station 1, Respiratory, Case 3)

Recurrent pulmonary emboli (signs of pulmonary hypertension without clinical evidence of other lung disease; ?DVT)

Primary pulmonary hypertension (signs of pulmonary hypertension without clinical evidence of other lung disease; usually a female)

Non-pulmonary causes of alveolar hypoventilation (kyphoscoliosis, obesity (see Station 1, Respiratory, Case 18), neuromuscular weakness)

Lung diseases which only occasionally result in cor pulmonale include:

Progressive massive fibrosis (?coal dust tattoos on the skin; chronic bronchitis is the most common cause of cor pulmonale in miners)

Bronchiectasis (especially cystic fibrosis; ?clubbing, cyanosis, full sputum pot, productive cough, crepitations; see Station 1, Respiratory, Case 4)

Cryptogenic fibrosing alveolitis (?clubbing, cyanosis, basal crackles; see Station 1, Respiratory, Case 1)

Systemic sclerosis (hands, facies; see Vol. 3, Station 5, Locomotor, Case 3)

Sarcoidosis (?lupus pernio; see Vol. 3, Station 5, Skin, Case 19)

Asthma (severe and chronic; may be missed if the reversibility is not checked in chronic small airways obstruction).

---

*These findings, which may be prominent in cor pulmonale due to other causes, may be difficult to elicit in cor pulmonale where a barrel-shaped chest and hyperinflation are present, and the heart is enfolded by overinflated lungs.

Case 21 | Collapsed lung/atelectasis

Frequency in survey: main focus of a short case or additional feature in 0.2% of attempts at PACES Station 1, Respiratory.

Survey note: see Vol. 2, Section F, Anecdote 93.

Record 1

There is no clubbing. On inspection of the chest from the front and the back, there is a *decrease* in *right-sided chest expansion*. This is confirmed on *palpation for chest expansion* and there is *displacement of cardiac apex* to the right. The percussion note is *dull* below the scapula. Tactile vocal fremitus is unreliable except in large pleural effusions; hence I have replaced it with auscultation for *vocal resonance,** which is *increased* below the scapula on the right where *bronchial breath sounds* are also present.

This all suggests a diagnosis of right†-sided lower lobe lung collapse, most likely to be due to focal chronic lung pathology such as postpneumonic scarring. (Check the *sputum pot* is empty as copious sputum production is compatible with chronic infection of a collapsed pulmonary lobe). I would like to investigate it further to rule out a proximal obstructive lesion of the large airways, most importantly a neoplasm, with a *chest X-ray* in the first instance proceeding, if required, to a *CT scan* of the thorax and/or a *bronchoscopy*.

Record 2

There is no clubbing. On inspection of the chest from the front and the back, there is a decrease in *right-sided chest expansion*. This is confirmed on *palpation for chest expansion* and there is *tracheal deviation* to the right. The percussion note is *dull* over the anterior upper chest on the right. Tactile vocal fremitus is unreliable except in large pleural effusions; hence I have replaced it with auscultation for *vocal resonance,** which is *increased* over the anterior upper chest on the right; *bronchial breath sounds* are also present.

This all suggests a diagnosis of right†-sided upper lobe lung collapse, most likely to be due to focal chronic lung pathology such as postpneumonic scarring. (Check the *sputum pot* is empty as copious sputum production is compatible with chronic infection of a collapsed pulmonary lobe). I would like to investigate it further to rule out a proximal obstructive lesion of the large airways, most importantly a neoplasm, with a *chest X-ray* in the first instance proceeding, if required, to a *CT scan* of the thorax and/or a *bronchoscopy*.

***A note on the examination for vocal resonance:** Early German physicians (18th century: pre-stethoscope era) asked patients to say *neun-und-neunzig* to evoke fremitus over the thorax, the English translation of which is *ninety-nine*. However, it is recommended that patients use the sound 'oy' (as in 'boy') because normal lung is believed to better transmit low-pitched vibrations than '99' when auscultating for vocal resonance. This improves the detection of not only increased resonance but also distortion of the transmitted sound to a bleating nature ('aegophony') in the presence of consolidation, which is often associated with collapsed lung. Eliciting vocal resonance is of paramount importance when trying to distinguish between the causes of dullness to percussion: a reduced vocal resonance suggesting pleural effusion and an increased vocal resonance suggesting collapse/consolidation.

†You should be able to work out from this what the equivalent signs would be on the left.

Causes of collapsed lung

Atelectasis is a collapse of lung tissue affecting part or all of one lung. In clinical practice the acute and sub-acute causes are common but less likely to be presented in an examination setting.

Acute:

1 Mucous plugging, particularly in asthma patients with sudden deterioration
2 Inhaled foreign body (mainly in children)
3 Chest wall injury/rib fractures causing atelectasis due to locally reduced movement

Subacute:

1 Proximal obstructing lesion of the large airways (e.g. neoplasm)
2 Postoperative patients/prolonged bed rest (much more common in patients with chronic lung disease who undergo specific risk assessment for postoperative atelectasis as part of their anaesthetic assessment for thoracoabdominal surgery in many centres)

Chronic:

1 Postpneumonic focal fibrosis
2 Bronchiectasis (usually associated with recurrent infection/excessive secretions)
3 Chronic aspiration (usually associated with recurrent infection/excessive secretions)
4 Diaphragmatic palsy
5 Pulmonary fibrosis
6 Trapped lung due to pleural thickening

Case 22 | Superior vena cava obstruction

Frequency in survey: main focus of a short case or additional feature in 0.1% of attempts at PACES Station 1, Respiratory.

Record
There is (may be) stridor. The face and upper extremities are *oedematous* (puffy) and *cyanosed*, and the eyes are *suffused*. The *superficial veins* over these areas are *dilated* and there is *fixed engorgement* of the *neck veins*. The undersurface of the tongue is covered with multiple venous angiomata. There is (may be) a radiation burn on the chest wall.

The diagnosis is superior vena cava obstruction, most likely due to carcinoma* of the bronchus, particularly small cell carcinoma (?lymph nodes, chest signs, clubbing, etc; see Station 1, Respiratory, Case 13). It has been treated by radiotherapy.†

The patient may complain of headaches (may be severe on coughing), difficulty in breathing, dysphagia, dizziness or blackouts. Physical signs are frequently absent or minimal.

Other causes of superior vena cava obstruction
Lymphoma
Aortic aneurysm
Mediastinal fibrosis
Mediastinal goitre

*The compression may either be by the tumour or by involved lymph nodes.
†Radiotherapy, or chemotherapy, is required urgently in this condition. A stent can sometimes be placed in the superior vena cava as a palliative procedure. Dexamethasone is also used.

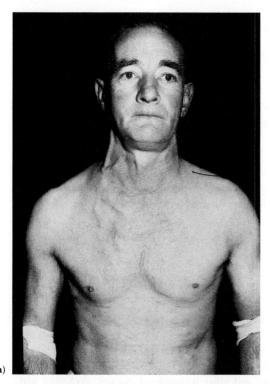
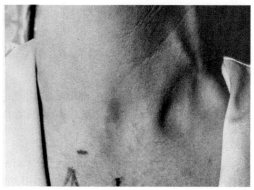

Figure C1.6 (a,b) Superior vena cava obstruction. Note the radiotherapy ink marks in (b).

Case 23 | Tuberculosis/apical consolidation

Frequency in survey: main focus of a short case or additional feature in 0.1% of attempts at PACES Station 1, Respiratory.

Record

The trachea in this Asian patient is central (may be deviated*) and the expansion is normal (may be reduced at the apex*). The percussion note is *dull* at the R/L apex with *diminished tactile fremitus*. There is *bronchial breathing* with *inspiratory crackles* over the area of dullness.

The diagnosis is R/L apical consolidation, with tuberculosis being a serious contender as the underlying cause.†

Principal varieties of tuberculosis

Primary pulmonary tuberculosis. The first infection with the tubercle bacillus (primary TB) usually includes involvement of the draining lymph node (the Ghon focus). All other TB lesions are regarded as post primary and are not accompanied by major involvement of the draining lymph nodes (in Europeans), though sometimes in immigrants gross enlargement of the lymph nodes may be seen. *Erythema nodosum, phlyctenular conjunctivitis* and *pleural effusion* may accompany primary pulmonary tuberculosis.

Miliary tuberculosis. Acute dissemination of tubercle bacilli via the bloodstream may occur if the initial infection is an overwhelming one or the patient's defences are poor due to malnutrition, corticosteroid or immunosuppressive drug therapy, HIV or intercurrent disease. This condition should be borne in mind in at-risk groups (see below).

Tuberculous meningitis. May occur at any age but is particularly common in small children as a complication of the primary infection.

Postprimary pulmonary tuberculosis. This form may arise as direct progression of a primary lesion, reactivation of an old lesion, haematogenous spread or from contact with a patient with *open* (sputum-positive) TB. The predisposing factors for reactivation are malnutrition, poor and overcrowded housing conditions, silicosis and other occupational diseases, alcoholism and cigarette smoking, immunosuppressive drugs, and diseases associated with impaired cellular immunity (e.g. Hodgkin's disease, leukaemia, lymphoma, AIDS). Complications of postprimary pulmonary TB include *empyema, laryngitis, aspergillomata* (colonization of a cavity), *amyloidosis, TB of the organs* and *adult respiratory syndrome.*

Bone and joint tuberculosis. There is a high rate in immigrants of Asian origin. Usually of haematogenous origin. The most common site for skeletal TB is the spine followed by the weight-bearing joints. AFB may be obtained from synovial fluid or bone but diagnostic exploration may have to be undertaken. Patients with TB can also have a reactive arthritis known as *Poncet's disease*; this usually settles with control of the TB.

Urinary tract tuberculosis. Results from haematogenous spread to the kidney with subsequent spread

---

*In the examination setting there are usually elicitable signs, even though in clinical practice one often encounters patients with pulmonary TB, sometimes with excessive radiological changes, who have no physical signs. The patient may have signs of fibrosis (e.g. deviated trachea), as seen in advanced cases, but the candidate should consider the diagnosis of pulmonary TB when there is only a dull percussion note, or a few crepitations at the apex of the lung.

†The differential diagnosis should include *carcinoma of the bronchus*, atypical pneumonia especially due to *Klebsiella pneumoniae*, pulmonary infarction and fungal infection.

down the ureteric tract. The patient may present with dysuria, nocturia, loin pain or may have painless haematuria, though many patients with positive urine cultures are asymptomatic. A history of recurrent urinary tract infection or *pyuria with negative bacterial cultures* should be regarded with suspicion for urinary tract TB.

Genital tuberculosis. A large majority of patients have evidence of tuberculosis at extragenital sites. Females present with infertility, pelvic inflammatory disease or amenorrhoea. Adnexal masses are palpable on pelvic examination in about half the cases.

Tuberculous peritonitis. Usually haematogenous. Often associated with weight loss, abdominal pain and gross ascites. Diagnosis can be made at laparoscopy when the peritoneum studded with whitish granulomata can be seen. Peritoneal fluid is rarely positive for AFB by stained smear and even by culture is positive in somewhat less than 50% of cases. May occur in the alcoholic with cirrhosis (see Footnote, Station 1, Abdominal, Case 7).

Tuberculous lymphadenitis. Mostly seen in patients of Afro-Asian origin. The patient may present with painless swelling of cervical lymph glands, or sometimes with pyrexia and lymphadenopathy. Untreated swelling may form a 'cold' abscess or sinus.

Cutaneous tuberculosis. This may present in one of many ways including a *primary complex* (an ulcerating papule on the face), *miliary* TB (particularly in immunocompromised children), *verrucous* TB (warty lesions as an occupational hazard in patients working with infected material), *scrofuloderma* (breakdown of skin over a tuberculous focus) and *lupus vulgaris* (see Vol. 3, Station 5, Skin, Case 38).

At-risk groups

Contacts – should be screened by tuberculin testing and chest X-ray

Immigrants from the Asian subcontinent have a high notification rate

Inhabitants of some institutions – prisons, lodging houses, hostel dwellers and mental institutions

Nursing homes – outbreaks of TB among the elderly in nursing homes have been reported

Medical laboratory workers – the incidence is high among staff in hospital pathology departments

Other groups – doctors, dentists, hospital employees, schoolteachers and those carers who work with children are potentially exposed to the risks for contracting TB

Treatment (see also Station 1, Respiratory, Case 7) Most patients can be treated at home. Patients are advised to avoid making new contacts for 2 weeks. Treatment regimens should last for 6 months except in those who have tuberculous meningitis; they should be treated for 12 months.

Drug therapy should be given as combination tablets to aid compliance. The initial phase of 2 months should include four drugs (see Station 1, Respiratory, Case 7). Treatment should be continued for 4 more months with rifampicin and isoniazid. Regular checks by nurses and health visitors are necessary to ensure compliance. The rifampicin in the combination tablets produces a pink/orange discoloration of the urine which will aid these checks.

Case 24 | Normal chest

Frequency in survey: has still not occurred in our surveys of PACES Station 1, Respiratory.

The College have made it clear that 'normal' is an option in PACES. To have no findings on clinical examination is common in real clinical medicine and so this must be a possibility in the exam. In terms of the practical reality of the exam, in order for PACES to proceed there must be a chest case in Station 1, Respiratory. If, at the last minute, neither of the scheduled chest cases turns up on the day, or if in the middle of a carousel the only one who did turn up decides not to continue or is too ill to continue, a substitute case has to be found at short notice. In this situation, one option is to proceed with a patient with a chest which is normal and make up an appropriate scenario. One simply has to imagine oneself as the invigilating registrar to think what that might be. One would first look amongst any surplus cases in the other stations for a patient with something relating to the chest. Failing that, one might look for someone who is a smoker or a member of the nursing, portering or other support staff who smokes and come up with a scenario such as:

> 'You have been asked to see this . . . -year-old smoker for insurance purposes. Please examine the chest . . .'

There may be a clue in the case scenario and the fact that the scenario has been hurriedly hand-scribbled. As it turns out, we have never yet heard through our surveys of this happening in the case of PACES Station 1, Respiratory. This is likely to be because at any one time, there are so many chest cases in the hospital that the case found at short notice is more likely to be one with COPD. Nevertheless, it could happen if time were short.

From our surveys, it is clear that the most common reason for finding no abnormality is missing the physical signs that are present (see probably both Anecdotes 1 and 2, Station 3, Cardiovascular, Case 24; possibly Anecdote 5, Station 1, Abdominal, Case 11; and Vol. 2, Section F, Experience 158). Other reasons for cases of 'normal' will be either because the physical signs are no longer present by the time the patient comes to the examination (see Anecdote 1, Station 3, CNS, Case 28) or that the examiners and candidate disagree with the selectors of the cases about the presence of physical signs (this may have happened in Anecdote, Vol. 3, Station 5, Eyes, Case 21; see also Vol. 2, Section F, Experience 198 and Anecdote 303).

Station 1
Abdominal

Short case	Checked and updated as necessary for this edition by
1 Transplanted kidney	Dr Fouad Albaaj*
2 Polycystic kidneys	Dr Fouad Albaaj*
3 Chronic liver disease	Dr Brian Cooper and Dr Chris Fegan*
4 Hepatosplenomegaly	Dr Brian Cooper*
5 Hepatomegaly (without splenomegaly)	Dr Brian Cooper*
6 Splenomegaly (without hepatomegaly)	Dr Brian Cooper and Dr Chris Fegan*
7 Ascites	Dr Brian Cooper*
8 Abdominal mass	Dr Brian Cooper*
9 Crohn's disease	Dr Brian Cooper*
10 Polycythaemia rubra vera	Dr Chris Fegan*
11 Normal abdomen	Dr Bob Ryder
12 PEG tube	New short case for this edition by Dr Matthew Lewis*
13 Single palpable kidney	Dr Brian Cooper*
14 Generalized lymphadenopathy	Dr Chris Fegan*
15 Hereditary spherocytosis	Dr Chris Fegan*
16 Idiopathic haemochromatosis	Dr Brian Cooper*
17 Primary biliary cirrhosis	Dr Brian Cooper*
18 Carcinoid syndrome	Dr Brian Cooper and Professor Hugh Jones*
19 Motor neurone disease	Dr Steve Sturman*
20 Nephrotic syndrome	Dr Fouad Albaaj*
21 Pernicious anaemia	Dr Chris Fegan*
22 Pyoderma gangrenosum	Dr Brian Cooper and Dr Malobi Ogboli*
23 Felty's syndrome	Dr David Carruthers*

*All suggested changes by these specalty advisors were considered by Dr Bob Ryder and were either accepted, edited, added to or rejected with Dr Ryder making the final editorial decision in every case.

Dr Fouad Albaaj, Consultant Nephrologist, City Hospital, Birmingham, UK
Dr Brian Cooper, Consultant Gastroenterologist, City Hospital, Birmingham, UK
Dr Chris Fegan, Consultant Haematologist, University Hospital of Wales, Cardiff, UK
Dr Matthew Lewis, Consultant Gastroenterologist, City Hospital, Birmingham, UK
Professor Hugh Jones, Consultant Physician and Endocrinologist and Honorary Professor of Andrology, Barnsley Hospital and University of Sheffield, UK
Dr Steve Sturman, Consultant Neurologist, City Hospital, Birmingham, UK
Dr Malobi Ogboli, Consultant Dermatologist, City Hospital, Birmingham, UK
Dr David Carruthers, Consultant Rheumatologist, City Hospital, Birmingham, UK

Case 1 | Transplanted kidney

Frequency in survey: main focus of a short case or additional feature in 16% of attempts at PACES Station 1, Abdominal.

Survey note: although in real life the majority of patients who have a renal transplant have other causes, it is noteworthy that our surveys suggested that most cases who appeared as MRCP short cases had polycystic kidney disease. There may be a parathyroidectomy scar present (see Vol. 2, Section F, Anecdote 101).*

Record

There is fullness in the flanks and an impression of a swelling under the scar in the right iliac fossa. On palpation, there are bilateral masses in the flanks that are bimanually ballotable (there may be one ballotable mass and one nephrectomy scar) and suggestive of *polycystic kidneys*. There is also an easily palpable rounded *mass under the scar in the right iliac fossa* which feels like a kidney. Look for evidence of kidney disease – AV fistula, peritoneal dialysis scar, parathyroidectomy scar.

I suspect this patient has had a renal transplant for renal failure due to polycystic kidney disease (see Station 1, Abdominal, Case 2).

Three most common diseases leading to referral for transplantation†

Diabetes mellitus with renal failure (transplantation offered earlier than in other forms of renal disease – posttransplant rehabilitation is more satisfactory if the damage due to other diabetic complications is minimal)

Hypertensive renal disease (incidence of end-stage renal failure not decreasing despite 'better' treatment of hypertension – reason not clear; occurs more often in the Afro-Caribbean than in the Caucasian patient)

Glomerulonephritis

Sickle cell disease (increased incidence of sickle crises may result from the improved haematocrit)

Systemic sclerosis (posttransplant rehabilitation may be limited by the chronic vascular and gastrointestinal manifestations)

Focal glomerulosclerosis (recurrence within the graft is common)

Oxalosis (there may be severe recurrence of stone disease)

Cystinosis and Fabry's disease (see Vol. 3, Station 5, Skin, Case 45) (continued disease activity)

Diseases in which renal transplantation is a particular problem

Haemolytic-uraemic syndrome (disease can recur and cyclosporin can increase the risk of this; rapid graft failure may ensue)

---

*Calcium metabolism in renal failure. Vitamin D is converted to its active form (1,25-dihydroxycholecalciferol = calcitriol) in the kidney. In renal failure there is decreased excretion of phosphate (leads to hyperphosphataemia) and low calcitriol (leads to hypocalaemia) and these combine to cause secondary hyperparathyroidism and renal osteodystrophy. Arterial calcification may occur with increased cardiovascular morbidity and mortality. Tertiary hyperparathyroidism occurs when the hyperstimulation of the parathyroids is prolonged, leading to autonomous (unregulated) hyperparathyroid tissue and this results in hypercalcae-mia. The aim of treatment is to prevent renal bone disease, arterial disease and the development of tertiary hyperparathyroidism by vitamin D replacement (e.g. alfacalcidol), restriction of dietary phosphate, phosphate binders (e.g. sevelamer hydrochloride and lanthanum carbonate). Calcimimetics (e.g. Cinacalcet) cause the parathyroids to perceive that extracellular calcium levels are higher than they are leading to a reduction in parathormone levels.

†These three causes of end-stage renal failure account for 75% of referrals for renal transplantation.

Table C1.1 Renal transplant outcomes

	5 year	10 year
HLA-identical living donor	88%	73%
Other living donor	74%	56%
HLA-matched cadaver	70%	56%

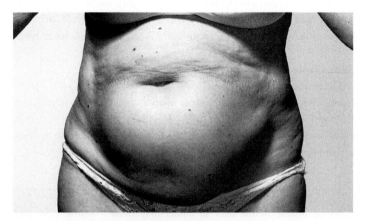

Figure C1.7 Renal transplant in right iliac fossa.

Case 2 | Polycystic kidneys

Frequency in survey: main focus of a short case or additional feature in 14% of attempts at PACES Station 1, Abdominal.

Record

There are *bilateral masses* in the *flanks* which are *bimanually ballotable*. I can *get above* them and the percussion note is *resonant* over them.* I suspect, therefore, that they are renal masses and a likely diagnosis is polycystic kidneys (*?uraemic facies*; the *blood pressure* may be raised). The *arteriovenous fistula/shunt* on his arm indicates that the patient is being treated with haemodialysis (about 50% develop renal failure†).

Other causes of bilateral renal enlargement include:

1 Bilateral hydronephrosis
2 Amyloidosis (?underlying chronic disease, hepatosplenomegaly, etc; see Station 1, Abdominal, Case 4)
3 Tuberous sclerosis (?adenoma sebaceum; see Vol. 3, Station 5, Skin, Case 9)
4 Von Hippel–Lindau disease.‡

Polycystic disease of the liver in adults may cause a nodular liver enlargement (liver function may be normal despite massive hepatomegaly). About 50% have renal involvement. Cystic liver is a major feature of autosomal recessive polycystic kidney disease (ARPKD, previously called infantile polycystic disease), but a minor feature of autosomal dominant polycystic kidney disease (ADPKD, previously called adult polycystic disease).

Other features of ADPKD

Cysts may also occur in other organs – most important are saccular aneurysms (berry aneurysms) of the cerebral arteries§ which, in combination with the hypertension, leads to serious risk of intracranial haemorrhage (cause of death in 10% of cases according to some authorities). There may be focal defects

Mitral valve prolapse (see Station 3, Cardiovascular, Case 10) may occur in 25% as a further manifestation of the systemic collagen defect. Patients often have palpitations and atypical chest pain. Other valvular abnormalities are also more common and echocardiography should be undertaken if a murmur is detected

It may present with flank pains, bleeding, urinary tract infection, nephrolithiasis, obstructive uropathy or obstruction of the surrounding structures

Renal cell carcinoma is not more common than in the general population, but it can be difficult to diagnose – CT and MRI may be useful

Presymptomatic screening by USS criteria and gene identification† is deferred to 20 years of age as it is not conclusive before this. The exceptions to this are if there is a family history of aneurysm or if hypertension or other signs of renal disease are present

---

*Look for abdominal scars from previous peritoneal dialysis or cyst aspiration. The latter is performed to relieve obstruction of the outflow tract by the cyst, intractable pain or haematuria.
†There are at least three gene mutations that can lead to ADPKD; the most common (85%), PKD1 (chromosome 16), is associated with a greater risk of renal failure than PKD2 (15% – chromosome 4). PKD3 is rare and has not been mapped.
‡An autosomal dominant condition caused by a defective tumour suppressor gene and characterized by retinal angiomata,

brain and spinal cord haemangiomata, renal cell carcinomata, endolymphatic sac tumours, phaeochromocytomata, papillary cystadenomata of the epididymis, angiomata of the liver and kidney, and cysts of the pancreas, kidney, liver and epididymis.
§Five percent of patients with ADPKD overall, but prevalence increases to 20% in individuals with a family history of brain aneurysm.

Case 3 | Chronic liver disease

Frequency in survey: main focus of a short case or additional feature in 12% of attempts at PACES Station 1, Abdominal.

Record

The patient is *icteric, pigmented* and (rarely) *cyanosed* (due to pulmonary venous shunts). He has *clubbing, leuconychia, palmar erythema, Dupuytren's contracture** and there are several *spider naevi*. He has a flapping tremor of the hands (suggesting some portosystemic encephalopathy). There are scratch marks on the forearms and back, and there is purpura. There is *gynaecomastia, scanty body hair* and his *testes* are *small*. There is 5 cm *hepatomegaly* and 3 cm *splenomegaly*. He has *ascites* and *ankle oedema*, and there are *distended abdominal veins* in which the flow is away from the umbilicus.

The diagnosis is likely to be cirrhosis of the liver with portal hypertension.

Possible causes

1 Alcohol

2 Viral hepatitis:

   (a) hepatitis B (?health or clinical laboratory worker, IV drug abuser, risky sexual practices)

   (b) hepatitis C† (the major cause of posttransfusion hepatitis; also transmitted between IV drug users)

   (c) hepatitis D (unusual; the D virus requires the presence of hepatitis B virus (HBV) for its replication and expression)

3 Autoimmune chronic active hepatitis (pubertal or menopausal female, steroid responsive; associated with diabetes, inflammatory bowel disease, thyroiditis and pulmonary infiltrates; ?smooth muscle antibodies)

4 Primary biliary cirrhosis (middle-aged female, scratch marks, xanthelasma; ?antimitochondrial antibody; see Station 1, Abdominal, Case 17)

---

*Twenty signs which may be present in the hands of the patient with chronic liver disease are clubbing, Dupuytren's contracture, palmar erythema, spider naevi, flapping tremor, leuconychia, scratch marks, icterus, pallor, pigmentation, cyanosis, xanthomata, purpura, koilonychia, paronychia, abscesses, oedema, muscle wasting, tattoos (?HBsAg positive), needle marks (intravenous drug abuse – more likely in antecubital fossa).

†In the management of *hepatitis C virus* (HCV), alcohol intake should be reduced as it hastens disease progression. Antiviral therapy with ribavarin and interferon can be tried if the patient is viraemic with abnormal liver histology. The cirrhotic patient should be considered for liver transplantation. There is a high incidence of hepatoma with HCV and patients should be screened for this (α-fetoprotein and USS of abdomen).

5 Haemochromatosis (male, slate-grey pigmentation; see Station 1, Abdominal, Case 16)
6 Non-alcoholic fatty liver disease (NAFLD), (?obesity, diabetes mellitus, hypertension, hyperlipidaemia)*
7 Cryptogenic

Other causes

Cardiac failure (?JVP ↑, *v* waves, S3 or a valvular lesion, tender pulsatile liver if tricuspid incompetence)

Constrictive pericarditis† (JVP raised, abrupt *x* and *y* descent, loud early S3 ('pericardial knock' – a valuable sign but only present in <40% of cases) though heart sounds often normal, slight 'paradoxical pulse', *no signs in lung fields*, chest X-ray may show calcified pericardium; rare but important cause of ascites as response to treatment may be dramatic)

Budd–Chiari syndrome (in the acute phase ascites develops rapidly with pain, there are no cutaneous signs of chronic liver disease and the liver is smoothly enlarged and tender; if the inferior vena cava is involved there is no hepatojugular reflux)

Biliary cholestasis (bile obstruction with or without infection), which leads to secondary biliary cirrhosis

Toxins and drugs (methotrexate, methyldopa, isoniazid, carbon tetrachloride, amiodarone, aspirin, phenytoin, propylthiouracil, sulphonamides)

Wilson's disease (?Kayser–Fleischer rings, tremor, rigidity, dysarthria)

α1-Antitrypsin deficiency (?lower zone emphysema)

Other metabolic causes (galactosaemia, tyrosinaemia, type IV glycogenolysis)

*Non-alcoholic fatty liver disease (NAFLD) is an increasingly common cause of asymptomatic abnormal liver blood tests. It is considered to be the manifestation of the metabolic syndrome (see Station 1, Respiratory, Case 18) in the liver. NAFLD defines a spectrum of liver disease from benign simple fatty liver disease (NAFL) to non-alcoholic steatohepatitis (NASH), with fibrosis leading to cirrhosis. The prevalence of NAFLD is as high as 20%, with about 2% of the population having the more serious NASH. Five percent to 20% of patients with NASH will progress to cirrhosis within 10 years. The histology is indistinguishable from alcoholic liver disease. The diagnosis is usually made on the basis of elevated serum transaminases and features of the metabolic syndrome (type 2 diabetes, hypertension, hyperlipidaemia and obesity) in the presence of a negative chronic liver disease screen.

Ultrasound can identify fat but not differentiate NAFL from NASH – a liver biopsy is required for this. Treatment is gradual weight loss which improves both inflammation and fibrosis and treatment of risk factors associated with the increased cardiovascular mortality of the metabolic syndrome. Bariatric surgery, metformin, thiazolidinediones and incretin-based therapies (GLP1 agonists and DPP4 inhibitors) are all potential treatments in need of long-term, well-controlled clinical trials.

†The spleen may be palpable. In the absence of evidence of *bacterial endocarditis* or *tricuspid valve disease*, the presence of splenomegaly in a patient with congestive heart failure should arouse suspicion of *constrictive pericarditis* or *pericardial effusion with tamponade*.

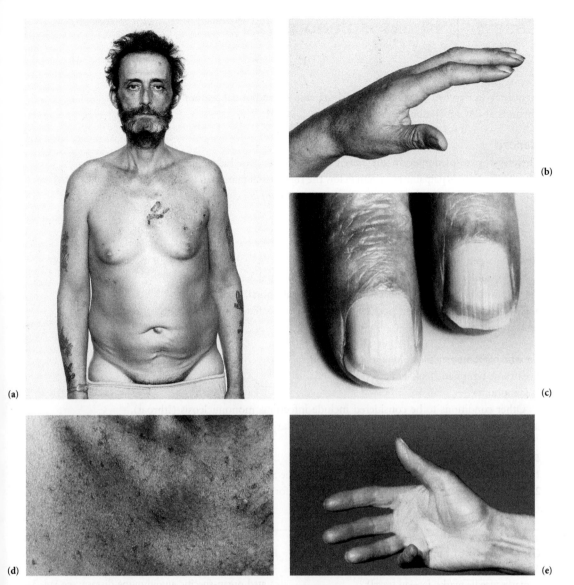

Figure C1.8 (a) Note from above downwards: spider naevi, herpes zoster (debilitated patient), gynaecomastia, tattoo marks, everted umbilicus, swelling of the flanks, abdominal wall veins and paucity of hair. (b) Clubbing of the fingers and leuconychia (same patient as (a)). (c) Leuconychia. (d) Spider naevi (close up). (e) Dupuytren's contracture.

Case 4 | Hepatosplenomegaly

Frequency in survey: main focus of a short case or additional feature in 12% of attempts at PACES Station 1, Abdominal.

Record

There is hepatosplenomegaly, the *spleen* is enlarged . . . cm below the left costal margin. The *liver* is palpable at . . . cm below the right costal margin; it is non-tender, firm and smooth (now look for clinical *anaemia, lymphadenopathy* and signs of *chronic liver disease*).

Likely causes to be considered are:

No other signs or clinical anaemia only

1 Myeloproliferative disorders (see Station 1, Abdominal, Case 6)
2 Lymphoproliferative disorders (see Station 1, Abdominal, Case 6)
3 Cirrhosis of the liver with portal hypertension* (less likely if there are no other signs of chronic liver disease)

Hepatosplenomegaly plus palpable lymph nodes†

1 Chronic lymphatic leukaemia
2 Lymphoma

Other conditions to be considered include infectious mononucleosis (?throat), infective hepatitis (?icterus), sarcoidosis and secondary syphilis.

Signs of chronic liver disease

1 Cirrhosis of the liver with portal hypertension (see Station 1, Abdominal, Case 3)
2 Chronic autoimmune liver disease (can occur before cirrhosis develops)

Other causes of hepatosplenomegaly

Acute viral hepatitis A, B or C or E‡ (?icterus, tattoo marks, needle marks, foreign travel)
Brucellosis ('Examine this farmer's abdomen')
Weil's disease (?icterus, sewerage worker or fell into canal)
Toxoplasmosis (glandular fever-like illness)
Cytomegalovirus infection (glandular fever-like illness)
Pernicious anaemia and other megaloblastic anaemias (NB: SACD; see Station 3, CNS, Case 37. NB: associated organ-specific autoimmune disease; see Vol. 3, Station 5, Skin, Case 8)
Storage disorders (e.g. Gaucher's – spleen is often huge; glycogen storage disease)
Amyloidosis (?underlying chronic disease)§

---

*The cirrhotic liver is often small and impalpable. The exceptions are alcoholic liver disease, primary biliary cirrhosis and cirrhosis complicated by hepatoma (bruit).
†These conditions can also occur without palpable lymph nodes.
‡NB: Hepatitis serology heads the list of investigations of icterus of uncertain cause.
§Though hepatosplenomegaly can occur in primary and myeloma-associated amyloidosis, it is more common in the secondary form. Other organs particularly involved in secondary amyloidosis are kidneys (nephrotic syndrome), adrenals (clinical adrenocortical failure may occur) and alimentary tract (rectal biopsy). Conditions associated with secondary amyloidosis include rheumatoid arthritis (including juvenile type), TB, leprosy, chronic sepsis, Crohn's disease, ulcerative colitis, ankylosing spondylitis, paraplegia (bedsores and urinary infection), malignant lymphoma and carcinoma. See also Footnote, Station 3, CNS, Case 1.

Other causes of portal hypertension (e.g. Budd–Chiari syndrome = hepatic vein thrombosis; see Station 1, Abdominal, Cases 3 and 7)

Infantile polycystic disease (in some variants of this, children have relatively mild renal involvement but hepatosplenomegaly and portal hypertension; they rarely survive to adulthood)

Common causes on a worldwide basis

Malaria

Kala-azar

Schistosomiasis

Tuberculosis

Case 5 | Hepatomegaly (without splenomegaly)

Frequency in survey: main focus of a short case or additional feature in 10% of attempts at PACES Station 1, Abdominal.

Record

The liver is palpable at . . . cm below the right costal margin (*?icterus, ascites,* signs of *cirrhosis* (do not miss gynaecomastia), *pigmentation, lymph nodes*).

Common causes

Cirrhosis – usually alcoholic (?spider naevi, gynaecomastia, etc; see Station 1, Abdominal, Case 3)

Secondary carcinoma (?hard and knobbly, cachexia, evidence of primary)

Congestive cardiac failure (?JVP ↑, ankle oedema, *S3* or cardiac murmur; tender pulsatile liver with giant *v* waves in the JVP in tricuspid incompetence)

Other causes of hepatomegaly

Infections such as glandular fever, Weil's disease and acute viral hepatitis (e.g. A,B,E) (remember hepatitis serology heads list of investigations in icterus of uncertain cause)

Primary tumours, both malignant (hepatoma may complicate cirrhosis) and benign (liver cell adenoma is associated with oral contraceptive use)

Lymphoproliferative disorders (?lymph nodes)

Primary biliary cirrhosis (?middle-aged female, scratch marks, xanthelasma, etc; see Station 1, Abdominal, Case 17)

Haemochromatosis (?male, slate-grey pigmentation, etc; see Station 1, Abdominal, Case 16)

Hepatic steatosis (alcohol, NAFLD; see Station 1, Abdominal, Case 3)

Sarcoidosis (?erythema nodosum or history of, lupus pernio, chest signs)

Amyloidosis (?rheumatoid arthritis or other underlying chronic disease; see Footnote, Station 1, Abdominal, Case 4)

Hydatid cyst (?Welsh connection – NB: patient's name)

Amoebic abscess (?tropical connection – name, appearance)

Budd–Chiari syndrome (?icterus, ascites, tender hepatomegaly)

Riedel's lobe (5th liver lobe – anatomical variant)

Emphysema (apparent hepatomegaly)

Hard and knobbly hepatomegaly – possible causes

Malignancy – primary or secondary

Polycystic liver disease (?kidneys; see Station 1, Abdominal, Case 2)

Macronodular cirrhosis (following hepatitis B with widespread necrosis)

Hydatid cysts (may be eosinophilia; rupture may be associated with anaphylaxis)

Syphilitic gummas (late benign syphilis; there is usually hepatosplenomegaly and anaemia; rapid response to penicillin)

Case 6 | Splenomegaly (without hepatomegaly)

Frequency in survey: main focus of a short case or additional feature in 9% of attempts at PACES Station 1, Abdominal.

Record

The spleen is palpable at . . . cm.

or

There is a *mass* in the *left hypochondrium*. On palpation I *cannot get above* the mass, it has a *notch*, and on inspiration moves diagonally across the abdomen. The *percussion note* is *dull* over the left lower lateral chest wall and over the mass.

I think this is the spleen enlarged at . . . cm. Likely causes* to be considered are:

Very large spleen†

1 Chronic myeloid leukaemia (Philadelphia (Ph) chromosome positive in 90%‡)
2 Myelofibrosis
and in other parts of the world
3 Chronic malaria
4 Kala-azar

Spleen enlarged 4–8 cm (2–4 finger breadths)

1 Myeloproliferative disorders§ (e.g. CML and myelofibrosis)

---

*To help you remember some common causes to mention in the examination, we have given the three or four most common causes of a spleen of a particular size. An alternative way of dividing up splenomegaly which can be found in many textbooks is:
1 Infectious and inflammatory splenomegaly (e.g. SBE, infectious mononucleosis, sarcoidosis)
2 Infiltrative splenomegaly:
  (a) benign (e.g. Gaucher's, amyloidosis)
  (b) neoplastic (e.g. leukaemias, lymphoma)
3 Congestive splenomegaly (e.g. cirrhosis, hepatic or portal vein thrombosis)
4 Splenomegaly due to reticuloendothelial hyperplasia (e.g. haemolytic anaemias).
†*Gaucher's* disease and *rapidly progressive lymphoma* (especially high-grade lymphoma) may also cause a huge spleen. *Chronic congestive splenomegaly* (Banti's syndrome = splenomegaly, pancytopenia, portal hypertension and gastrointestinal bleeding) may also cause massive splenomegaly. A huge spleen developing in a patient with *polycythaemia rubra vera* is usually due to the development of myelofibrosis.

‡In Ph-positive CML, the Ph chromosome (9:22 translocation; first described in 1973) is present in all dividing cells of the myeloid series and in some B lymphocytes. In the early 1980s, interferon-α was shown to reduce WBC count and induce haematological remission in some patients, inducing Ph-negativity in about 10% and a 1–3-year longer survival than treatment with hydroxyurea. Glivec, which is a tyrosine kinase inhibitor, is targeted at the molecular product of the Ph chromosome – 85% 8-year survival.
§When listing the causes of splenomegaly or hepatosplenomegaly in the limited time of the examination, to use the term 'myeloproliferative disorders' in its broadest interpretation is a useful way of covering several conditions in one phrase. If asked to explain it (unlikely), one strict definition covers a group of related disorders of haemopoietic stem cell proliferation: CML, myelofibrosis, polycythaemia rubra vera and essential thrombocythaemia. The term can be used more broadly to cover acute myeloid leukaemia as well. A small spleen is more likely to be due to acute leukaemia than CML or myelofibrosis because splenic enlargement in the latter conditions is often already marked at the time of presentation.

2 Lymphoproliferative disorders* (e.g. lymphoma and chronic lymphatic leukaemia)

3 Cirrhosis of the liver with portal hypertension (spider naevi, icterus, etc; see Station 1, Abdominal, Case 3)

Spleen just tipped or enlarged 2–4 cm (1–2 finger breadths)

1 Myeloproliferative disorders†

2 Lymphoproliferative disorders* (?palpable lymph nodes)

3 Cirrhosis of the liver and other causes of portal hypertension (e.g. congenital hepatic fibrosis, portal vein thrombosis)

4 Infections such as:

  (a) glandular fever (?throat, lymph nodes)

  (b) infectious hepatitis (?icterus)

  (c) subacute bacterial endocarditis (?heart murmur, splinter haemorrhages, etc.)

Other causes of splenomegaly

Polycythaemia rubra vera (?plethoric, middle-aged man)

Brucellosis ('Examine this farmer's abdomen')

Sarcoidosis (?erythema nodosum or history of; lupus pernio; chest signs)

Haemolytic anaemia (?icterus)

Pernicious anaemia and other megaloblastic anaemias (?pallor; NB: SACD; see Station 3, CNS, Case 37; NB: associated organ-specific autoimmune diseases, especially autoimmune thyroid disease, diabetes, Addison's, vitiligo, hypoparathyroidism; see Vol. 3, Station 5, Skin, Case 8)

Idiopathic thrombocytopenic purpura (?young female, purpura)

Paroxysmal nocturnal haemoglobinuria (rare 3rd–4th decade, caused by an acquired defect in the cell membrane)

Felty's syndrome (?hands, nodules)

Amyloidosis (?underlying chronic disease, other organ involvement; see Station 1, Abdominal, Case 4)

SLE (?typical rash)

Lipid storage disease (spleen may be enormous, e.g. Gaucher's)

Myelomatosis

Chronic iron deficiency anaemia

Thyrotoxicosis

Other infections (subacute septicaemia, typhoid, disseminated TB, trypanosomiasis, echinococcosis)

Other causes of congestive splenomegaly* (hepatic vein thrombosis, portal vein obstruction, schistosomiasis, congestive heart failure)

*The lymphoproliferative disorders are chronic lymphatic leukaemia, lymphoma, myelomatosis, Waldenström's macroglobulinaemia, acute lymphatic leukaemia and hairy cell leukaemia. Of these, the first two and Waldenström's macroglobulinaemia are usually associated with lymphadenopathy and hepatomegaly. Multiple myeloma seldom causes palpable splenomegaly. Hairy cell leukaemia typically presents in men as pancytopenia and splenomegaly.

†When listing the causes of splenomegaly or hepatosplenomegaly in the limited time of the examination, to use the term 'myeloproliferative disorders' in its broadest interpretation is a useful way of covering several conditions in one phrase. If asked to explain it (unlikely), one strict definition covers a group of related disorders of haemopoietic stem cell proliferation: CML, myelofibrosis, polycythaemia rubra vera and essential thrombocythaemia. The term can be used more broadly to cover acute myeloid leukaemia as well. A small spleen is more likely to be due to acute leukaemia than CML or myelofibrosis because splenic enlargement in the latter conditions is often already marked at the time of presentation.

Case 7 | Ascites

Frequency in survey: main focus of a short case or additional feature in 6% of attempts at PACES Station 1, Abdominal.

Survey note: occurred in the examination: (i) as part of cirrhosis; (ii) on its own without a clearly defined underlying cause, in which case it was the main focus and possible causes were often discussed; and (iii) in association with an obvious mass or the irregular liver of malignancy.

Record

There is *generalized swelling* of the abdomen and the umbilicus is *everted.** The flanks are *stony dull* to percussion but the centre is resonant (floating, gas-filled bowel). The dullness is *shifting* and a *fluid thrill* can be demonstrated (only in tense, large ascites).
   This is ascites.

Usual causes

1 Cirrhosis with portal hypertension (?hepatomegaly, icterus, spider naevi, leuconychia, etc; see Station 1, Abdominal, Case 3); treatment consists of salt restriction, diuretic therapy (spironolactone or amiloride); paracentesis is increasingly used as initial treatment

2 Intraabdominal malignancy (especially ovarian and gastrointestinal – ?hard knobbly liver, mass, cachexia, nodes, e.g. Troisier's sign also called Virchow's node)

3 Congestive cardiac failue (?JVP ↑, ankle and sacral oedema, hepatomegaly (pulsatile if tricuspid incompetence), large heart, tachycardia, S3 or signs of the cardiac lesion)

Other causes

Nephrotic syndrome (?young, underlying diabetes (fundi), evidence of chronic disease underlying amyloid, evidence of collagen disease, etc; see Station 1, Abdominal, Case 20)

Other causes of hypoalbuminaemia (e.g. malabsorption)

Tuberculous peritonitis† (?ethnic origin, chest signs)

Constrictive pericarditis (JVP raised, abrupt *x* and *y* descent, loud early S3 ('pericardial knock'), though heart sounds often normal, slight 'paradoxical' pulse, *no signs in lung fields*; chest X-ray may show calcified pericardium; rare but important as response to treatment may be dramatic)

Budd–Chiari syndrome (ascites develops rapidly with pain, icterus but no signs of chronic liver disease, smoothly enlarged tender liver; causes include tumour infiltration, oral contraceptives, polycythaemia rubra vera, ulcerative colitis and severe dehydration)

Myxoedema (?facies, ankle jerks, etc; very rare)

Meigs' syndrome (ovarian fibroma; important as easily correctable by surgery)

Pancreatic ascites (complication of acute pancreatitis)

Chylous ascites (due to lymphatic obstruction; milky fluid)

---

*An umbilical hernia may be present.
†NB: Tuberculous peritonitis may attack debilitated alcoholics. Therefore it should always be considered when ascites is present in a cirrhotic. Fever or abdominal pain are suggestive but may not be present. Examination of the ascitic fluid may help – an exudative protein content ($>25\,g\,L^{-1}$) with lymphocytes is also suggestive. Staining of the fluid for AFB is rarely positive and culture is only positive in somewhat less than 50%. Diagnostic procedures include peritonoscopy (bowel adhesions may cause difficulty) and open peritoneal biopsy. Cirrhotic patients should also have ascites tapped to rule out spontaneous bacterial peritonitis as well as TB.

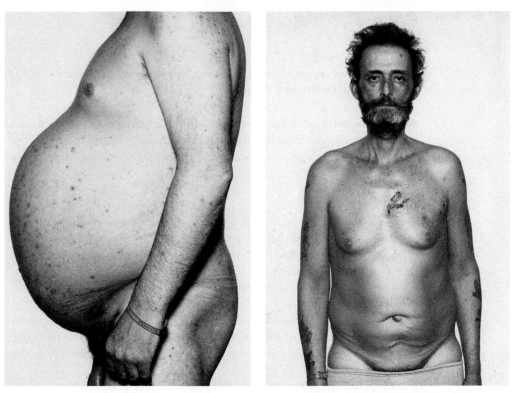

Figure C1.9 (a) Gross ascites. (b) Residual ascites in another patient on treatment with diuretics (see also Station 1, Abdominal, Case 3).

Case 8 | Abdominal mass

Frequency in survey: main focus of a short case or additional feature in 3% of attempts at PACES Station 1, Abdominal.

Survey note: discussion usually concerned differentiation from/of enlarged organs (spleen, kidney, liver) or differential diagnosis.

Record 1

In this young (?somewhat pale-looking) adult patient there is a freely mobile 5 × 4 cm (measure) firm tender mass in the *right iliac fossa*. None of the abdominal organs is enlarged, and there are no fistulae.

The diagnosis could be Crohn's disease (Station 1, Abdominal, Case 9).

Other causes of a mass in the right iliac fossa

1 Ileocaecal tuberculosis (?ethnic origin, chest signs)
2 Carcinoma of the caecum (?older person, non-tender and hard mass, lymph nodes; investigate with colonoscopy)
3 Amoebic abscess (?travelled abroad)
4 Lymphoma (?hepatosplenomegaly, lymph nodes elsewhere; investigate with CT scan)
5 Appendicular abscess (investigate with USS)
6 Neoplasm of the ovary (investigate with USS/CT scan)
7 Ileal carcinoid (rare)
8 Transplanted kidney
9 Faecal matter in caecum (especially in constipation)

Record 2

A mobile tender 6 × 5 cm mass is palpable in the *left iliac fossa* in this elderly patient. None of the other organs is palpable.

It is probably a diverticular abscess (usually tender; investigate with USS/CT scan).

Other causes of a mass in the left iliac fossa

1 Carcinoma of the colon (?non-tender, hepatomegaly; investigate with colonoscopy)
2 Neoplasm of the left ovary (investigate with USS/CT scan)
3 A faecal mass (no other signs)
4 Amoebic abscess

Record 3

In this thin and pale patient there is a round, hard 8 × 6 cm non-tender mass with ill-defined edges in the *epigastrium*. It does not move with respiration. Neither the liver nor the spleen is enlarged (check neck for lymph nodes).

The probable diagnosis is a neoplasm such as:
1 Carcinoma of the stomach (?Troisier's sign also called Virchow's node; investigate with upper GI endoscopy)

2 Carcinoma of the pancreas (?icterus; NB: Courvoisier's sign; investigate with CT scan)

3 Lymphoma (?generalized lymphadenopathy, spleen; investigate with CT scan).

Record 4

In this elderly patient there is a *pulsatile* (pulsating anteriorly as well as transversely), 6 × 4 cm firm mass* palpable 2 cm above the umbilicus and reaching the epigastrium. Both femoral pulses are palpable just before the radials (no evidence of dissection) and there are no bruits heard either over the mass or over the femorals. (Look for evidence of peripheral vascular insufficiency in the feet.)

This patient has an aneurysm of his abdominal aorta (the most common cause is arteriosclerosis†).

If you find a mass in either upper quadrant you should define:

Its size

Its shape

Its consistency

Whether you can get above it

Whether it is bimanually ballotable

Whether it moves with respiration

Whether it is tender.

In either upper quadrant it has to be differentiated from a renal mass (see Station 1, Abdominal, Case 2); if in the left hypochondrium, it has to be differentiated from a spleen (see Station 1, Abdominal, Case 6) and in the right hypochondrium from a liver (see Station 1, Abdominal, Case 5). Other causes of an upper quadrant mass include:

Carcinoma of the colon

Retroperitoneal sarcoma

Lymphoma (?generalized lymphadenopathy, spleen)

Diverticular abscess (?tender).

---

*Pulsations without a mass may be transmitted from a normal aorta. A mass from a neighbouring structure may overlie the aorta and transmit (only anterior) pulsations.

†Mycotic aneurysms (see Vol. 2, Section F, Anecdote 277) are a major complication (2.5% of patients with valvular infections) of infective endocarditis and are most commonly associated with relatively non-invasive organisms such as *Streptococcus viridans*. They may occur at any age, either during the active phase or months (sometimes years) after the endocarditis has been successfully treated. More common sites of mycotic aneurysms are the brain (2–6% of all aneurysms in the brain), sinuses of Valsalva, and ligated ductus arteriosus. Clinical manifestations of abdominal aortic aneurysms (e.g. backache) appear after the lesions have started to leak slowly. Surgical treatment is almost always indicated.

Case 9 | Crohn's disease

Frequency in survey: main focus of a short case or additional feature in 3% of attempts at PACES Station 1, Abdominal.

Survey note: there were several different presentations: as a right iliac fossa mass, as multiple scars and sinuses on the abdomen, as perianal Crohn's disease (only one case) and as Crohn's disease of the lips. In one-third of cases the clue was given that the patient had diarrhoea.

Record 1

The *multiple laparotomy scars* suggest a chronic, relapsing, abdominal condition which has led to crises requiring surgical intervention on several occasions. In view of the associated *fistula* formation, Crohn's disease is likely.

Record 2

The chronically *swollen lips* (granulomatous infiltration) and history of chronic diarrhoea are suggestive of Crohn's disease (examine inside the *mouth* for *ulcers* which vary in size).

Record 3

There is a (characteristic) *dusky blue discoloration* of the perianal skin. There are *oedematous skin tags* (which look soft but are very firm), there is *fissuring, ulceration* and *fistula* formation.

The diagnosis is perianal Crohn's disease (may antedate disease elsewhere in the bowel).

Record 4

Right iliac fossa mass (see Station 1, Abdominal, Case 8).

Other physical signs in Crohn's disease

Fever
Anaemia (malabsorption, chronic disease and GI blood loss)
Clubbing
Arthritis (including sacroiliitis)
Erythema nodosum (see Vol. 3, Station 5, Skin, Case 23)
Pyoderma gangrenosum (see Vol. 3, Station 5, Skin, Case 50)
Iritis
Ankle oedema (hypoproteinaemia)
Aphthous ulcers
Angular stomatitis

Treatment of Crohn's disease

Remember that as well as the usual treatment with corticosteroids and immunosuppressives (e.g. azathioprine), anti-TNF-α antibodies (infliximab, adalimumab) can completely heal the intestinal inflammation (c. 65% of cases) and heal fistulae. However eventual relapse is usual.

Other causes of anal fistulae (rare)

Simple fistula from an abscess of anal gland crypts
Tuberculosis
Ulcerative colitis
Carcinoma of the rectum
Trauma
Radiation
Lymphogranuloma venereum

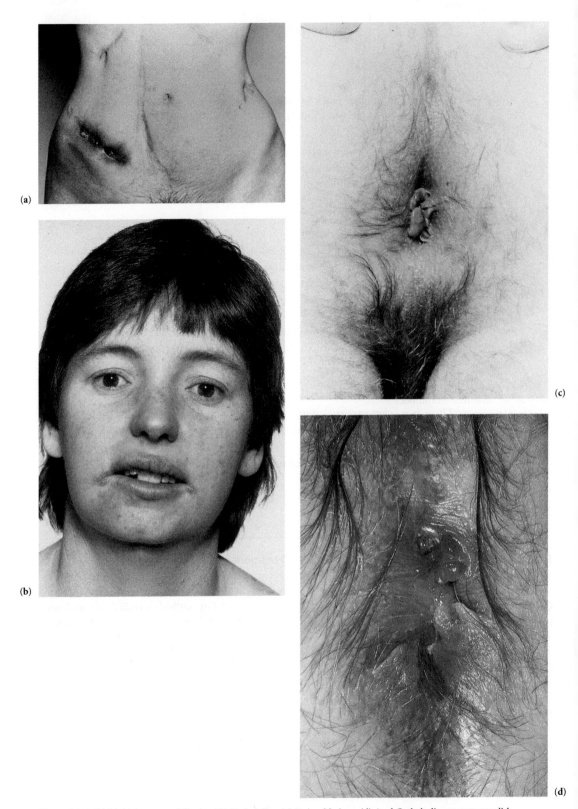

Figure C1.10 (a) Multiple scars and fistulae. (b) Crohn's lips. (c) Perianal lesions. (d) Anal Crohn's disease, note purplish discoloration of the perianal skin, oedematous skin tags, fissuring, ulceration and fistula formation.

Case 10 | Polycythaemia rubra vera

Frequency in survey: main focus of a short case or additional feature in 3% of attempts at PACES Station 1, Abdominal.

Record

This patient has *facial plethora* and a *dusky cyanosis* of the face, hands, feet and (look at the lips and ask the patient to protrude his/her tongue) mucous membranes. There are (may be) ecchymoses (spontaneous bruising) and *scratch marks* (pruritus). (Ask the patient's permission to gently pull down the lower eyelids.) The conjunctival vessels are markedly engorged. (If allowed, look at the fundi for markedly dilated retinal veins, and ask to feel the abdomen for splenomegaly* and to take the blood pressure which may be raised.)

These features suggest a diagnosis of polycythaemia rubra vera.

The diagnosis of primary polycythaemia is based upon demonstration of raised red cell mass and the presence of the V617F mutation in the JAK II gene (also present in 50% of essential thrombocythaemia patients). *Pseudopolycythaemia* (reduced plasma volume) is associated with alcohol abuse, smoking, diuretic use and dehydration.

In primary polycythaemia, the characteristic laboratory findings reveal the consequences of increased bone marrow activity. Typically, the red cell, white cell and platelet counts are elevated. The haemoglobin and the haematocrit are raised. The mean corpuscular volume is reduced, suggestive of iron deficiency erythropoiesis. Being a primarily malignant disorder, red cell proliferation continues until the iron stores are exhausted, giving an iron deficiency picture with a high haemoglobin level.

Causes of secondary polycythaemia

Physiologically appropriate increased erythropoietin production

Arterial hypoxaemia – chronic pulmonary disease, right-to-left shunt, Pickwickian syndrome (see Station 1, Respiratory, Case 18), etc.

Abnormal release of oxygen from haemoglobin – congenitally decreased red cell 2,3-DPG; smokers – carboxyhaemoglobinaemia

Interference with tissue oxygen metabolism – cobalt poisoning

Physiologically inappropriate erythropoietin production

Neoplasms – renal, adrenal, hepatocellular, ovarian, cerebellar haemangioblastoma, phaeochromocytoma, etc.

Non-neoplastic renal disease – cysts, hydronephrosis

---

*Splenomegaly occurs in over 70% of patients and hepatomegaly may be present in about 40% of patients.

Case 11 | Normal abdomen

Frequency in survey: main focus of a short case or additional feature in 2% of attempts at PACES Station 1, Abdominal.

The College has made it clear that 'normal' is an option in PACES. No findings on examination is common in real clinical medicine and so this must be a possibility in the exam. In terms of the practical reality of the exam, in order for PACES to proceed there must be an abdominal case in Station 1, Abdominal. If, at the last minute, neither of the scheduled abdo cases turn up on the day or if, in the middle of a carousel, the only one who did turn up decides not to continue or is too ill to continue, a substitute case has to be found at short notice. In this situation, one option is to proceed with a patient with an abdomen which is normal and make up an appropriate scenario. One simply has to imagine oneself as the invigilating registrar to think what that might be. One would first look amongst any surplus cases in the other stations for a volunteer or one might ask a member of the nursing, portering or other support staff. At the planning meetings for PACES when it was first launched, the College came up with the following scenario as an example of one that might be used:

'This . . . -year-old patient presented with haematemesis. Please examine the abdomen.'

There may thus be a clue in the case scenario and the fact that the scenario has been hurriedly hand-scribbled.

From our surveys it is clear that the most common reason for finding no abnormality is missing the physical signs that are present – possibly Anecdote 5 below (see probably both Anecdotes 1 and 2, Station 3, Cardiovascular, Case 24 and Vol. 2, Section F, Experience 158). Other reasons for cases of 'normal' will be either because the physical signs are no longer present by the time the patient comes to the examination (see Anecdote 1, Station 3, CNS, Case 28) or that the examiners and candidate disagree with the selectors of the cases about the presence of physical signs (this may have happened in Anecdote, Vol. 3, Station 5, Eyes, Case 21; see also Vol. 2, Section F, Experience 198 and Anecdote 303).

The following are anecdotes from our surveys.

Anecdote 1

A candidate was asked to examine the abdomen of a patient he was told had presented with epigastric pain. His findings were a tender epigastrium but nothing else. They asked him what he had found other than tenderness but he could not find any other signs. They asked him whether he wanted to examine the patient again. He did so but he still didn't find anything else. They asked him how he would investigate someone with epigastric pain. The candidate passed PACES and is fairly confident that this was a case of 'normal abdomen'.

Anecdote 2

A candidate was asked to examine a lady's abdomen. She found a nephrectomy scar in the otherwise normal abdomen of a lady who had some purpura. At the time she reported the case to us, she did not know whether or not she had passed but she was fairly confident that there were no other signs.

Anecdote 3

A candidate was asked to examine a lady's abdomen. The patient was an obese lady and he could not find any abnormality. The discussion focused on the management of polycystic kidney disease. He passed PACES on that attempt and is fairly confident that it may have been polycystic kidneys that he could not find because of her obesity.

Anecdote 4

A candidate was asked to examine the abdomen. She could find no abnormality and told the examiner she thought the abdomen was normal. She was asked to demonstrate the 'tests' for splenic enlargement. She passed the examination and in retrospect she still feels that it was a normal abdomen.

Anecdote 5

A candidate was asked to examine a man's abdomen. He could find no abnormality and diagnosed a normal abdomen. In retrospect, he is not sure if he missed something. Though he failed the clinical, he felt he had passed the short case section (pre PACES case).

Case 12 | PEG tube

Frequency in survey: main focus of a short case or additional feature in 2% of attempts at PACES Station 1, Abdominal.

Survey note: see Vol. 2, Section F, Anecdotes 94–97.

Record

The patient has a *tube in the epigastrium*. (Now look for evidence of *underlying neurological disease* [hemiparesis, tremor, muscle wasting] *or surgery* [head and neck cancer, intestinal resections].)*

This is a percutaneous endoscopic gastrostomy (PEG) tube.

Indications for PEG feeding

Head and neck cancer (risk of cancer seeding with standard peroral pull-through technique – percutaneous PEG placement preferred)

Neurological conditions:

(a) Stroke (NG feed for 14 days, then consider PEG)

(b) Cerebral palsy and congenital neurological deficits

(c) Head injury

(d) Brain tumours

Neuromuscular conditions:

(a) Multiple sclerosis

(b) Parkinson's disease

(c) Motor neurone disease

Dementia is generally considered a poor indication for PEG feeding as there is no evidence that it improves the quality or duration of life. Current advice is to persevere with careful hand feeding, varying the size and timing of meals and considering modified flavour, temperature and consistency to improve intake (Peterborough Palliative Care in Dementia Group).

Alternative types of tube

Nasogastric (NG) tubes: suitable for short-term feeding especially

Nasojejunal (NJ) tubes (often actually sited in duodenum): preferred in patients with impaired gastric emptying

Radiologically inserted gastrostomy (RIG): inserted under imaging guidance (useful in patients with atypical anatomy, e.g. large hiatus hernia)

Surgically placed jejunostomies: frequently used in upper GI cancer

Complications of PEG insertion

Procedure related: visceral perforation, intraabdominal haemorrhage, peritonitis, stomal sepsis, colonic perforation, pneumonia, death

Subsequent: occlusion, displacement,† 'buried bumper syndrome' (traction on internal flange causes migration into the gastric mucosa), pneumonia

---

*Consider commenting on nutritional status (patient's weight, muscle bulk, subcutaneous fat and any evidence of specific nutritional deficiencies, e.g. stomatitis, easy bruising, osteoporotic fractures).

†Be aware that PEG tubes that become displaced within the first 14–28 days should not be reinserted at the bedside as the track will not be securely established – endoscopic replacement is necessary.

Case 13 | Single palpable kidney

Frequency in survey: main focus of a short case or additional feature in 2% of attempts at PACES Station 1, Abdominal.

Record

There is a mass (describe consistency, edges, size, etc.) on the R/L side* of the abdomen in the midzone. It is *bimanually ballotable*, I can *get above it*, and the percussion note is *resonant* over it.

It is, therefore, likely to be renal in origin (check for the pale, brownish-yellow tinge of uraemia, dialysis fistula/shunt/scars, etc.).

Possible causes

1 Polycystic disease (see Station 1, Abdominal, Case 2) with only one kidney palpable
2 Carcinoma (?weight loss, evidence of secondaries, anaemia, polycythaemia, pyrexia)
3 Hydronephrosis
4 Hypertrophy of a single functioning kidney (unilateral renal agenesis (1:500–1000 births) may predispose in the long term to proteinuria, hypertension and glomerular sclerosis)

Features of renal cell carcinoma

Accounts for 2% of adult malignancies
Increased risk with smoking
Spreads to the aortic and para-aortic nodes
Distant metastases may occur in the lung (50%), bone (49%), skin (11%), liver (8%) and brain (3%)
Haematuria is the most frequent presenting symptom. Pain and abdominal mass are also common but the classic triad of haematuria, pain and abdominal mass occurs in <10% of patients
Treatment is with nephrectomy and immunotherapy – interferon-α and interleukin 2

*NB: A palpable right kidney may be normal in a thin person.

Case 14 | Generalized lymphadenopathy

Frequency in survey: main focus of a short case or additional feature in 0.9% of attempts at PACES Station 1, Abdominal.

Record

There is generalized lymphadenopathy with/without . . . cm *splenomegaly* (or hepatosplenomegaly).

The likeliest causes would be a *lymphoreticular disorder* (Hodgkin's and non-Hodgkin's lymphoma, etc.) or *chronic lymphatic leukaemia*.

Other causes

Infectious mononucleosis* (?sore throat)
Sarcoidosis (?erythema nodosum or history of)
Tuberculosis (?ethnic origin, lung signs)
Brucellosis (?farm worker)
Toxoplasmosis* (glandular fever-like illness)
Cytomegalovirus* (glandular fever-like illness)
Thyrotoxicosis (?exophthalmos, goitre, tachycardia, etc; see Vol. 3, Station 5, Endocrine, Case 3)
Progressive generalized lymphadenopathy (HIV; see Vol. 3, Station 5, Skin, Case 36)
Secondary syphilis

Diagnosis and staging of non-Hodgkin's lymphoma

The precise histological subtype needs to be established according to the current WHO/REAL classification and the extent of the disease:

Lymph node biopsy – fine needle aspirate is not adequate for histological subtyping
CT scan – usually chest, abdomen and pelvis; occasionally neck
Bone marrow aspirate and trephine
Other less frequently used staging investigations – PET scanning, LP, CT or MRI of the head (in certain subtypes, e.g. lymphoblastic lymphoma where the risk of CNS disease is high)
ENT examination of the postnasal space

*Lymph nodes likely to be tender in acute infectious cases.

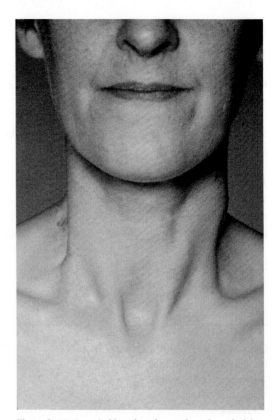

Figure C1.11 A cervical lymph node seen from the end of the bed.

Case 15 | Hereditary spherocytosis

Frequency in survey: main focus of a short case or additional feature in 0.9% of attempts at PACES Station 1, Abdominal.

Survey note: some candidates were shown a pale adult of about 30 years of age and asked to examine the abdomen.

Record

This patient has *splenomegaly* (sometimes there may also be hepatomegaly), *pale skin* and conjunctivae* and *icteric sclerae.* The spleen is enlarged (say by how much) below the left costal edge (there may be a splenectomy scar† instead).

The underlying cause of this triad of jaundice, anaemia and splenomegaly may be haemolytic anaemia.‡

Causes of haemolytic anaemias

Hereditary haemolytic anaemias:
   hereditary spherocytosis
   hereditary elliptocytosis
   thalassaemia
   sickle cell anaemia
Acquired haemolytic anaemia:
   acquired autoimmune haemolytic anaemia
   primary or idiopathic haemolytic anaemia

Secondary haemolytic anaemia:
   lymphoproliferative disorders
   SLE
   chronic inflammatory disease (e.g. ulcerative colitis)
   drugs (e.g. methyldopa, mefenamic acid)
   infections (e.g. brucellosis, infectious mononucleosis, etc.)
   non-lymphoid neoplasms (e.g. ovarian tumours)

---

*Jaundice may be barely detectable or absent in some cases but anaemia is a regular feature of hereditary spherocytosis.

†Splenectomy is advisable in severe cases of hereditary spherocytosis and in mild cases with complications such as gallstones. Splenectomy removes a protective blood-filtering bed and renders patients, especially the young ones, more vulnerable to infections. This tendency can be minimized, but not completely eliminated, by immunization and careful attention to all infections. Recommendations for postsplenectomy prophylaxis include vaccinations for *Pneumococcus, Haemophilus influenzae* B and *Meningococcus* C, annual flu vaccine and lifelong penicillin prophylaxis.

‡The other contender for this triad is a group of systemic conditions (e.g. infective endocarditis, SLE, pernicious anaemia, infectious mononucleosis, etc.). The absence of various stigmata of

these and the presence of some for hereditary spherocytosis (e.g. leg ulcers), the hint of a family history (autosomal dominant) from the examiner, and a relatively young age may give you enough confidence to suggest the diagnosis. However, the definitive diagnosis of this condition cannot be made without laboratory help (low mean corpuscular volume, high mean corpuscular haemoglobin concentration, because the red cells tend to be dehydrated, spherocytosis on the blood film, increased osmotic fragility and, in most cases, a decreased spectrin content of the red cells). Anaemia, jaundice and splenomegaly are also present in other varieties of hereditary and acquired haemolytic anaemias. They may also, of course, occur together in chronic liver disease but then one would expect other diagnostic clues (see Station 1, Abdominal, Case 3).

Case 16 | Idiopathic haemochromatosis

Frequency in survey: main focus of a short case or additional feature in 0.8% of attempts at PACES Station 1, Abdominal.

Record

There is (in this thin patient) *slate-grey pigmentation,* decreased body hair and gynaecomastia* (and testicular atrophy* – iron deposition affecting hypothalamic-pituitary function). The *liver** is *enlarged* at . . . cm (in 95% of symptomatic patients; spleen is present in 50%).

The diagnosis is haemochromatosis.

Males > females.

In males it may present at any time in adult life. In females it usually presents after the menopause (physiological iron loss protects).

Autosomal recessive – association with HLA-A3. The HFE gene was identified in 1996 as the gene whose mutations give rise to genetic haemochromatosis. The gene is located on the short arm of chromosome 6 and the most important mutation is C282Y, in which a substitution of cysteine by tyrosine occurs at position 282 of the mature protein (others are H63D and S65C). Homozygous C282Y mutation is responsible for about 90% of genetic haemochromatosis in northern Europe. Haemochromatosis is a common genetic disorder – the carrier rate is about 1/10 in populations of northern European origin. Homozygote rates vary between 1/200 and 1/600.

Other features which may be present

Spider naevi

Palmar erythema

Ascites

Jaundice

Diabetes mellitus* (not entirely due to iron deposition in the pancreas because insulin levels may be normal and there is a higher incidence of diabetes in relatives without iron overload; high incidence of insulin resistance and fat atrophy)

Arthropathy* (pseudogout – especially the second and third MCP joints, wrists, hips and knees)

Cardiac involvement* (large heart, dysrhythmias, congestive cardiac failure; it is the presenting manifestation in 15% – sometimes young adults; it may be *misdiagnosed* as idiopathic cardiomyopathy)

Hepatocellular carcinoma (develops in 33% of cirrhotic patients; it does not appear to occur if the disease is treated in the precirrhotic stage; hence the importance of *family screening*)

Addison's disease, hypothyroidism and hypoparathyroidism are exceedingly rare

Treatment

Weekly *phlebotomy* (500 mL) until the haemoglobin concentration falls below $11\,g\,dL^{-1}$ and the patient is marginally iron deficient (serum ferritin $<10\,\mu g\,L^{-1}$ – this usually takes 2–3 years), then maintenance phlebotomy to keep the serum iron and ferritin in the low normal range (about once every 3 months). When phlebotomy is initiated before cirrhosis develops, survival is normal. If anaemia and hypoproteinaemia preclude

*The association of hepatomegaly, skin pigmentation, diabetes mellitus, heart disease, arthritis and evidence of hypogonadism should always suggest haemochromatosis. These days, the precirrhotic condition is often diagnosed in young relatives by family screening. The diagnosis should be considered in any patient with unexplained hepatomegaly, idiopathic cardiomyopathy, abnormal pigmentation or loss of libido (may antedate other clinical manifestations of the disease). Ninety percent of patients show bronzing of the skin due to excess melanin. In half, haemosiderin is also present, giving the skin the classic slate-grey appearance.

phlebotomy, *desferrioxamine* may be indicated. This is most practicably administered by high-dose subcutaneous infusion using a portable pump. *Ascorbic acid* given concurrently improves iron excretion.

NB: Patients with alcoholic liver disease may have increased stainable iron on liver biopsy and increased serum ferritin levels. It is necessary to check HFE status to identify those with genetic haemochromatosis who abuse alcohol. In those without haemochromatosis, ferritin levels often fall into the normal range with abstention from alcohol. If ferritin levels remain high, venesection may be necessary.

Case 17 | Primary biliary cirrhosis

Frequency in survey: main focus of a short case or additional feature in 0.8% of attempts at PACES Station 1, Abdominal.

Record

This middle-aged lady is *icteric* (may not be) with *pigmentation* of the skin. There are *excoriations* (due to scratching) and she has *xanthelasma* (other xanthomata frequently occur over joints, skinfolds and at sites of trauma). The liver is enlarged . . . cm (may be very large; there may be splenomegaly).

The clinical diagnosis is primary biliary cirrhosis (PBC) (there may be *clubbing*). The scratch marks are due to *pruritus* (the predominant presenting symptom).

HLA phenotypes DR8 and C4B2 = threefold increase in risk

Serum antimitochondrial antibody positive in 95–99%

Smooth muscle antibody positive in 66%

Antinuclear antibody positive in 35%

Rheumatoid factor positive in 70%

Antithyroid antibody positive in 40%

Diagnosis is established by liver biochemistry (raised hepatic alkaline phosphatase, raised bilirubin (late)), positive antimitochondrial antibody and compatible liver biopsy histology. Twenty-five percent of cases are asymptomatic at diagnosis.* In some patients, there are overlapping features between PBC and autoimmune liver disease. The only approved drug therapy for PBC is oral ursodeoxycholic acid, which eases pruritus, improves liver biochemistry and histology and delays the onset of advanced liver disease, partial hypertension and the need for transplantation. Corticosteroids, penicillamine, colchicine, azathioprine, methotrexate, cyclosporin and chlorambucil have been tried in PBC but are no longer used because of lack of efficacy and/ or unacceptable side-effects. Because of the risk of malabsorption, patients may need a low-fat diet, fat-soluble vitamin supplements and treatment for osteomalacia.

The pruritus may respond to cholestyramine (taken before and after meals) or ursodeoxycholic acid, though phenobarbitone, rifampicin, opiate antagonists (e.g. naloxone) or propofol may also help. Resistant pruritus can respond to norethandrolone but this deepens jaundice. Liver transplantation is the treatment of choice for advanced disease with jaundice or hepatic failure. Severe pruritis may be an indication for transplantation. The disease may recur in the transplanted liver.

The patient is at risk of

Bleeding oesophageal varices (late feature)

Steatorrhoea and malabsorption, leading to Osteomalacia

Associated conditions*

Sjögren's syndrome

Systemic sclerosis

CREST syndrome

Rheumatoid arthritis

Hashimoto's thyroiditis

Renal tubular acidosis

Coeliac disease

Dermatomyositis

Cutaneous disorders (e.g. discoid LE, pemphigoid, lichen planus)

---

*The incidental finding of a raised alkaline phosphatase in patients with the conditions on this list should raise the suspicion of an associated primary biliary cirrhosis.

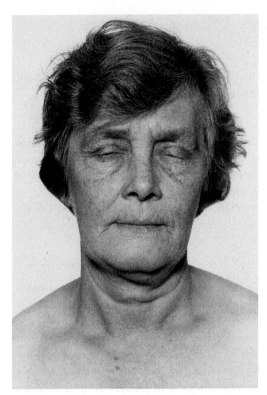

Figure C1.12 Note xanthelasma, pigmentation and spider naevi.

Case 18 | Carcinoid syndrome

Frequency in survey: main focus of a short case or additional feature in 0.7% of attempts at PACES Station 1, Abdominal.

Record

There is *cutaneous flushing*,* facial *telangiectasiae* and the *liver is palpable* . . . cm below the right costal margin (may be irregular).

In view of the history of *diarrhoea*,† these features are suggestive of the carcinoid syndrome.

Carcinoid tumours arise from enterochromaffin cells and are most commonly found in the appendix or rectum but these rarely give rise to the carcinoid syndrome. The actual carcinoid syndrome is produced by carcinoid tumours (usually ileal, but also from the stomach, bile duct, duodenum, pancreas, lung and gonads) which have metastasized to the liver, presumably because the metastatic tumour impedes hepatic clearance of mediators (including *serotonin (5-HT)*, bradykinin, histamine and tachykinins, as well as prostaglandins) released from the tumour. The flush (head and upper thorax) is red initially but then becomes purple and commonly lasts only a few minutes but may continue for hours.* Frequent flushing may lead to telangiectasiae. During a flush, the heart rate increases and the blood pressure falls.‡

Other features of carcinoid syndrome

Fibrotic lesions (probably due to chronic 5-HT excess):
  Right-sided endocardial fibrosis (33% of patients; heart failure due to *pulmonary stenosis*, tricuspid incompetence or both is less common but implies a poor prognosis)
  Pleural, peritoneal and retroperitoneal fibroses

Bronchoconstriction (20% of patients; wheezing occurs during episodes of flushing and is probably not due to 5-HT)
Abdominal pain,† weight loss and cachexia
Diagnosis confirmed by the finding of a very high urinary 5-HIAA
Imaging to localize lesions may include octreoscan,§ CT, MRI and PET scanning§
Somatostatin analogues, cyproheptadine (may ameliorate the diarrhoea) and leucocyte interferon may be beneficial in treatment. Surgical debulking may be required. Radiotherapy or chemotherapy with streptozocin, cisplatin, etoposide and doxorubicin alone or in combination can lead to benefit in 20–30% of cases.

Ectopic humoral syndromes in histological carcinoid tumours¶

Cushing's syndrome (ACTH in bronchial carcinoid)
Dilutional hyponatraemia (antidiuretic hormone in bronchial carcinoid)
Gynaecomastia (HCG in gastric carcinoid)
Acromegaly (GHRH in foregut carcinoid)
Hypoglycaemia (insulin in pancreatic carcinoid)

---

*Flushing tends to be more intense and longer lasting with bronchial carcinoids and more patchy (anywhere on the body) with gastric carcinoids. Headache commonly follows the flush. It may be precipitated by alcohol, food, stress, palpation of the liver, or it may follow administration of catecholamines, pentagastrin or reserpine. The mediator of the flush is uncertain and is probably not 5-HT. Conversely, the diarrhoea does seem to be mediated by 5-HT as it can be reduced by inhibition of 5-HT synthesis. Nevertheless, the diarrhoea is typically exacerbated during episodes of flushing.

†This important clue may be in the written instruction. Diarrhoea (2–30 stools per day), frequently accompanied by abdominal cramping, is not usually disabling but can occasionally be voluminous with malabsorption and fluid and electrolyte imbalance.
‡Cf. pallor and hypertension with phaeochromocytoma.
§Octreoscan: ^{111}Indium-labelled octreotide (a somatostatin analogue) used in scintigraphy to detect tumours expressing somatostatin receptors. PET scanning detects the increased metabolism of glucose in the carcinoid lesions.
¶Typically such patients do not have carcinoid syndrome.

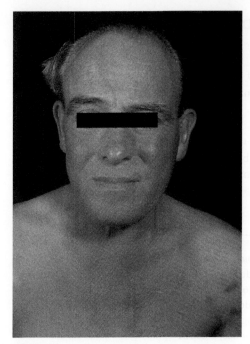

Figure C1.13 Cutaneous flush in the carcinoid syndrome.

Case 19 | Motor neurone disease

Frequency in survey: main focus of a short case or additional feature in 0.7% of attempts at PACES Station 1, Abdominal.

Survey note: see Vol. 2, Section F, Anecdote 97.

Motor neurone disease is dealt with in Station 3, CNS, Case 11.

Case 20 | Nephrotic syndrome

Frequency in survey: main focus of a short case or additional feature in 0.7% of attempts at PACES Station 1, Abdominal.

Record
There is *extensive oedema* affecting the ankles, lower legs and periorbital tissues (especially in the morning) of this (may be young*) patient. The skin is pale (oedema in the skin). There are (may be) white bands across the nails (from chronic hypoalbuminaemia). There are (may be) bilateral *pleural effusions* and *ascites*.

This patient's extensive oedema could be due to nephrotic syndrome.†

Most common cause
Glomerulonephritis (77% – usually minimal change in childhood but membranous in adults)

Causes of nephrotic syndrome
1 *Minimal change disease*
   (a) Primary (idiopathic):
   with atopy HLA-B12
   without atopy
   (b) Secondary:
   lymphoma
   carcinoma (renal, lung, pancreas)
   IgA nephropathy
   diabetes mellitus
   AIDS
2 *Focal and segmental glomerulosclerosis*
   (a) Primary:
   idiopathic
   superimposed on minimal change
   (b) Secondary:
   infection – HIV
   drugs – heroin abuse, NSAIDs, analgesic abuse
   reduced renal cell mass – cortical necrosis, renal dysplasia
   normal renal cell mass – diabetes mellitus, hypertension, Alport's syndrome, sickle cell disease, cystinosis, sarcoidosis

3 *Membranous glomerulonephritis*
   (a) Primary (idiopathic)
   (b) Secondary:
   infection – hepatitis B (75% of cases), hepatitis C, malaria, schistosomiasis
   multisystem – SLE, mixed connective tissue disease, dermatomyositis, Sjögren's syndrome
   neoplastic (lung, colon, stomach, breast), lymphoma
   drugs – gold, mercury, penicillamine
   familial – sickle cell disease
   miscellaneous – *de novo* in renal allograft, bullous pemphigoid, Fanconi's syndrome
4 *Mesangiocapillary glomerulonephritis*
   (a) Primary (idiopathic):
   type 1 – subendothelial deposits
   type 2 – dense deposit disease
   (b) Secondary – SLE, cryoglobulinaemia, scleroderma, light and heavy chain disease
5 *Fibrillary glomerulonephritis*
Amyloidosis, multiple myeloma, cryoglobulinaemia, lupus nephritis

Malaria due to *Plasmodium malariae* is an important cause in areas where it is endemic. There are about 70 rare causes.

---

*The oedema of the acute poststreptococcal glomerulonephritis (proteinuria, haematuria, oliguria, oedema, hypertension, renal failure), which mainly affects children and young adults, is usually due to salt and water retention. Only in a small proportion does heavier proteinuria leading to nephrotic syndrome develop.

†Defined as proteinuria $>3.5\,g/1.75\,m^2$ of body surface per 24 h, hypoalbuminaemia and oedema. Hypercholesterolaemia is often present.

Investigations for nephrotic syndrome

Urine microscopy (?red cells, casts, lipid deposits), 24-h urinary protein

Urinary protein selectivity (clearance ratio of IgG to transferrin below 0.15 in minimal change disease, which carries a good prognosis)

Renal profile, eGFR

Specific tests for the causal diseases (glucose, antinuclear factors, etc.)

Renal biopsy

Complications

Acute kidney injury (due to aggressive diuresis, renal vein thrombosis, drug-induced interstitial nephritis)

Thrombosis (deep venous, arterial, pulmonary, renal vein) due to dehydration, immobility and a hypercoagulable state (urinary loss of antithrombin and increased hepatic production of fibrinogen)

Malnutrition (normal protein diet unless marked uraemia)

Atheroma and ischaemic heart disease (hypercholesterolaemia*)

Infection

Treatment

General and supportive measures (low-salt diet, diuretics and lipid-lowering agents) should be given to all patients. Specific therapy with corticosteroids in minimal change disease has a successful outcome, especially in children. Corticosteroids with cytotoxic therapy are also given to other varieties with variable outcomes. Prolonged anticoagulation is required if thromboembolic episodes occur.

*Most nephrotic patients have elevated total and LDL cholesterol levels with low or normal HDL cholesterol. Xanthelasmata accumulate rapidly in nephrotic syndrome.

Case 21 | **Pernicious anaemia**

Frequency in survey: main focus of a short case or additional feature in 0.7% of attempts at PACES Station 1, Abdominal.

Survey note: see Vol. 2, Section F, Anecdote 98.

Pernicious anaemia is dealt with in Vol. 3, Station 5, Other, Case 6.

Case 22 | Pyoderma gangrenosum

Frequency in survey: main focus of a short case or additional feature in 0.7% of attempts at PACES Station 1, Abdominal.

Survey note: see Vol. 2, Section F, Anecdote 99.

Pyoderma gangrenosum is dealt with in Vol. 3, Station 5, Skin, Case 50.

Case 23 | Felty's syndrome

Frequency in survey: main focus of a short case or additional feature in 0.1% of attempts at PACES Station 1, Abdominal.

Record

There is a *symmetrical deforming arthropathy* with *spindling* and *ulnar deviation* of the fingers, and *nodules* at the elbows. The *spleen* is enlarged at . . . cm. (Check for anaemia.)

If *neutropenia** is present (?evidence of secondary infection) this, in combination with rheumatoid arthritis and splenomegaly, would constitute Felty's syndrome.†

Occurs in older patients with long-standing rheumatoid disease (5%).

Other signs and features of Felty's syndrome

Lymphadenopathy
Skin pigmentation
Vasculitic leg ulceration
Keratoconjunctivitis sicca
Thrombocytopenia
Haemolytic anaemia
Lack of relationship between the degree of haematological abnormality and the size of spleen
Tests for antinuclear factor are often positive as well as rheumatoid factor which is invariably positive

---

*Splenectomy may correct the neutropenia and prevent further infections in some patients, but many do not improve.

†Felty's syndrome is very rare in the UK these days because current trends for early aggressive disease-modifying antirheumatic drugs (DMARD) and biological therapies in patients who fail to respond to methotrexate have meant that most extraarticular manifestations have reduced significantly (e.g. rheumatoid vasculitis and Felty's syndrome).

Station 3
Cardiovascular

Short case	Checked and updated as necessary for this edition by
1 Prosthetic valves (mechanical)	Dr Teri Millane*
2 Mitral incompetence (lone)	Dr Teri Millane*
3 Mixed mitral valve disease	Dr Teri Millane*
4 Aortic incompetence (lone)	Dr Teri Millane*
5 Aortic stenosis (lone)	Dr Teri Millane*
6 Mixed aortic valve disease	Dr Teri Millane*
7 Mitral stenosis (lone)	Dr Teri Millane*
8 Irregular pulse	Dr Teri Millane*
9 Other combinations of mitral and aortic valve disease	Dr Teri Millane*
10 Mitral valve prolapse	Dr Teri Millane*
11 Tricuspid incompetence	Dr Teri Millane*
12 Ventricular septal defect	Dr Teri Millane*
13 Marfan's syndrome	Dr David Carruthers*
14 Pulmonary stenosis	Dr Teri Millane*
15 Ankylosing spondylitis	Dr David Carruthers*
16 Atrial septal defect	Dr Teri Millane*
17 Ebstein's anomaly	New short case for this edition by Dr Chetan Varma*
18 Raised jugular venous pressure	Dr Teri Millane*
19 Down's syndrome	Dr Bob Ryder
20 Hypertrophic cardiomyopathy	Dr Teri Millane*
21 Dextrocardia	Dr Teri Millane*
22 Rheumatoid arthritis	Dr David Carruthers*
23 Fallot's tetralogy with a Blalock shunt	Dr Teri Millane*
24 Normal heart	Dr Bob Ryder
25 Cannon waves	Dr Teri Millane*
26 Coarctation of the aorta	Dr Teri Millane*
27 Eisenmenger's syndrome	Dr Teri Millane*
28 Infective endocarditis	Dr Teri Millane*
29 Patent ductus arteriosus	Dr Teri Millane*
30 Pulmonary incompetence	Dr Teri Millane*
31 Slow pulse	Dr Teri Millane*

*All suggested changes by these specialty advisors were considered by Dr Bob Ryder and were either accepted, edited, added to or rejected with Dr Ryder making the final editorial decision in every case.

Dr Teri Millane, Consultant Cardiologist, City Hospital, Birmingham, UK
Dr David Carruthers, Consultant Rheumatologist, City Hospital, Birmingham, UK
Dr Chetan Varma, Consultant Cardiologist, City Hospital, Birmingham, UK

Case 1 | Prosthetic valves (mechanical)

Frequency in survey: main focus of a short case or additional feature in 17% of attempts at PACES Station 3, Cardiovascular.

Survey note: both mitral and aortic prostheses occurred (often leaking). There may also be murmurs from the unreplaced valve.

Record 1

There is a *midline sternotomy scar*. There is a *click at the first heart sound* (closing of the mitral prosthesis) and an *opening click** in diastole (this may occasionally be followed by a mid-diastolic flow murmur, particularly with the older ball and cage valves).

These clicks represent the opening and closing of a *mitral valve prosthesis*. (The pansystolic murmur ± signs of heart failure suggest it is leaking.†)

(Check for left submammary thoracotomy scar suggesting previous mitral valve surgery.)

Record 2

There is a *midline sternotomy scar*. The first heart sound is normal (unless there is accompanying mitral stenosis) and is followed by a soft *ejection click** (opening of the prosthesis often inaudible in newer prosthesis), an *ejection systolic murmur* (flow murmur through prosthesis) and a *click at* (as part of) *the second sound* (closing of the prosthesis).

These clicks suggest an *aortic valve prosthesis*. (The early diastolic murmur and collapsing pulse (?wide pulse pressure) suggest it is leaking.†)

Complications of prosthetic valves

Thromboembolic disease (anticoagulants or antiplatelet agents reduce but do not abolish)

Haemorrhage due to inadvertent overanticoagulation

Infective endocarditis (always consider when leakage develops)‡

Leakage due to wear of the valve (rare in mechanical valves)

Leakage due to inadequacy or infection (bacterial endocarditis) of valve siting

Near total or even total dehiscence of the valve from its siting (the valve will be seen to rock on X-ray screening when there is serious leakage)

Valve obstruction from thrombosis/fibrosis clogging up the valve mechanics – usually older mitral valve replacements

Haemolysis (rare with modern devices)

NB: Bioprosthetic§ porcine heterografts and cadaveric homografts do not cause clicks. They last on average 8–10 years and are therefore only used nowadays in the elderly or are seen in adult survivors of congenital heart disease (where they are often calcified, producing signs of valve/conduit obstruction). Regurgitation is not uncommon in the aortic position.

*Clicks can be audible without a stethoscope. Their cessation or diminution can be a harbinger of serious valve dysfunction, and should always be taken seriously if reported by the patient or a relative.
†Transoesophageal echocardiography (TOE) is usually required to assess the function of prosthetic valves in detail, particularly if malfunction is suspected (the metal causes artefactual echoes which can be a serious problem when dealing with the limited echo windows available to the transthoracic echocardiographer; multiple views are available with TOE).
‡See Station 3, Cardiovascular, Case 28.
§Signs may be very subtle, or even absent, if the prosthetic valve is biological.

Case 2 | Mitral incompetence (lone)

Frequency in survey: main focus of a short case or additional feature in 9% of attempts at PACES Station 3, Cardiovascular.

Record

The pulse is regular (give rate). The venous pressure is not raised and there is no ankle or sacral oedema (unless in cardiac failure). The apex beat is *thrusting* (volume overload) in the sixth intercostal space in the anterior axillary line, and there is (may be) a systolic thrill. There is a left *parasternal heave*. The *first heart sound* is *soft* with a loud pulmonary second sound. There is a loud *pansystolic murmur* at the apex, *radiating* to the *axilla*.

The diagnosis is significant mitral incompetence with signs of pulmonary hypertension.

Causes of mitral incompetence*

1 Degenerative mitral valve disease
2 Severe left ventricular dilation (due to any cause, resulting in lateral displacement of the papillary muscles and dilation of the mitral annulus† interfering with coaptation of the valve leaflets to produce *functional* regurgitation)
3 Papillary muscle dysfunction (ischaemia, infarction or other degenerative disease of the chordae tendinae)
4 Rheumatic heart disease (affects males more commonly than females; contrast with mitral stenosis which affects females more commonly than males)
5 Mitral valve prolapse (see Station 3, Cardiovascular, Case 10)
6 Previous mitral valvotomy for mitral stenosis (left thoracotomy scar)

Other physical signs (which may occur in severe mitral incompetence)
Mid-diastolic rumbling murmur‡ (brief and rare)
Sharp and abbreviated peripheral pulse (lack of sustained forward stroke volume because of the regurgitant leak)
Wide splitting of the second sound (early closure of the aortic valve because the regurgitant loss shortens the left ventricular ejection time)
Fourth heart sound (acute severe regurgitation with sinus rhythm)

---

*Regardless of the aetiology, mitral incompetence is a condition which gradually worsens spontaneously ('mitral incompetence begets mitral incompetence'), enlargement of the left atrium and left ventricle both worsen the incompetence and a vicious circle is set up.

†Left ventricular dilation is an increasingly common cause of significant mitral regurgitation in NYHA III and IV heart failure. If associated with ischaemia, valve repair with an annuloplasty ring is usually undertaken at the time of coronary bypass surgery.

‡A short mid-diastolic murmur in the context of mitral incompetence could indicate associated mitral stenosis or it could represent a flow (left atrium to left ventricle) murmur. The presence of an opening snap in such cases indicates mitral stenosis. In the absence of an opening snap, the mid-diastolic murmur has two possible causes: (i) severe mitral incompetence with an increased flow murmur; or (ii) associated mitral stenosis and a calcified mitral valve. In the former there is often a third heart sound. In the latter the murmur is usually longer.

Other causes of mitral incompetence*

Infective endocarditis (fever, splenomegaly, petechiae, splinter haemorrhages, clubbing, Osler's nodes, Janeway lesions, Roth's spots, etc.)

Annular calcification (especially in the elderly female)

Hypertrophic cardiomyopathy (see Station 3, Cardiovascular, Case 20)

Rupture of the chordae tendinae* (usually causes acute severe mitral incompetence; causes include infective endocarditis, rheumatic mitral valve disease, mitral valve prolapse, trauma)

Connective tissue disorders:

(a) SLE (Libman–Sachs endocarditis; see Vol. 3, Station 5, Locomotor, Case 16)

(b) rheumatoid arthritis (?hands, ?nodules)

(c) ankylosing spondylitis (?male with fixed kyphosis and stooped posture; aortic valve more commonly affected; see Vol. 3, Station 5, Locomotor, Case 6)

Congenital with or without other abnormalities:

(a) Marfan's syndrome (?tall with long extremities, arachnodactyly, high-arched palate, etc; see Station 3, Cardiovascular, Case 13)

(b) Ehlers–Danlos syndrome (?hyperextensible skin and joints, thin scars, etc; see Vol. 3, Station 5, Skin, Case 28)

(c) pseudoxanthoma elasticum (?loose skin or 'chicken skin' appearance in antecubital fossae, inguinal regions, neck, etc; see Vol. 3, Station 5, Skin, Case 10)

(d) osteogenesis imperfecta (?blue sclerae, deformity from old fractures, etc; see Vol. 3, Station 5, Other, Case 4)

(e) ostium primum atrial septal defect (see Station 3, Cardiovascular, Case 16)

Endomyocardial fibrosis (10% of cardiac admissions in East Africa; also occurs in West Africa, southern India and Sri Lanka; the aetiology is unknown)

Indications for surgery

Improvements in surgical techniques, particularly valve repair, and the reduction in operative mortality have reduced the threshold of physicians for considering surgery. Surgery is indicated if there are echocardiographic features of increasing left ventricular dimensions (suggesting volume overload) with or without symptoms. A left ventricular end-systolic dimension of ≥45 mm (in the parasternal long-axis view on the echocardiogram) is used as an index of dilation.† Repair and reconstruction of the valve (valvuloplasty) and its ring (annuloplasty), if feasible, are preferable because of the low perioperative mortality and lack of requirement for long-term anticoagulation. As for other volume-loading pathology, signs of progressive left ventricular dilation (demonstrated by serial echocardiography) are the key to decisions relating to timing of surgery. Acute severe mitral incompetence (e.g. infective endocarditis, ruptured chordae tendinae) may require emergency valve replacement.

---

*If the posterior leaflet is predominantly involved, the systolic murmur is best heard at the left sternal edge whereas if the anterior leaflet is involved, the murmur is best heard over the spine.

†Concomitant atrial fibrillation or pulmonary hypertension lowers the threshold for surgery, as does poor left ventricular function at any stage.

Case 3 | Mixed mitral valve disease

Frequency in survey: main focus of a short case or additional feature in 9% of attempts at PACES Station 3, Cardiovascular.

Record 1

There is a *malar flush* and a *left thoracotomy scar*. The pulse is irregularly irregular (give rate) in rate and volume and the venous pressure is not raised. The cardiac impulse is *tapping* and the apex beat is *not displaced*. There is a *left parasternal heave*. On auscultation, there is a *loud* first heart sound, a *pansystolic murmur** radiating to the axilla, a loud pulmonary second sound, and an *opening snap* followed by a *mid-diastolic rumbling murmur* localized to the apex.

The patient has mixed mitral valve disease. In view of the tapping cardiac impulse, the loud first heart sound and the undisplaced apex, I think this is predominant mitral stenosis. There are signs of pulmonary hypertension.

Record 2

There is a left thoracotomy scar. The pulse is irregularly irregular (give rate) in rate and volume and the venous pressure is not raised. The apex beat is *thrusting* (volume loaded) and *displaced* to the sixth intercostal space in the anterior axillary line and there is a *left parasternal heave*. On auscultation, the first heart sound is *soft* and there is a loud *pansystolic murmur* at the left sternal edge and/or apex radiating to the axilla. There is a loud pulmonary second sound and, with the patient in the left lateral position, I could hear a *mid-diastolic rumbling murmur* following an opening snap.†

The patient has mixed mitral valve disease with pulmonary hypertension. In view of the soft first heart sound and displaced and vigorous apex beat, I think this is predominant mitral incompetence.

If it is not clear clinically which lesion is predominant (e.g. loud first heart sound but enlarged left ventricle) and the examiners want your opinion, point out the factors in favour of each (see Table C3.1) then come down in favour of the one you think most likely, but point out that in this case echocardiography‡ would be required to be certain, e.g. 'It is difficult in this case. The loud first heart sound would suggest predominant mitral stenosis; however, the enlarged left ventricle suggests mitral incompetence as the more important lesion. I think echocardiography would be required to resolve the issue'.

---

*In the patient with severe pulmonary hypertension when a very large right ventricle displaces the left ventricle posteriorly, the murmur of tricuspid incompetence (see Station 3, Cardiovascular, Case 11) can mimic that of mitral incompetence. The murmur of tricuspid incompetence is ordinarily heard best at the lower left sternal border, increases with inspiration and is not heard in the axilla or over the spine posteriorly. In tricuspid incompetence giant *v* waves will be present.

†In severe mitral incompetence without mitral stenosis, a mid-diastolic flow murmur may be heard without an opening snap. The presence of a third heart sound (due to rapid ventricular filling in severe mitral incompetence) is incompatible with any significant degree of mitral stenosis.

‡Cardiac catheter studies are rarely indicated in the assessment of valvular heart disease if full 2-dimensional echocardiographic imagings (including TOE) are available.

Table C3.1 Factors pointing to a predominant lesion in mixed mitral valve disease

	Mitral stenosis	Mitral incompetence
Pulse	Small volume	Sharp and abbreviated
Apex	Not displaced; tapping impulse present	Displaced, thrusting
First heart sound	Loud	Soft
Third heart sound	Absent	Present

Case 4 | Aortic incompetence (lone)

Frequency in survey: main focus of a short case or additional feature in 8% of attempts at PACES Station 3, Cardiovascular.

Record

The pulse is regular* (give rate), of large volume and *collapsing* in character. The venous pressure is not raised but *vigorous arterial pulsations* can be seen in the neck (Corrigan's sign†). The apex beat is *thrusting* (volume overload) in the anterior axillary line, in the sixth intercostal space. There is a high-pitched *early diastolic murmur* audible down the left sternal edge and in the aortic area; it is *louder* in *expiration* with the patient *sitting forward*. (The blood pressure may be wide with a high systolic and low diastolic. In severe cases it may be 250–300/30–50.)

The diagnosis is aortic incompetence. Now consider looking for *Argyll Robertson pupils, high-arched palate* or *marfanoid* appearance, or obvious features of an arthropathy especially *ankylosing spondylitis*. If these are not present the aortic incompetence is likely to be rheumatic in origin – rheumatic fever and infective endocarditis are the most common identifiable causes, although hypertension-induced aortic root dilation with secondary aortic incompetence is increasingly common.

The early diastolic murmur can be difficult to hear and is easily overlooked (see Vol. 2, Section F, Anecdote 276). It should be specifically sought with the patient sitting forward in expiration. Listen for the 'absence of silence' in the early part of diastole. The murmur is usually best heard over the mid-sternal region or at the lower left sternal edge. In some cases, particularly syphilitic aortitis, it is loudest in the aortic area. There is often an accompanying systolic murmur due to increased flow which does not necessarily indicate coexistent aortic stenosis (see Station 3, Cardiovascular, Case 6).

If there is a mid-diastolic murmur at the apex, it may be an Austin Flint murmur‡ or it may represent some associated mitral valve disease. These two may be clinically indistinguishable, though the presence of a loud first heart sound and an opening snap suggest the latter. Though the first heart sound in the Austin Flint may be loud, it is never palpable (i.e. no tapping impulse).

Causes of aortic incompetence

Rheumatic fever

Infective endocarditis

Long-standing hypertension (by causing aortic dilation; complications of hypertension such as ascending aortic aneurysm or dissecting aneurysm may also cause aortic incompetence)

Marfan's syndrome (?tall with long extremities, arachnodactyly and high-arched palate, etc; see Station 3, Cardiovascular, Case 13)

Ankylosing spondylitis (?male with fixed kyphosis and stooped 'question mark' posture; see Vol. 3, Station 5, Locomotor, Case 6; aortic incompetence may also occur in the other seronegative arthropathies – psoriatic, ulcerative colitis and Reiter's sydrome)

Rheumatoid arthritis (?hands, nodules)

Coarctation of the aorta (in association with a bicuspid aortic valve)

---

*The pulse is usually regular unless there is associated mitral valve disease.

†Other physical signs which result from a large pulse volume and peripheral vasodilation include de Musset's sign (the head nods with each pulsation) and Quincke's sign (capillary pulsation visible in the nail beds).

‡The Austin Flint murmur occurs in severe aortic incompetence. It is probably attributable to: (i) the regurgitant jet interfering with the opening of the anterior mitral valve leaflet; and (ii) the left ventricular diastolic pressure rising more rapidly than the left atrial diastolic pressure.

Associated perimembranous ventricular septal defect (loss of support of valve – not a feature of muscular VSDs)

Syphilitic aortitis (?Argyll Robertson pupils; there may be an aneurysm of the ascending aorta)

Hurler's syndrome

Indications for surgery

Although patients tolerate aortic incompetence longer than aortic stenosis (see Station 3, Cardiovascular, Case 5), the clinician's aim is to replace the valve *before* serious left ventricular dysfunction occurs. Every effort should be made to recognize any reduction in left ventricular function or reserve as early as possible (i.e. before symptoms appear). Serial echocardiograms will show a gradual increase in left ventricular dimensions.* Vasodilators, particularly ACE inhibitors and calcium antagonists, are thought to reduce the rate of deterioration in mild to moderate aortic incompetence, and should be considered even in asymptomatic patients. The left ventricular ejection fraction, though normal at rest, may show a subnormal rise during exercise. Aortic valve replacement may have to be undertaken as a matter of urgency in patients with infective endocarditis in whom the leaking valve causes rapidly progressive left ventricular dilation.

*Echocardiographic assessment of severity of AR is based on a range of echo features, including end-diastolic dimension >70 mm or an end-systolic dimension >50 mm.

Case 5 | Aortic stenosis (lone)

Frequency in survey: main focus of a short case or additional feature in 7% of attempts at PACES Station 3, Cardiovascular.

Record 1

The *pulse* is regular (give rate), of *small volume* and *slow rising*. The venous pressure is not raised (unless there is cardiac failure). The apex beat is palpable 1 cm to the left of the mid-clavicular line in the fifth intercostal space (the apex position is normal or only slightly displaced in pure aortic stenosis unless the left ventricle is starting to fail) as a forceful *sustained heave* (pressure overload).* There is a *systolic thrill* palpable over the aortic area and the carotids (may be felt over the apex). Auscultation reveals a *harsh ejection systolic murmur* in the aortic area *radiating* into the *neck*, and the *aortic second sound* is *soft* (or absent). (An associated ejection click is usually present if the valve is bicuspid.) (The blood pressure is usually low normal with a decreased difference between systole and diastole – pulse pressure.)

The diagnosis is aortic stenosis.

Possible causes

1 Degenerative calcification (in the elderly; the stenosis is usually relatively mild)
2 Rheumatic heart disease (mitral valve is usually involved as well and aortic incompetence is often present)
3 Bicuspid aortic valve (more common in males; typically presents in the sixth decade)
4 Congenital (may worsen during childhood and adolescence due to calcification)

In the late stages of aortic stenosis when cardiac failure with low cardiac output supervenes, the murmur may become markedly diminished in intensity. The murmur of associated mitral stenosis should be carefully sought, particularly in the female patient, because the association of these two obstructive lesions tends to diminish the physical findings of each. Mitral stenosis is easily missed and the severity of aortic stenosis underestimated. As with all valvular heart diseases, echocardiography is of great value in a situation like this.

Indications for surgery

In the adult patient valve replacement is indicated for symptoms if left ventricular function is preserved. Asymptomatic patients should be investigated further with carefully supervised exercise testing to determine true 'asymptomatic' status. In patients with poor left ventricular function, decision making is difficult. Functional imaging, such as dobutamine stress echocardiography, can be helpful in assessment of left ventricular reserve. Critical coronary lesions which can exacerbate

---

*There may also be a presystolic impulse due to left atrial overactivity (this is also felt in moderately severe cases of hypertrophic obstructive cardiomyopathy). The result is a double apical impulse best felt in the left lateral recumbent position.

Other signs which may be present include: a fourth heart sound; a single second sound or even paradoxical splitting of the second sound, which are both due to prolonged left ventricular ejection.

the symptoms of aortic stenosis (and vice versa) should be managed at the same time. Asymptomatic children and young adults can be treated with valvotomy if the obstruction is severe, as the operative risk appears to be less than the risk of sudden death. This is only temporary but may postpone the need for valve replacement for many years. Valve repair is increasingly advocated, particularly in younger patients. Recent advances include percutaneous transcatheter aortic valve implantation (TAVI) currently indicated in patients unsuitable for standard aortic surgery.

β-Blockers, to slow the heart rate and hence increase ejection time, can be used in symptomatic patients pending surgery or in those unfit for surgery. β-Blockers also reduce cardiac work by reducing the rate of rise of systolic pressure and thus the effective valve gradient.

Calcific aortic stenosis is increasingly common and, due to the proximity of the atrioventricular node (and its subsequent involvement in the calcific process), may be associated with atrioventricular nodal block, par-ticularly in the postsurgical population. Look for the small scar(s) of pacemaker implantation inferior to either clavicle.

Record 2

The *carotid pulses* are *normal*, the apical impulse is just palpable and not displaced. There are *no thrills*. There is an *ejection systolic murmur* which is not (usually) harsh or loud and is audible in the aortic area but only faintly in the neck. The aortic component of the second sound is well heard. The blood pressure is normal (or may be hypertensive – there may be a resultant ejection click).

These findings suggest aortic sclerosis* (or minimal aortic stenosis) rather than significant aortic stenosis. (NB: The differentiation of this from the other causes of a short systolic murmur is: prolapsing mitral valve, see Station 3, Cardiovascular, Case 10; trivial mitral incompetence and hypertrophic cardiomyopathy, see Station 3, Cardiovascular, Case 20.)

---

*Aortic sclerosis on echocardiography, even without haemody-namically significant obstruction to left ventricular outflow, is associated with a 50% increased risk of death from cardiovascular causes and risk of myocardial infarction.

Case 6 | Mixed aortic valve disease

Frequency in survey: main focus of a short case or additional feature in 5% of attempts at PACES Station 3, Cardiovascular.

Record 1

The pulse is regular (give rate) and *slow rising* (may have a *bisferiens* character). The venous pressure is not raised. The apex beat is palpable 1 cm to the left of the mid-clavicular line as a *forceful, sustained heave* (*pressure loaded*). There is a *systolic thrill* palpable at the apex, in the aortic area and also in the carotid. There is a *harsh ejection systolic murmur* in the aortic area radiating into the neck, the *aortic component* of the second sound is *soft*, and there is an *early diastolic murmur* down the *left sternal edge* audible when the patient is sitting forward in expiration.

The diagnosis is mixed aortic valve disease. Since the pulse is slow rising rather than collapsing, there is a systolic thrill, the second sound is soft and the apex has a forceful heaving quality, I think there is predominant aortic stenosis. (Systolic blood pressure will be low with a low pulse pressure.)

Record 2

The pulse is regular (give rate), of *large volume* and *collapsing* (may have a *bisferiens* character). The venous pressure is not raised. The apex beat is *thrusting* (*volume loaded*) in the *anterior axillary line* in the sixth intercostal space. There is a harsh *ejection systolic murmur* in the aortic area radiating into the neck and an *early diastolic murmur* down the *left sternal edge* (loudest with the patient sitting forward in expiration).

The diagnosis is mixed aortic valve disease. Since the pulse is collapsing rather than plateau in character and the apex is displaced and thrusting, I think the predominant lesion is aortic incompetence. (Blood pressure will show a wide pulse pressure.)

Often mixed aortic murmurs will be due to either aortic stenosis with incidental aortic incompetence or severe aortic incompetence with a systolic flow murmur.* In such cases commenting on dominance is easy. If it is not clear clinically which lesion is predominant and the examiners request your opinion, point out the factors in favour of each (see Table C3.2), stress that you would like to measure the blood pressure and how this would help and lean towards or, if possible, come down in favour of the one you think most likely, giving the reasons (see Station 3, Cardiovascular, Case 3 for an example of how this might be done in the case of mixed mitral valve disease). Echocardiography will be very helpful but be aware that Doppler valve gradient is inaccurate in the presence of significant aortic incom-

petence; TOE may be helpful in more precisely delineating the anatomy of the aortic valve.

Treatment

There is a trend towards aortic valve *repair* if at all possible, particularly in younger patients with congenital aortic valve disease.

As for any valve lesion, surgery is generally indicated for *symptoms* in stenotic lesions (pressure overload) and for signs of *left ventricular compromise* in regurgitant lesions (volume overload). Exercise testing is advocated in all but severe aortic stenosis to objectively assess exercise tolerance. Echocardiography is vital for follow-up for subtle signs of deteriorating function of the volume-loaded ventricle.

*NB: The causes of aortic incompetence in this latter case (see Station 3, Cardiovascular, Case 4).

Table C3.2 Factors pointing to a predominant lesion in mixed aortic valve disease

	Aortic incompetence	Aortic stenosis
Pulse	Mainly collapsing	Mainly slow rising
Apex	Thrusting, displaced (volume loaded)	Heaving, not displaced much (pressure loaded)
Systolic thrill	Absent	Present
Systolic murmur	Not loud, not harsh	Loud, harsh
Blood pressure:		
systolic	High	Low
pulse pressure	Wide	Narrow

Case 7 | Mitral stenosis (lone)

Frequency in survey: main focus of a short case or additional feature in 5% of attempts at PACES Station 3, Cardiovascular.

Record

There is a *malar flush* and a *left thoracotomy scar*. The pulse is *irregularly irregular* (give rate) in rate and volume (if sinus rhythm, the volume is usually small). The venous pressure is not raised, and there is no ankle or sacral oedema (unless in cardiac failure). The cardiac impulse is *tapping* (palpable first heart sound) and the apex is not displaced. There is a *left parasternal heave*. The *first heart sound* is *loud*, there is a loud pulmonary second sound and an *opening snap* followed by a *mid-diastolic rumbling murmur* (with *presystolic accentuation* if the patient is in sinus rhythm) *localized* to the apex and heard most loudly with the patient in the *left lateral* position.*

The diagnosis is mitral stenosis. The patient has had a valvotomy in the past. There are signs of pulmonary hypertension.

Other signs which may be present

Giant *v* waves (tricuspid incompetence – usually secondary; may be primary; Station 3, Cardiovascular, Case 11)

Graham Steell† murmur – rare (secondary pulmonary incompetence; a high-pitched, brief, early diastolic whiff in the presence of marked signs of pulmonary hypertension and a pulse which is not collapsing)

The opening snap soon after the second sound‡ in tight mitral stenosis (<0.09 sec – mean left atrial pressure above 20 mmHg); longer after the second sound in mild mitral stenosis (>0.1 sec – mean left atrial pressure below 15 mmHg); absent if the mitral valve is calcified (first heart sound soft).

Indications for intervention (surgery or percutaneous transcatheter valvuloplasty)

Significant symptoms which limit normal activity

An episode of pulmonary oedema with or without a precipitating cause

Recurrent emboli§

Pulmonary oedema in pregnancy (emergency transcatheter valvuloplasty)

Criteria for valvotomy (open or transcatheter)¶

Mobile valve (loud first heart sound, opening snap, absence of calcium in submitral apparatus on TOE)**

Absence of mitral incompetence

---

*If unsure about the presence of the murmur, it can be accentuated by exercise; get the patient to touch her toes and then recline 10 times.

†Though associated eponymously with Graham Steell, the original source of the observation was probably George Balfour of Edinburgh, for whom Steell worked as house physician. *Journal of the Royal College of Physicians* 1991, **25**: 66–70.

‡The interval from the second sound to the opening snap varies with heart rate. If the interval is ≤0.07 sec with the heart rate <100, the mitral stenosis is usually of haemodynamic significance.

§Anticoagulation is recommended in all but very mild mitral stenosis, even if in sinus rhythm (particularly if the left atrium is enlarged on transthoracic echo).

¶Should be considered, particularly in the young female who is planning a pregnancy. Sometimes it can be performed before the development of significant symptoms.

**Transoesophageal echo (TOE) is by far the best way to image the mitral valve. It is possible to perform transcatheter mitral valvuloplasty using TOE alone, obviating the need for ionizing radiation – particularly useful in pregnancy.

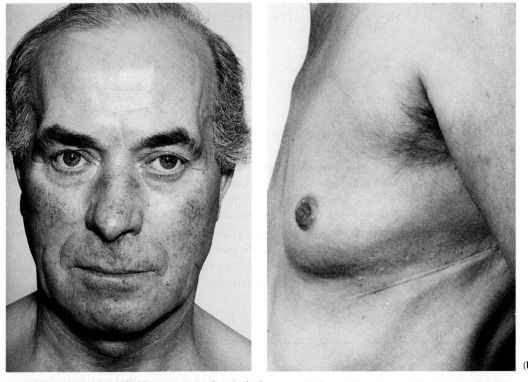

(a)

(b)

Figure C3.1 (a) Mitral facies. (b) Thoracotomy scar for mitral valvotomy.

Case 8 | Irregular pulse

Frequency in survey: main focus of a short case or additional feature in 5% of attempts at PACES Station 3, Cardiovascular.

Survey note: though an irregular pulse was usually encountered in the examination as a feature in the common valvular short cases, occasionally it was itself the main focus of a short case. This was often because the patient had a goitre.

Record

The pulse is . . . /min and *irregularly irregular* in rate and volume, suggesting atrial fibrillation with a controlled* ventricular response (uncontrolled if the rate is >90/min). Now look at the *neck* (goitre), *eyes* (exophthalmos), *face* (mitral facies, hypothyroidism† or hemiplegia due to an embolus) and *chest* (thoracotomy scar).‡

Differential diagnosis

The differentiation of an irregular pulse due to controlled atrial fibrillation from that of multiple extrasystoles will depend upon the observation that only in atrial fibrillation do long pauses occur in groups of two or more (with ectopic beats, the compensatory pause follows a short pause because the ectopic is premature). Furthermore, exercise may abolish extrasystoles but worsen the irregularity of atrial fibrillation. Without recourse to an electrocardiogram, atrial fibrillation can be difficult to distinguish from atrial flutter with variable block, from multiple atrial ectopics due to a shifting pacemaker, and sometimes from paroxysmal atrial tachycardia with block. Only in atrial fibrillation is the ventricular rhythm truly *chaotic*.

Causes of atrial fibrillation

Ischaemic heart disease (especially myocardial infarction)

Sinoatrial (sick sinus syndrome) disease with primary involvement of the conduction tissue

Rheumatic heart disease

Hypertensive heart disease

Thyrotoxicosis

Cardiomyopathy§

Acute infections (especially lung)

Constrictive pericarditis

Local neoplastic infiltration (particularly lymphoma)

---

*Though controlled atrial fibrillation may sometimes feel regular initially, if you concentrate there is a definite irregular variation in the beat-to-beat time interval (see Vol. 2, Section F, Experience 189).

†Previously treated Graves' disease now on inadequate thyroxine replacement – pulse rate slow, ankle jerk relaxation slow, etc.

‡If allowed, follow up any positive findings from this *visual survey* by appropriate examination of the relevant system. If there is no visible abnormality proceed, if allowed, to examine the heart, the neck for a goitre, and thyroid status.

§In many patients with cardiomyopathy no cause can be found ('idiopathic'). It is thought that most of these are a result of viral myocarditis. Often the index event cannot be recalled by the patient, and may have occurred some decades earlier. Occult ischaemic heart disease is the most common form of 'dilated cardiomyopathy' and the label 'idiopathic' should only be used after coronary artery disease has been excluded by angiography.

Sometimes the causal disorder can be identified. Some of the usual causes can be grouped as follows:

1. Toxic (alcohol, adriamycin, cyclophosphamide, emetine, corticosteroids, lithium, phenothiazines, etc.)
2. Metabolic (thiamine deficiency, kwashiorkor, pellagra, obesity, porphyria, uraemia, electrolyte imbalance)
3. Endocrine (thyrotoxicosis, acromegaly, myxoedema, Cushing's, diabetes mellitus)
4. Collagen diseases (SLE, polyarteritis nodosa, etc.)
5. Infiltrative (amyloidosis, haemochromatosis, neoplastic, glycogen storage disease, sarcoidosis, mucopolysaccharidosis, Gaucher's disease, Whipple's disease)
6. Infective (viral, rickettsial, mycobacterial)
7. Genetic (hypertrophic cardiomyopathy, muscular dystrophies)
8. Fibroplastic (endomyocardial fibrosis, Löffler's endocarditis, carcinoid)
9. Miscellaneous (postpartum, incessant atrial tachycardia).

Treatment

Oral anticoagulants and atrial fibrillation: the advice relating to this topic is changing rapidly. It is, however, a *perfect* subject for PACES so make sure you are up to date!* Likewise, the best management of atrial fibrillation. If asked, choose a scenario to discuss, e.g. acute-onset atrial fibrillation in an elderly person associated with a chest infection or paroxysmal atrial fibrillation in an otherwise fit 40-year-old, etc. Do not forget the role of cardioversion, and remember that management depends on the treatment aim, i.e. restoration and maintenance of sinus rhythm *or* control of the resulting irregular ventricular rate.

*www.nice.org.uk

Case 9 | Other combinations of mitral and aortic valve disease

Frequency in survey: main focus of a short case or additional feature in 4% of attempts at PACES Station 3, Cardiovascular.

Survey note: patients with any combination of aortic and mitral valve disease may be found in the examination (including, very rarely, lesions of one valve in combination with a prosthetic valve; see Station 3, Cardiovascular, Case 1). Whenever you are examining the heart it is essential that, having found some obvious murmurs, you go in search of the others which may be present and less obvious, before presenting your findings (see Vol. 2, Section F, Experience 185 and Anecdote 276).

If the examiner seeks an opinion as to which are the main lesions, or if you feel confident to offer one, the criteria used are the same as those described under mixed mitral valve disease (see Station 3, Cardiovascular, Case 3) and mixed aortic valve disease (see Station 3, Cardiovascular, Case 6). The example here is of a *record* of mixed mitral and aortic valve disease.

Record

There is a left thoracotomy scar and the patient has a malar flush. The pulse is irregularly irregular (give rate) and *slow rising* (can be difficult to assess if the patient is in atrial fibrillation) in character. The venous pressure is not elevated. The apex is . . . (give appropriate word on the basis of what you find, e.g. thrusting, heaving, lifting, etc.) in the anterior axillary line and there is a *left parasternal heave*. There is a *systolic thrill* at the apex, in the aortic area and in the neck. The first heart sound is *loud*, there is a harsh *ejection systolic murmur* in the aortic area radiating into the neck, a *pansystolic murmur* at the lower left sternal edge radiating to the *apex* and to the *axilla*, an *early diastolic murmur* just audible in the aortic area and down the *left sternal edge* with the patient *sitting forward in expiration*, and an *opening snap* followed by a *mid-diastolic rumbling murmur* localized to the apex.

The findings suggest mixed aortic and mitral valve disease. The slow rising pulse suggests that aortic stenosis is the dominant aortic valve lesion. It is not possible to ascertain clinically which is the major mitral valve lesion.* Further investigation involving transthoracic echocardiography, probably leading on to transoesophageal echo and/or cardiac catheterization with left ventricular angiography, would be required to assess the haemodynamic significance of each lesion.

---

*In the case of severe mitral stenosis, the signs of significant aortic stenosis may be underestimated. A displaced apex in the above setting would tend to suggest that mitral incompetence is haemodynamically dominant.

Case 10 | Mitral valve prolapse

Frequency in survey: main focus of a short case or additional feature in 3% of attempts at PACES Station 3, Cardiovascular.

Record

The pulse (in this well-looking patient) is regular (give rate) and the venous pressure is not raised. The apex beat is palpable in the fifth intercostal space in the mid-clavicular line. There are no heaves or thrills. On auscultation, the heart sounds are normal but there is a *mid-systolic click** (which is usually but not always) followed by a late *systolic crescendo-decrescendo murmur* loudest at the left sternal edge (as the condition progresses the murmur develops the characteristics of mitral incompetence; see Station 3, Cardiovascular, Case 2).

These findings suggest mitral valve prolapse (floppy posterior mitral valve leaflet – echocardiography is useful for confirmation).

The prolapse is increased by anything which decreases cardiac volume (standing position, Valsalva manoeuvre) and as a result the click and murmur occur earlier during systole and the murmur is prolonged. Increasing cardiac volume (squatting position, propranolol) has the reverse effect. Phonocardiography documents these effects well. Mitral valve prolapse (said to occur in 5–10% of the population,† more commonly in females) is usually asymptomatic but may be associated with atypical chest pain, palpitation, fatigue and dyspnoea. The symptoms may become worse once the patient knows there is a murmur. The prognosis is good† but complications can include infective endocarditis, atrial and ventricular dysrhythmias, worsening mitral incompetence, embolic phenomena (transient ischaemic attacks, amaurosis fugax, acute hemiplegia), rupture of the mitral valve (age-related degenerative changes) and sudden death. The condition may be familial and there may be a family history of sudden death. There is a serious risk of precipitating cardiac neurosis which may, at least in part, contribute to the association with atypical chest pain. There is often myxomatous degeneration of the mitral valve, deposition of acid mucopolysaccharide material and redundant valve tissue.

Causes and associations

Marfan's syndrome
Polycystic kidney disease
Congenital heart disease
Congestive cardiomyopathy
Hypertrophic cardiomyopathy
Myocarditis
Mitral valve surgery
Fabry's disease
Ehlers–Danlos syndrome
Osteogenesis imperfecta
Systemic lupus erythematosus (after Libman–Sachs endocarditis)
Muscular dystrophy
Turner's syndrome
Primary mitral valve prolapse

---

*The click is characteristic but easily missed if you have not heard one before. This may be because of the distraction of the murmur. Concentrate on listening for other sounds at different frequencies from the murmur and you will hear it.

†It may be that the clinically silent, echocardiographic mitral valve prolapse which is common in thin, young women is a variant of normal, distinct from the floppy valve or complication of chordal lengthening or rupture needing mitral valve replacement, which is most common in elderly men. It seems likely that 'echo only' mitral valve prolapse carries a good prognosis whereas complications are associated with the clinical variety. Endocarditis chemoprophylaxis is not required (see Station 3, Cardiovascular, Case 28).

Other points of note

Mitral valve prolapse (MVP) can be an incidental finding during echocardiography.

Indications for surgery are as for mitral regurgitation (see Station 3, Cardiovascular, Case 2); surgical repair rather than valve replacement is favoured.

Palpitations are usually due to benign ventricular ectopy and generally respond well to β-blockade if symptoms are troublesome.

Other causes of a short systolic murmur audible at the apex should always be thought of and excluded. These are:

Trivial mitral incompetence (the usual cause – the murmur may not be pansystolic but there is no click)

Aortic stenosis/sclerosis (see Station 3, Cardiovascular, Case 5)

Hypertrophic cardiomyopathy (see Station 3, Cardiovascular, Case 20).

Case 11 | Tricuspid incompetence

Frequency in survey: main focus of a short case or additional feature in 3% of attempts at PACES Station 3, Cardiovascular.

Record

The JVP is elevated (say height*) and shows *giant v waves*† which oscillate the earlobe (if the venous pressure is high enough) and which are diagnostic of tricuspid incompetence. (Now, if allowed, examine the heart, respiratory system and abdomen.‡)

The most common cause of tricuspid incompetence is *not* organic but dilation of the right ventricle and of the tricuspid valve ring due to right ventricular failure§ in conditions such as:

Mitral valve disease
Cor pulmonale
Eisenmenger's syndrome
Right ventricular infarction (rare)
Primary pulmonary hypertension.

Causes of primary tricuspid incompetence

Infective endocarditis (especially intravenous drug addicts – recurrent septicaemia with pulmonary infiltrates should raise suspicion)

Congenital heart disease (e.g. Ebstein's anomaly)
Carcinoid syndrome (flushing, diarrhoea, hepatomegaly, sometimes asthma; fibrous plaques on the endothelial surface of the heart are associated with tricuspid incompetence and pulmonary stenosis)
Myxomatous change (may be associated with mitral valve prolapse or atrial septal defect)
Rheumatic heart disease (extremely rare and usually associated with tricuspid stenosis; almost invariably associated with other valvular disease – if there is pulmonary hypertension it may not be possible to differentiate organic from functional tricuspid incompetence on clinical grounds alone)
Trauma

---

*In centimetres vertically above the sternal angle, not the suprasternal notch or supraclavicular fossa. In tricuspid incompetence which is secondary to right ventricular dilation, the venous pressure is usually of the order of 8–10 cm or more.

†These *v* waves are in fact *cv* waves because systole spans the time between *c* and *v* waves of the normal jugular pulse.

‡In the *heart* you would expect to find the pansystolic murmur of tricuspid incompetence which may be louder on inspiration (Carvallo's sign) and augmented by the Müller manoeuvre (attempted inspiration against a closed glottis). The murmur is only audible (at the lower right sternal edge) if the right-sided pressures are very high. Very rarely, there may be murmurs of associated or underlying disease of the heart valves, especially mitral. There may be a tricuspid diastolic murmur louder on inspiration and augmented by the Müller manoeuvre. This could be due to increased flow across the tricuspid valve or to concomitant tricuspid stenosis. In the *respiratory system* you would be looking for signs of the condition leading to underlying cor pulmonale. In the *abdomen* you may find forceful epigastric pulsations and hepatomegaly which is tender and pulsatile. In severe, long-standing tricuspid incompetence, ascites and signs of chronic liver disease (see Station 1, Abdominal, Case 3) can occur.

§The importance of a functional tricuspid valve in maintaining normal right ventricular function is increasingly recognized and a surgeon will often place an annuloplasty ring for secondary tricuspid regurgitation when operating for the primary condition. Tricuspid valve replacement is rarely indicated or performed.

Case 12 | Ventricular septal defect

Frequency in survey: main focus of a short case or additional feature in 2% of attempts at PACES Station 3, Cardiovascular.

Survey note: youthfulness of patient is sometimes a clue to the diagnosis.

Record

The pulse is regular (give rate) and the venous pressure is not raised. The apex beat is (may be) palpable halfway between the mid-clavicular line and the anterior axillary line, and there is a *left parasternal heave* (there may be a systolic thrill). There is a *pansystolic murmur* at the lower left sternal edge which is also audible at the apex. (The pulmonary second sound may be loud due to pulmonary hypertension and there may be an early diastolic murmur of secondary pulmonary incompetence.)*

The diagnosis is ventricular septal defect.

Other features of ventricular septal defect

Maladie de Roger (small haemodynamically insignificant hole, loud murmur, normal heart size, etc.; tends to close spontaneously)

Development of Eisenmenger's complex (see Station 3, Cardiovascular, Case 27) if a significant defect is left untreated

Susceptibility to subacute bacterial endocarditis (defects of all sizes†)

Association with aortic incompetence in 5% of cases (10% in Japan)‡

Possibility of a mitral mid-diastolic flow murmur if shunt is large

May occur following acute myocardial infarction with septal rupture

Sometimes associated with Down's syndrome and Turner's syndrome

Newer technology allows percutaneous transcatheter closure of suitable VSDs, including those secondary to acute myocardial infarction

---

*Although cases like the one presented here are occasionally seen in the exam, it is very unlikely that there would be a haemodynamically significant VSD, as this would have been operated upon in childhood. There may be no evidence of right ventricular overload and the P2 may be normal. Candidates are advised to present the signs as they find them, and conclude whether there is/is not a haemodynamically significant VSD. Generally, defects that have been 'allowed' to persist into adult life are likely to be small. The smaller the hole, the greater the pressure difference between the two ventricles, and the louder the murmur.

†Defects in the membranous region (just under the aortic valve) persist and are associated with late aortic incompetence which may require surgery; echocardiography is mandatory during follow-up. Defects in the muscular part of the septum may close spontaneously during childhood.

‡See Station 3, Cardiovascular, Case 28 for antibiotic prophylaxis.

Case 13 | Marfan's syndrome

Frequency in survey: main focus of a short case or additional feature in 1% of attempts at PACES Station 3, Cardiovascular.

Survey note: see Vol. 2, Section F, Experience 26.

Marfan's syndrome is dealt with in Vol. 3, Station 5, Locomotor, Case 9.

Case 14 | Pulmonary stenosis

Frequency in survey: main focus of a short case or additional feature in 1% of attempts at PACES Station 3, Cardiovascular.

Record

The pulse is regular and the JVP is not elevated (prominent *a* wave in severe cases).* The cardiac apex is not palpable but there is (may be) a *left parasternal heave*. A *systolic thrill* is palpable over the left second and third interspaces. An *ejection click* and a *systolic murmur* (and may be also a fourth heart sound) are heard over the *pulmonary area*. The murmur is louder during inspiration and radiates to the suprasternal notch. The second sound is (may be) split (the pulmonary component is soft).†

The diagnosis is pulmonary stenosis.

Poststenotic dilation of the pulmonary arteries may be seen on the chest X-ray and, in the severe case, right ventricular hypertrophy and diminution of pulmonary vascular markings. A minor degree of pulmonary stenosis is compatible with a normal life span. Surgical relief is required in symptomatic cases or if there is a gradient of more than 50 mmHg across the pulmonary valve. Balloon valvotomy is becoming the technique of choice in children and young adults, especially if the valve is not dysplastic. If treatment is delayed too long in severe pulmonary stenosis, an irreversible fibrotic change can take place in the hypertrophied right ventricle.

Pulmonary stenosis may occur in the setting of surgically corrected tetralogy of Fallot. In this case there will usually be a left or right thoracotomy scar associated with a previous Blalock shunt (see Station 3, Cardiovascular, Case 23) *and* a midline scar from the later complete Fallot repair. The dysplastic pulmonary valve was often replaced with a valved conduit which can calcify and obstruct in later life. If there is a single mid-line scar, the patient may have had an open pulmonary valvotomy in childhood, which often leaves a loudish murmur without any objective evidence of obstruction. Echocardiography is the key investigation.

*A patient with severe pulmonary stenosis may have cyanosis (check buccal mucosa) if the foramen ovale is unsealed and this may be intermittent.
†Pulmonary incompetence is commonly associated with many causes of pulmonary stenosis (particularly after repair of tetral-ogy of Fallot and after pulmonary valvuloplasty). One should specifically listen for the tell-tale early diastolic murmur radiating from the pulmonary area down the left sternal edge. Like the murmur of aortic incompetence, it is easily missed unless specifically sought.

Case 15 | Ankylosing spondylitis

Frequency in survey: main focus of a short case or additional feature in 0.8% of attempts at PACES Station 3, Cardiovascular.

Survey note: see Vol. 2, Section F, Anecdote 102.

Ankylosing spondylitis is dealt with in Vol. 3, Station 5, Locomotor, Case 6.

Case 16 | Atrial septal defect

Frequency in survey: main focus of a short case or additional feature in 0.8% of attempts at PACES Station 3, Cardiovascular.

Record 1

The pulse in this middle-aged female is irregularly irregular (onset of atrial fibrillation is usually the cause of symptoms after the third or fourth decade, otherwise asymptomatic). The JVP is not elevated (unless in right heart failure). The apex beat is just palpable and not displaced. The second heart sound is widely split and the two-component split is not influenced by respiration (*fixed splitting*). There is an *ejection systolic murmur* (due to increased flow across the pulmonary valve) over the pulmonary area. (Occasionally there may be an ejection click due to pulmonary artery dilation.)

The diagnosis is atrial septal defect of little haemodynamic significance.

Record 2

The pulse is irregularly irregular (atrial fibrillation) in this middle-aged woman. There is no oedema and the JVP is not elevated. The apex beat is just palpable in the left fifth intercostal space just outside the mid-clavicular line, there is a *left parasternal heave* (right ventricular volume overload), and there is (may be) a systolic thrill over the pulmonary area (large left-to-right shunt). The second sound is *widely split*. There is an *ejection systolic murmur*, and an *ejection click* (may be palpable) over the pulmonary area, and a *mid-diastolic rumble* over the tricuspid area (a large left-to-right shunt causes increased flow through the tricuspid valve).

The diagnosis is a haemodynamically significant atrial septal defect.

Male-to-female ratio is 1/3.

Other features of atrial septal defect

Ostium secundum defect is the most common type and may be multiple (fenestrated ASD) – small defects can easily pass unnoticed clinically

Ostium primum defect is common in Down's syndrome (see Vol. 3, Station 5, Other, Case 5) and is associated with mitral regurgitation (due to the cleft in the anterior leaflet of the mitral valve)

rSR in the right precordial leads on ECG. Right-axis deviation is associated with an ostium secundum defect, left-axis deviation suggests an ostium primum defect

Dilated proximal pulmonary arteries and an enlarged right heart with pulmonary plethora* on chest X-ray. The aortic knuckle is small and left heart border is straight. The peripheral pulmonary vascularity is replaced by clear lung fields with the advent of pulmonary hypertension. The superior vena cava is enlarged in the sinus venosus type

*The main differential diagnosis of *pulmonary plethora* due to a left-to-right shunt is atrial septal defect, ventricular septal defect (see Station 3, Cardiovascular, Case 12), patent ductus arteriosus (see Station 3, Cardiovascular, Case 29). It may be possible to differentiate these on chest X-ray by looking at the left atrium and aorta. Small left atrium and normal aorta suggest atrial septal defect, large left atrium and normal aorta suggest ventricular septal defect, large left atrium and large or abnormal aorta suggest patent ductus arteriosus.

Diagnosis is confirmed by TOE. If performed, cardiac catheterization will show a step-up in oxygen saturation in the mid right atrium, suggestive of a left-to-right shunt

Surgical closure for ostium secundum defect is recommended if the pulmonary to systemic flow ratio is 2/1 or more, or if the patient is symptomatic. Anatomically suitable defects can be closed using percutaneous transcatheter technology. At present, surgical closure is required for ostium primum and sinus venosus ASDs, although some of the newer devices are encouraging. Closure does not seem to prevent the early development of atrial fibrillation

There is a risk of paradoxical emboli in patients, even with small ASDs. Anticoagulation should be considered, particularly if there is echocardiographic evidence of bidirectional shunting

Patients with pulmonary hypertension are cyanosed and may have clubbing of the fingers (Eisenmenger's syndrome; see Station 3, Cardiovascular, Case 27). The systolic murmur becomes faint and an early diastolic murmur with a loud P2 appears. Operative repair is contraindicated

Usual causes of death in large, untreated defects: right heart failure, arrhythmias, pulmonary embolism, brain abscess, rupture of the pulmonary artery

Case 17 | Ebstein's anomaly

Frequency in survey: main focus of a short case or additional feature in 0.8% of attempts at PACES Station 3, Cardiovascular.

Survey note: see Vol. 2, Section F, Anecdote 103.

Record

There is prominence (or *asymmetry*) of the chest (due to dilated right heart). The *JVP is elevated* (say height)* and shows *giant v waves*† which are diagnostic of tri-cuspid incompetence.‡ On auscultation, there is a widely split first heart sound (due to loud and delayed tricuspid component of the first heart sound) and the second heart sound is also widely split (due to delayed closure of the pulmonary valve sec-ondary to right bundle branch block). Prominent third or fourth sounds are (may be) present (may occur even in the absence of heart failure). A low-intensity *pan-systolic murmur increasing on inspiration* is best heard at the lower left sternal edge.

The giant *v* waves suggest tricuspid incompetence and the other features suggest that it is a chronic primary tricuspid incompetence most likely due to congenital heart disease such as Ebstein's anomaly.

Other features of Ebstein's anomaly

It is a rare abnormality of the tricuspid valve with a variable degree of displacement of the leaflets of the tricuspid valve towards the apex away from the atrio-ventricular ring, i.e. there is a portion of the right ventricle that is 'atrialized' (see Figure C3.2)

Associated lesions include intraatrial connection (patent foramen ovale/atrial septal defect >50%), pulmonary stenosis and ventricular septal defect (<5%). There may therefore be other murmurs as a result of these lesions

In cases with associated lesions, there may be a signifi-cant right-to-left shunt with associated cyanosis and clubbing. A malar flush may be seen

Presentation is variable depending upon the degree of displacement of the valves and presence of associated malformations, varying from early neonatal death to an incidental finding in an asymptomatic adult. Typical presentation in adolescence is with arrhyth-mia, usually as the result of an associated accessory pathway and/or atrial fibrillation or flutter (>30%)

Hepatomegaly from hepatic congestion due to raised right atrial pressure may be present with associated abnormalities in liver function tests

The cause is usually thought to be genetic but case–control studies suggest that maternal exposure in the first trimester to lithium carbonate increases risk

ECG is usually abnormal:

Tall P waves reflect right atrial enlargement

---

*In centimetres vertically above the sternal angle, not the suprasternal notch or supraclavicular fossa.

†These *v* waves are in fact *cv* waves because systole spans the time between *c* and *v* waves of the normal jugular pulse.

‡In fact, the jugular venous pressure is often unimpressive despite severe tricuspid regurgitation owing to the large and compliant right atrium/atrialized right ventricle.

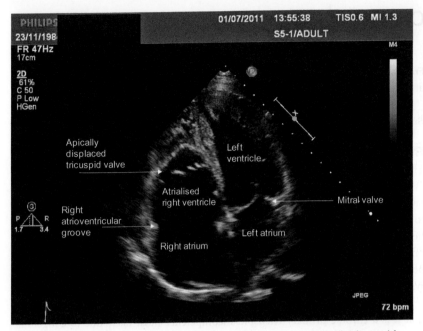

Figure C3.2 Echocardiogram in a patient with Ebstein's anomaly showing 'atrialized' right ventricle.

Look for an accessory pathway (short PR interval/δ waves) with left bundle branch block (right side origin of accessory pathway)

No accessory pathway with right bundle branch block is common

Complications

Haemodynamic deterioration occurs due to degree of tricuspid regurgitation, right-to-left shunting at atrial level and sustained arrhythmia.

Surgical interventions

Vary from repair of the valve to creation of arterial circuits to bypass the right ventricle (Fontan type operations). Arrhythmias are managed with medication and/or ablation procedures.

Case 18 | Raised jugular venous pressure

Frequency in survey: main focus of a short case or additional feature in 0.8% of attempts at PACES Station 3, Cardiovascular.

Record

The JVP is elevated (measure) at . . . cm above the sternal angle (look for individual waves and time against the opposite carotid artery). The predominant wave is the systolic *v* wave which reaches the ear lobes. (If there is no oscillation of the blood column, sit the patient up to find the upper level. Make sure that there is no superior vena caval obstruction with congestion of the face and neck, and prominent veins on the upper chest; see Station 1, Respiratory, Case 22.) The carotid pulsation is irregularly irregular and the rhythm is atrial fibrillation (look for the evidence of congestive cardiac failure: ankle and sacral oedema, hepatomegaly, which may be pulsatile in tricuspid incompetence).

The large *v* wave suggests tricuspid incompetence either organic or due to congestive cardiac failure (see Station 3, Cardiovascular, Case 11).

Causes of a raised JVP (if venous obstruction is excluded)

Congestive cardiac failure (ischaemic heart disease, valvular heart disease, hypertensive heart disease, cardiomyopathy)

Cor pulmonale (?signs of chronic small airways obstruction, cyanosis, etc; see Station 1, Respiratory, Case 20)

Pulmonary hypertension (large *a* wave in the JVP when in sinus rhythm – primary (young females) and sec- ondary to mitral valve disease or thromboobliterative disease)

Constrictive pericarditis (abrupt *x* and *y* descent, loud early *S3* ('pericardial knock') though heart sounds often normal, slight 'paradoxical' pulse, *no signs in the lungs*; chest X-ray may show calcified pericardium)

Large pericardial effusion (*x* descent, pulsus paradoxus, breathlessness, chest X-ray shows cardiomegaly, echocardiogram shows effusion)

Case 19 | Down's syndrome

Frequency in survey: main focus of a short case or additional feature in 0.7% of attempts at PACES Station 3, Cardiovascular.

Survey note: see Vol. 2, Section F, Anecdote 105.

Down's syndrome is dealt with in Vol. 3, Station 5, Other, Case 5.

Case 20 | Hypertrophic cardiomyopathy

Frequency in survey: main focus of a short case or additional feature in 0.7% of attempts at PACES Station 3, Cardiovascular.*

Record

The pulse is regular (may be irregular if patient is in atrial fibrillation) and of normal volume (in severe cases the carotid pulse has a '*jerky*' character) and the JVP is not elevated (may show a prominent *a* wave). The cardiac apex is forceful in the left fifth intercostal space just outside the mid-clavicular line, there is (may be) a strong *presystolic impulse* (*double apical impulse* caused by atrial systole), and a *systolic thrill* is palpable over the left sternal border. There is a *fourth heart sound*, and an *ejection systolic murmur* (may be harsh) over the left third interspace, which radiates widely to the base and to the axilla (perhaps because it merges with the pansystolic murmur of mitral incompetence which frequently accompanies hypertrophic cardiomyopathy). The intensity of the ejection murmur is enhanced by minimal exercise.

The findings suggest hypertrophic cardiomyopathy (HCM).

Other features of hypertrophic cardiomyopathy

Patients may be asymptomatic. Severe cases are marked by symptoms such as dyspnoea, palpitations, angina, dizziness and syncope (often after cessation of exercise due to temporary reduction in cardiac output or secondary to paroxysmal ventricular arrhythmia; cf. aortic stenosis where syncope usually occurs during exercise)

ECG: normal in 25%. ST–T and T wave changes, tall QRS in mid-precordial leads. Q wave in inferior and lateral precordial leads (due to septal hypertrophy). Sometimes left-axis deviation

Chest X-ray may be normal or it may show left atrial enlargement

Echocardiography is diagnostic and characteristically shows asymmetrical septal hypertrophy, and may show systolic anterior motion of the anterior mitral valve leaflet

HCM is an autosomal dominant condition associated with several genes coding for myosin (with hundreds of different mutations described). Many cases arise *de novo* and the condition may have variable penetrance, making genetic studies difficult. All first-degree relatives of an affected individual should be offered clinical screening for the condition

The risk of a poor outcome for any given individual can be assessed using the following criteria: history of syncope, family history of sudden cardiac death, poor blood pressure response to exercise, the presence of ventricular arrhythmias on Holter monitoring, outflow tract gradient of >40 mmHg at rest, and a septal thickness of >18 mm on echocardiography

Treatment options include β-blockers, rate-limiting calcium antagonists, septal ablation or myomectomy and pacing technologies, including implantable defibrillators for high-risk individuals

---

*Hypertrophic cardiomyopathy did not occur in our extensive pre PACES surveys. A case of hypertrophic obstructive cardiomyopathy (HOCM), as it was referred to, was included in one mock Membership examination. One of the examiners commented to us that none of his prospective candidates got the correct diagnosis. It is of course possible that conditions such as

HCM did occur in the examination sittings covered by our survey, but the candidates concerned did not get, or even suspect, the diagnoses and were not enlightened by their examiners. These days, the word 'obstructive' has been removed as it is not essential for the diagnosis, and the risk profile is the same for both the obstructive and non-obstructive forms of HCM.

Case 21 | Dextrocardia

Frequency in survey: main focus of a short case or additional feature in 0.6% of attempts at PACES Station 3, Cardiovascular.

Record

The pulse is regular (give rate) and of good volume. The JVP is not raised. The apex beat is *not palpable on the left side*, but can be felt in the fifth *right* intercostal space in the mid-clavicular line.

This patient has dextrocardia.* (If allowed, listen to the lung fields – Kartagener's syndrome – and feel the abdomen to see which side the liver is on – situs inversus.)

If situs inversus is present the patient is usually otherwise normal. Dextrocardia without situs inversus is usually associated with cardiac malformation. Dextrocardia may occur in Turner's syndrome.

Kartagener' syndrome: dextrocardia, bronchiectasis, situs inversus, infertility, dysplasia of frontal sinuses, sinusitis and otitis media. Patients have ciliary immotility.

*Consider the possibility of this diagnosis if you cannot feel the apex beat and then have difficulty hearing the heart sounds. As you gradually move the stethoscope towards the right side of the chest, they get louder.

Case 22 | Rheumatoid arthritis

Frequency in survey: main focus of a short case or additional feature in 0.6% of attempts at PACES Station 3, Cardiovascular.

Survey note: see Vol. 2, Section F, Anecdote 104.

Rheumatoid arthritis is dealt with in Vol. 3, Station 5, Locomotor, Case 1.

Case 23 | Fallot's tetralogy with a Blalock shunt

Frequency in survey: main focus of a short case or additional feature in 0.3% of attempts at PACES Station 3, Cardiovascular.

Survey note: the cases of Fallot's tetralogy in our survey all had a Blalock shunt.

Record

There is a thoracotomy scar. There is *central cyanosis* and *clubbing* of the fingers. The pulse is regular (give rate) and the *left pulse is weaker than the right* (or vice versa). The venous pressure is normal. The apex beat is (may be) palpable (say where), there is a *left parasternal heave* and a *systolic thrill* is palpable in the pulmonary area. There is a loud *ejection systolic murmur** (unless the stenosis is so severe that virtually no blood traverses it) in the *pulmonary area*. There is (may be) a soft early diastolic murmur of aortic regurgitation (common in adult survivors).

It is likely that this patient has had a Blalock shunt† for Fallot's tetralogy (pulmonary stenosis, ventricular septal defect,‡ right ventricular hypertrophy and overriding aorta).

The features that may be helpful in differentiating Fallot's tetralogy from Eisenmenger's are shown in Table C3.3 (see Station 3, Cardiovascular, Case 27).

---

*There may be a continuous murmur over the shunt (front or back of chest).

†Anastomosis of the subclavian artery to the pulmonary artery. This operation is not often performed nowadays as total correc-tion on cardiopulmonary bypass is usually the treatment of choice.

‡There is no murmur from the VSD as it is large and non-restrictive, i.e. both ventricles are at the same pressure.

Case 24 | Normal heart

Frequency in survey: main focus of a short case or additional feature in 0.2% of attempts at PACES Station 3, Cardiovascular.

The College has made it clear that 'normal' is an option in PACES. No findings on examination is common in real clinical medicine and so this must be a possibility in the exam. In terms of the practical reality of the exam, in order for PACES to proceed there must be a cardiovascular case in Station 3, Cardiovascular. If, at the last minute, neither of the scheduled heart cases turns up on the day; or if in the middle of a carousel the only one who did turn up decides not to continue or is too ill to continue, a substitute case has to be found at short notice. In this situation, one option is to proceed with a patient with a normal heart and make up an appropriate scenario. One simply has to imagine oneself as the invigilating registrar to think what that might be. One would first look amongst any surplus cases in the other stations for a volunteer or one might ask a member of the nursing, portering or other support staff, and come up with a scenario such as:

> 'This . . . -year-old patient complains of palpitations. Please examine the heart . . .'

There may thus be a clue in the case scenario and the fact that the scenario has been hurriedly hand-scribbled.

From our surveys it is clear that the most common reason for finding no abnormality is missing the physical signs that are present, as is likely in the two anecdotes below (possibly also Anecdote 5, Station 1, Abdominal, Case 11 and Vol. 2, Section F, Experience 158). Other reasons for cases of 'normal' will be either because the physical signs are no longer present by the time the patient comes to the examination (see Anecdote 1, Station 3, CNS, Case 28) or that the examiners and candidate disagree with the selectors of the cases about the presence of physical signs (this may have happened in Anecdote, Vol. 3, Station 5, Eyes, Case 21; see also Vol. 2, Section F, Experience 198 and Anecdote 303).

The following are anecdotes from our surveys.

Anecdote 1
A candidate was asked to examine a lady's cardiovascular system. The patient had cushingoid features and tachypnoea, but he could not decipher a murmur. The patient's general condition was very poor and instead of telling the truth by saying that he couldn't hear in view of her severe dyspnoea, the candidate made out that the patient had mixed aortic valve disease. He failed PACES on that attempt and reports that he had no clue what the case was as the patient was obese and extremely breathless and he couldn't make out the murmurs.

Anecdote 2
A candidate was asked to examine the heart. He could find no abnormality and said so because he thought he had to be honest. He has no idea what the diagnosis was. He failed (pre PACES case).

Case 25 | Cannon waves

Frequency in survey: main focus of a short case or additional feature in 0.1% of attempts at PACES Station 3, Cardiovascular.

Survey note: one candidate was asked to examine the heart only, another was asked to look at the patient's neck and then examine the heart, and a third was asked to take the patient's pulse.

Record

There are sharp *a* waves* (cannon waves*) visible in this patient's jugular veins. (Feel the carotid pulse on the opposite side.) These waves occur irregularly even though the pulse is regular but slow at 48/min.

As the waves are irregular and the pulse is slow, the explanation is that this patient has complete heart block.

If allowed to auscultate, you will hear an S1 of variable intensity; the sound coinciding with the cannon wave will be soft.

Causes of cannon waves

Regular cannon waves – nodal rhythm, paroxysmal nodal tachycardia, partial heart block with very long PR interval

Irregular cannon waves – complete heart block, multiple ectopic beats

---

*Candidates who have never seen cannon waves have been known to confuse them with giant *v* waves (see Station 3, Cardiovascular, Case 11). Cannon waves are seen like sharp flicks and are quite characteristic in appearance. You should attempt to see some in the pacemaker clinic of a cardiology unit. Cannon waves are giant *a* waves and these occur whenever the right atrium contracts against a closed tricuspid valve, and the whole of the energy released by the right atrial contraction is transmitted to the JVP, as forward flow is impossible (the ECG complex associated with a cannon wave shows that the P wave falls between the end of the QRS and the T wave or at the end of the T wave).

Case 26 | Coarctation of the aorta

Frequency in survey: main focus of a short case or additional feature in 0.1% of attempts at PACES Station 3, Cardiovascular.

Record 1

The radial pulses (in this young adult) are regular, equal* and of large volume (give rate). The *carotid pulsations* are *vigorous*,† and the JVP is not elevated (unless there is heart failure). The *femorals* are *delayed* and of *poor volume* (palpate the radial and femoral simultaneously). The *blood pressure* in the right arm is elevated at 190/110 mmHg (it will be *low in the legs*).There are *visible arterial pulsations*‡ and *bruits* can be heard over and around the *scapula, anterior axilla* and over the *left sternal border* (internal mammary artery). The cardiac impulse is heaving but not displaced (unless in failure). Systolic *thrills* are palpable over the collaterals and suprasternally. There is a *systolic murmur* which is loudest at the level of the *fourth intercostal space posteriorly* (the level of the coarctation), but is also audible in the *second intercostal space* close to the sternum (the murmur, if present, of the associated bicuspid aortic valve is often obscured by that from the coarctation).§

These findings suggest a diagnosis of significant coarctation of the aorta.

Record 2

There is a *left-sided thoracotomy scar*. The right radial *pulse* is normal, whilst the *left is diminished (or absent)*. The carotid pulses are normal and the JVP is not elevated. The femorals are palpable and there is no radiofemoral delay. The apex beat is normal, and there is an ejection click associated with a soft systolic murmur in the aortic area.

The left thoracotomy scar and absent/reduced left radial pulse suggest repaired coarctation of the aorta whilst the aortic signs are compatible with associated bicuspid aortic valve. (The left radial pulse is commonly reduced or absent as a result of the surgical repair – the origin of the left subclavian artery is in close proximity to the coarctation and the left subclavian can actually form part of the repair in some cases.)

Following repair

It can be useful to assess the brachial/ankle index with a Doppler probe to assess the functional state of the repair.

---

*Rarely (2%), the coarctation is proximal to the origin of the left subclavian artery and the left arm pulses will be weaker than the right; rib notching will be unilateral and right-sided.

†If you see vigorous carotid pulsations the likeliest cause is aortic incompetence (?collapsing pulse). The occasional patient, however, will have coarctation.

‡Collaterals are best observed with the patient sitting up and leaning forward with the arms hanging by the side.

§A continuous murmur in systole and diastole, arising from the dilated collaterals, may be heard over the back. An early diastolic murmur arising because of the dilated ascending aorta may be heard especially in older patients.

Echocardiography is a poor imaging modality after coarctation repair; MRI is much preferred and is recommended for follow-up.

Balloon dilation of the coarctation and/or recoarctation is useful in selected cases. Stent implantation is under assessment

Complications following repair

1 Aortic valve degeneration

2 Aneurysm formation at site of repair (can become infected – mycotic aneurysm)

3 Aneurysm rupture

4 Recoarctation

5 Aortic dissection in later life (anywhere from top to bottom)

Male-to-female ratio is 2/1.

Other features and associations of coarctation of the aorta

Rib notching* and poststenotic dilation on chest X-ray

Bicuspid aortic valve in 25% (site of infective endocarditis and may lead to coexisting aortic incompetence; diagnosis can be made by echocardiography)

Berry aneurysms of the circle of Willis (may cause death even in corrected cases)

Patent ductus arteriosus (?machinery murmur, etc; see Station 3, Cardiovascular, Case 29)

Turner's syndrome (check for features of Turner's if your patient is female – webbed neck, increased carrying angle, short stature, etc; see Vol. 3, Station 5, Endocrine, Case 11)

Marfan's syndrome (?tall, arachnodactyly, high-arched palate, lens dislocation, etc; see Vol. 3, Station 5, Locomotor, Case 9)

High mortality after the age of 40. Hypertension† may not be cured even in corrected cases (low perfusion of kidneys may involve the renin-angiotensin system)

Other causes of rib notching

Neurofibromatosis (multiple neuromata on the intercostal nerves)

Enlargement of nerves (amyloidosis, congenital hypertrophic polyneuropathy)

Inferior vena cava obstruction

Blalock shunt operation (left-sided unilateral rib notching)

Congenital

†Coarctation in adults usually presents clinically with hypertension.

Case 27 | Eisenmenger's syndrome

Frequency in survey: main focus of a short case or additional feature in 0.1% of attempts at PACES Station 3, Cardiovascular.

Record

There is *central cyanosis* and *clubbing* of the fingers (may be only in the toes in patent ductus arteriosus). The pulse (give rate) is regular (and small in volume). A large *a* wave is (may be) seen in the venous pulse (due to forceful atrial contraction in the face of the right ventricular hypertrophy). There is a marked *left parasternal heave* and (often) a palpable (pulmonary) second heart sound. On auscultation, (the signs of pulmonary hypertension are heard) the *second heart sound* is *loud* and single, there is (may be) a right ventricular fourth heart sound, (may be) a pulmonary early systolic ejection click, (may be) an early diastolic murmur (dilated pulmonary artery leads to secondary pulmonary incompetence), and (may be) a pansystolic murmur (secondary tricuspid incompetence – *v* wave in JVP).

These findings suggest Eisenmenger's syndrome with pulmonary hypertension.

Causes

1 Large, non-restrictive ventricular septal defect (VSD)* (cyanosis due to bidirectional shunt at the ventricular level)

2 Primary pulmonary hypertension (cyanosis due to intrapulmonary shunting)

3 Atrial septal defect (fixed and wide splitting of the second sound)

4 Patent ductus arteriosus† (normal splitting of the second sound – *P2* follows *A2* and the split widens with inspiration; only the lower limbs are cyanosed – differential cyanosis)

5 Other complex congenital heart disease (cyanosis usually due to bidirectional shunt at the ventricular level)

6 Fallot's tetralogy – palliated or untreated (see Station 3, Cardiovascular, Case 23)

Once Eisenmenger's syndrome has developed, it is too late (high mortality) for correction of the cardiac anomaly. A palliative procedure involving redirection of the venous return has been successful in the presence of transposition of the great arteries, VSD and severe pulmonary vascular disease. Heart/lung transplantation is an option but has a much poorer prognosis than heart transplantation alone. Death commonly occurs between the ages of 20 and 40 years and is usually due to pulmonary infarction, right heart failure, dysrhythmias and, less often, infective endocarditis or cerebral abscess.

With the advent of cardiopulmonary bypass in the 1960s, VSD repair was possible, and the prevalence of Eisenmenger's syndrome due to congenital heart disease in the adult population is falling all the time.

It is generally now agreed that untreated isolated atrial septal defect does *not* lead to Eisenmenger's

*When due to a VSD, it is termed Eisenmenger's complex. The classic pansystolic murmur of the VSD tends to disappear as the right and left ventricular pressures equalize. A pansystolic murmur in Eisenmenger's complex is more likely to be from tricuspid incompetence.

†Again, the classic patent ductus arteriosus murmur tends to shorten to a soft systolic murmur, and then disappear as the pressures in the pulmonary artery and descending aorta equalize. Untreated patent ductus arteriosus is very rare these days as it can be repaired surgically without the need for cardiopulmonary bypass.

Table C3.3 The features which may be helpful in differentiating Eisenmenger's syndrome from tetralogy of Fallot

	Eisenmenger's syndrome	Fallot's tetralogy
Pulmonary systolic thrill	Absent	Present
Pulmonary systolic murmur	Absent	Intense (unless such severe stenosis that there is no flow)
Right ventricle	Very hypertrophied	Hypertrophied
Chest X-ray	Large pulmonary arteries	Small pulmonary arteries

syndrome. The absence of chest signs helps to differentiate Eisenmenger's syndrome from the cyanosis and pulmonary hypertension of cor pulmonale. The features which may be helpful in differentiating Eisenmenger's syndrome from Fallot's tetralogy (the most common cause of central cyanosis in the adolescent or young adult) are shown in Table C3.3. Furthermore, the patient with Fallot's tetralogy in the examination may well have thoracotomy scars and a pulse which is weaker on the left than on the right, from a previous Blalock shunt operation (see Station 3, Cardiovascular, Case 23).

Case 28 | Infective endocarditis

Frequency in survey: main focus of a short case or additional feature in 0.1% of attempts at PACES Station 3, Cardiovascular.

Record

This patient has mitral incompetence* suggested by a pansystolic murmur over the precordium, radiating to the left axilla, a third heart sound, a dilated left ventricle with the point of maximum impulse in the left sixth intercostal space in the anterior axillary line, and a right ventricular lift. There are (may be) *splinter haemorrhages*, the conjunctivae are pale† and there is a *petechial haemorrhage* inside the right lower eyelid (look for *cutaneous manifestations* elsewhere on the body). There is no clubbing‡ (ask to look for *splenomegaly* and for *Roth's spots*§).

There is an infusion line and I strongly suspect that this patient has infective endocarditis.

Cutaneous manifestations of infective endocarditis

Four lesions involving the *skin* and *its appendages* have traditionally been considered as the peripheral manifestations of infective endocarditis: *petechiae, subungual* ('*splinter*') *haemorrhages, Osler's nodes* and *Janeway lesions*. Since the advent of effective antibiotic therapy and early diagnosis in most cases, these signs have become less frequent in real life but, whenever available, would be presented in the MRCP clinical examination.

Petechiae are often present in the *conjunctivae*, on the skin of the *dorsum* of the *hands* and *feet*, the anterior chest and abdominal wall and on the oropharynx. Petechiae are common in both acute and subacute endocarditis but are not specific and may occur in *thrombocytopenia, scurvy, renal failure, bacteraemia* without endocarditis (e.g. *meningococcaemia*) and after *cardiopulmonary bypass* in the absence of infection (presumably due to fat microemboli).

Subungual (*splinter*) *haemorrhages* are more commonly seen after trauma and in *psoriasis* but they are also seen in all forms of endocarditis.* A true splinter almost always occurs about 3–5 mm proximal to the free edge of the nail.

Osler's nodes are small, raised, red to purple, *tender* lesions that are most often seen on the pulps of the fingers and toes. They may also be seen on the soles and palms. Osler's nodes are not common, and they are almost always associated with a more protracted course of the disease.

Janeway lesions are small (1–4 mm in diameter), irregular, flat, erythematous, *non-tender macules* present most often on the palms, soles and around the ankles. They may appear on the tips of the fingers and toes and occasionally on the extremities and the trunk. These lesions *blanch on pressure*. They are not common and usually occur in acute fulminant endocarditis but seldom occur in bacteraemia without endocarditis.

---

*In the examination setting, one usually expects a valvular lesion when asked to examine the heart of a patient with infective endocarditis. However, murmurs are not essential for this diagnosis.
†*Pallor* in a patient with a *valvular lesion* (though uncommon these days when patients are diagnosed and treated early) should alert the candidate to look for other circumstantial evidence (e.g. temperature chart, intravenous line) and cutaneous manifestations of SBE.

‡Clubbing is rare in endocarditis and only occurs in the subacute variety.
§*Roth's spots* (infrequent; usually subacute variety) are seen on the retina as cotton-wool exudates, often surrounded by a haemorrhage. Histologically, these lesions are collections of lymphocytes in the nerve layer of the retina surrounded by oedema and/or haemorrhage. Roth's spots may occur in association with other infections.

Acute versus subacute bacterial endocarditis*

Many authorities now recommend abandoning the terms acute (ABE) and subacute (SBE) bacterial endocarditis and using 'infective endocarditis' instead. Nevertheless, a comparison between the two extremes of the spectrum does provide a useful reminder that very different presentations of infective endocarditis can occur. The clinical course in classic *acute bacterial endocarditis* (most common organism *Staphylococcus aureus* – 50–70% of cases) is usually measured in *days*, the associated systemic illness is more severe and *early mortality higher*, the patient is more likely to suffer rapid destruction of the valve and more likely to have one or more focal collections outside the heart. Treatment in the acute variety should not be delayed until blood culture results are available. Classic *subacute bacterial endocarditis* (most common organism *Streptococcus viridans*) may have a course measured in *weeks or months* with vague non-specific complaints of general malaise, anorexia, aches and pains, weakness and fatigue, low-grade fevers and night sweats.

Intravenous drug abuse is a common cause of either left- or right-sided endocarditis and commonly presents late and with staphylococcal infection. Paradoxically, the florid signs of acute endocarditis are thus becoming commonplace, as are the myriad infective complications of the condition (cerebral abscess, spinal abscess, mycotic pulmonary emboli, etc.).

Infective endocarditis can be a fatal complication of central line incision, particularly in the immunocompromised where endocarditic infection with fungal agents is a real risk.

Aortic root abscess may develop in association with aortic valve endocarditis. This can cause heart block (ask to see the ECG and examine the PR interval; the ward review should include serial ECGs).

Antimicrobial prophylaxis against infective endocarditis (NICE guidance, March 2008)

Antibacterial prophylaxis and chlorhexidine mouthwash are not recommended for the prevention of endocarditis in patients undergoing dental procedures

Antibacterial prophylaxis is not recommended for the prevention of endocarditis in patients undergoing procedures of the:

(a) upper and lower respiratory tract (including ear, nose and throat procedures and bronchoscopy)

(b) genitourinary tract (including urological, gynaecological and obstetric procedures)

(c) upper and lower gastrointestinal tract

Whilst these procedures can cause bacteraemia, there is no clear association with the development of infective endocarditis. Prophylaxis may expose patients to the adverse effects of antimicrobials when the evidence of benefit has not been proven

Any infection in patients at risk of endocarditis† should be investigated promptly and treated appropriately to reduce the risk of endocarditis

If patients at risk of endocarditis† are undergoing a gastrointestinal or genitourinary tract procedure at a site where infection is suspected, they should receive appropriate antibacterial therapy that includes cover against organisms that cause endocarditis

Patients at risk of endocarditis† should be:

(a) advised to maintain good oral hygiene

(b) told how to recognize signs of infective endocarditis, and advised when to seek expert advice

---

*Whilst endocarditis is associated with prior valve abnormalities, 50% of cases occur on structurally normal valves.
†Patients at risk of endocarditis include those with valve replacement, acquired valvular heart disease with stenosis or regurgitation, structural congenital heart disease (including surgically corrected or palliated structural conditions, but excluding isolated atrial septal defect, fully repaired ventricular septal defect, fully repaired patent ductus arteriosus, and closure devices considered to be endothelialized), hypertrophic cardiomyopathy, or a previous episode of infective endocarditis.

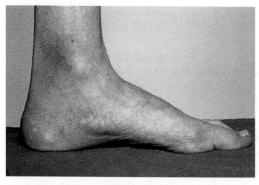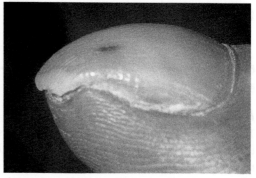

Figure C3.3 (a) Janeway lesions above the ankle. (b) Splinter haemorrhage.

Case 29 | Patent ductus arteriosus

Frequency in survey: main focus of a short case or additional feature in 0.1% of attempts at PACES Station 3, Cardiovascular.

Record

The *pulse* is *collapsing* (may be normal if the duct is narrow and the 'run-off' from the aorta to the left pulmonary artery is small) in character, regular (give rate) and the venous pressure is not raised. The apex is *thrusting* (volume overload) in the anterior axillary line (may be normal if the ductus is small), and there is (sometimes) a *left parasternal heave* (if there is associated pulmonary hypertension). On auscultation, there is a continuous *'machinery' murmur** with systolic *accentuation* heard in the second left intercostal space near the sternal edge (but maximal 5–7.5 cm above or to the left of this, *beneath the clavicle*, and also *heard posteriorly*).

The diagnosis is patent ductus arteriosus.

Male-to-female ratio is 1/3.

The incidence is higher in patients born at a high altitude. Spontaneous closure is rare except in premature infants. The diagnosis is made by echocardiography or MRI. Closure can usually be effected using percutaneous transcatheter technology although surgical repair is still advocated for large calcified ducts.

Other causes of a continuous murmur†
With collapsing pulse
Mitral incompetence and aortic incompetence
Ventricular septal defect and aortic incompetence

Without collapsing pulse
Venous hum (common in normal children – maximal to the right of the sternum – diminishes or disappears when the child lies flat or when the right JVP is compressed)
Pulmonary arteriovenous fistula or shunt (e.g. Blalock)

Complications of large‡ patent ductus arteriosus
Infective endocarditis
Heart failure
Eisenmenger's syndrome (see Station 3, Cardiovascular, Case 27)

---

*The murmur seldom lasts for the whole of systole and diastole. It may occupy only the latter part of systole and the early part of diastole. Occasionally, particularly in young children, it may occur as a crescendo in late systole only. The unwary may mistake the systolic component of this murmur for pulmonary stenosis – listen posteriorly: the murmur of a patent ductus will still be as loud as that anteriorly, whereas that of pulmonary stenosis will be much softer.

†NB: The murmur of patent ductus distinguishes itself by being loudest below the left clavicle. There should not usually be any diagnostic difficulty.
‡Small ducts detected in adult life with no haemodynamic sequelae do not require intervention.

Case 30 | Pulmonary incompetence

Frequency in survey: main focus of a short case or additional feature in 0.1% of attempts at PACES Station 3, Cardiovascular.

Record 1

There is a *mid-line sternotomy scar*. The first sound is normal. The pulmonary component of the second sound is soft. There is an *ejection systolic murmur* in the *pulmonary area* and a long *decrescendo diastolic murmur* audible along the *left sternal edge*.

The patient has signs of *mixed pulmonary valve disease* with predominant incompetence. The mid-line scar suggests that this may be associated with previous valvotomy surgery for *congenital pulmonary stenosis.**

Record 2†

This patient has features of *mitral stenosis* (state them; see Station 3, Cardiovascular, Case 7) combined with evidence of *pulmonary hypertension* and *pulmonary incompetence* suggested by a *palpable second sound* in the pulmonary area, followed by an *early diastolic murmur*, which has a sharp whiffing quality, most loudly heard in the pulmonary area but radiating only for a few centimetres down the left sternal edge. There is also an early ejection systolic murmur audible over the pulmonary area.

The patient has a Graham Steell murmur complicating mitral stenosis with pulmonary hypertension.

Record 3†

This patient has *cyanosis* and a weak peripheral pulse. The JVP is *elevated* with both *a* and *v* waves being prominent. The apex beat is not palpable, but there is a strong right ventricular heave. The auscultatory signs are a *gallop of the fourth heart sound*, a *pansystolic murmur* over the tricuspid area (sometimes associated with a *thrill*), a *pulmonary ejection click*, grade 2/6 mid-systolic murmur over the pulmonary area and an *early diastolic murmur* heard over the same region. In addition, she‡ also has ankle oedema.

These features suggest that she has *primary pulmonary hypertension* associated with pulmonary incompetence.

---

*This is the most common scenario in which stable pulmonary incompetence will be manifest in clinical practice. Increasingly, the importance of maintaining right ventricular function has been recognized, leading to greater investigation and surgical reintervention in this circumstance.

†The other scenario of a case where there is a focus on pulmonary incompetence is that of a patient who has established pulmonary hypertension and its associated features. Pulmonary hypertension results in dilation of both the main pulmonary artery and the valve ring; the valve cusps do not close completely and a regurgitant murmur, known as the Graham Steell murmur, is produced. In some cases this becomes the focus of the examiners' attention and your record should take account of it.

‡In primary pulmonary hypertension, the ratio of males to females is 1/4.

Record 4*

The JVP is elevated with a large *v* wave reaching the right earlobe (there may be secondary *tricuspid incompetence*). There is a right ventricular lift but the apex beat is not palpable. There is a pansystolic murmur heard over the left third interspace and a high-pitched mid-diastolic murmur.†

The patient has pulmonary incompetence and tricuspid incompetence.

Causes of pulmonary hypertension

Primary: primary pulmonary hypertension – rare, favours women with a female-to-male ratio of 4/1

Secondary:

Acquired heart disease: mitral valve disease, congestive cardiomyopathy (of any cause)

Congenital heart disease: atrial/ventricular septal defect, patent ductus arteriosus

Pulmonary vascular disease:

(a) vasoactive: autoimmune disease, high altitude

(b) obliterative: thromboembolic disease, schistosomiasis

Structural lung disease: emphysema, cystic fibrosis, etc.

---

*Rarely there may be a patient with a valvular pulmonary incompetence either caused by carcinoid (see Station 1, Abdominal, Case 18) involvement of the pulmonary valve or due to endocarditis (the patient may have been a drug addict). In patients with a valvular pulmonary incompetence, there is unlikely to be any evidence of pulmonary hypertension. Other possible causes of valvular incompetence are congenital malformation or a previous surgical procedure.

†The diastolic murmur of valvular pulmonary incompetence occurs after the delayed P2 which is more like mid-diastolic than early diastolic in timing.

Case 31 | Slow pulse

Frequency in survey: main focus of a short case or additional feature in 0.1% of attempts at PACES Station 3, Cardiovascular.

Record

The pulse rate is regular at 40/min (irregularly irregular pulse with beat-to-beat variation may be atrial fibrillation with a slow ventricular response) and there is *no increase* in the rate on *standing* (complete heart block; mostly in older patients). The JVP is not elevated (unless there is heart failure) but just visible, and there is a complete dissociation of *a* and *v* waves with frequent *cannon waves* (flicking *a* waves occurring during ventricular systole). (The pulse pressure is large and this may be evident clinically.)

This patient has complete heart block.

Other causes of bradycardia

β-Blocker therapy: about 2% of patients receiving β-blockers have excessive bradycardia (heart rate increases by a few beats on standing and during exercise)

Atrial fibrillation with a slow ventricular response (may be regular if there is associated complete heart block): the patient may be on β-blockers and/or digoxin

Hypothyroidism (?facies, ankle jerks, etc; see Vol. 3, Station 5, Endocrine, Case 5)

Sinoatrial disease: bradycardia–tachycardia syndrome

Digoxin toxicity

Cardiac pacing

Most patients with complete heart block will benefit from a demand pacemaker (even asymptomatic patients with a heart rate <40). Cardiac pacing is recommended for all symptomatic patients with bradycardia, and for those with brady–tachy syndrome who will need antiarrhythmic therapy to control episodes of tachycardia.

Most authorities would agree that all patients with complete heart block, and those with Mobitz type 2 block, should be offered cardiac pacing, even if the arrhythmia is intermittent (unless associated with acute ischaemia or other reversible events) and/or the patient is asymptomatic.

Station 3
Central Nervous System

Short case	Checked and updated as necessary for this edition by
1 Peripheral neuropathy	Dr Steve Sturman*
2 Myotonic dystrophy (dystrophia myotonica)	Dr Steve Sturman*
3 Parkinson's disease	Dr Saiju Jacob*
4 Charcot–Marie–Tooth disease (hereditary motor and sensory neuropathy)	Dr Steve Sturman*
5 Abnormal gait	Dr Saiju Jacob*
6 Spastic paraparesis	Dr Saiju Jacob*
7 Cerebellar syndrome	Dr Steve Sturman*
8 Hemiplegia	Dr Steve Sturman*
9 Muscular dystrophy	Dr Saiju Jacob*
10 Multiple sclerosis	Dr Saiju Jacob*
11 Motor neurone disease	Dr Steve Sturman*
12 Friedreich's ataxia	Dr Saiju Jacob*
13 Visual field defect	Dr Steve Sturman*
14 Ulnar nerve palsy	Dr Steve Sturman*
15 Old polio	Dr Steve Sturman*
16 Ocular palsy	Dr Saiju Jacob*
17 Spinal cord compression	Dr Saiju Jacob*
18 Ptosis	Dr Steve Sturman*
19 Guillain–Barré syndrome (acute inflammatory demyelinating polyradiculopathy)	Dr Steve Sturman*
20 Choreoathetosis	Dr Saiju Jacob*
21 Bulbar palsy	Dr Steve Sturman*
22 Lateral popliteal (common peroneal) nerve palsy	Dr Steve Sturman*
23 Proximal myopathy	Dr Saiju Jacob*
24 Absent ankle jerks and extensor plantars	Dr Steve Sturman*
25 Cerebellopontine angle lesion	Dr Steve Sturman*
26 Cervical myelopathy	Dr Steve Sturman*
27 Myasthenia gravis	Dr Steve Sturman*
28 Normal central nervous system	Dr Bob Ryder
29 Syringomyelia	Dr Steve Sturman*
30 Diabetic foot/Charcot's joint	Dr Bob Ryder
31 Holmes–Adie–Moore syndrome	Dr Steve Sturman*
32 Nystagmus	Dr Saiju Jacob*
33 Carpal tunnel syndrome	Dr Saiju Jacob*
34 Drug-induced extrapyramidal syndrome	Dr Saiju Jacob*
35 Lower motor neurone VIIth nerve palsy	Dr Saiju Jacob*
36 Dysarthria	Dr Steve Sturman*
37 Subacute combined degeneration of the cord	Dr Saiju Jacob*

Short case	Checked and updated as necessary for this edition by
38 Argyll Robertson pupils	Dr Steve Sturman*
39 Congenital syphilis	Dr Steve Sturman*
40 Dysphasia	Dr Steve Sturman*
41 Horner's syndrome	Dr Saiju Jacob*
42 Infantile hemiplegia	Dr Steve Sturman*
43 Jugular foramen syndrome	Dr Steve Sturman*
44 Lateral medullary syndrome (Wallenberg's syndrome)	Dr Steve Sturman*
45 Polymyositis	Dr Steve Sturman*
46 Pseudobulbar palsy	Dr Steve Sturman*
47 Psychogenic/factitious	Dr Steve Sturman*
48 Radial nerve palsy	Dr Steve Sturman*
49 Subclavian-steal syndrome	Dr Steve Sturman*
50 Tabes	Dr Steve Sturman*
51 Thalamic syndrome	Dr Steve Sturman*
52 Wasting of the small muscles of the hand	Dr Saiju Jacob*

*All suggested changes by these specialty advisors were considered by Dr Bob Ryder and were accepted, edited, added to or rejected with Dr Ryder making the final editorial decision in every case.

Dr Steve Sturman, Consultant Neurologist, City Hospital, Birmingham, UK
Dr Saiju Jacob, Consultant Neurologist, Queen Elizabeth Neurosciences Centre, Birmingham, UK

Case 1 | Peripheral neuropathy

Frequency in survey: main focus of a short case or additional feature in 10% of attempts at PACES Station 3, CNS.

Record

There is *impairment* of *sensation* to light touch, vibration sense, joint position sense and pinprick over a *stocking* and, to a lesser extent, a *glove distribution* (much less common).

　　The patient has a peripheral neuropathy.

Most likely causes

1 Diabetes mellitus (?fundi, amyotrophy)
2 Carcinomatous neuropathy (?evidence of primary, cachexia, clubbing)
3 Vitamin B_{12} deficiency (subacute combined degeneration not always present; ?plantars)
4 Vitamin B deficiency (alcoholics*)
5 Drugs (e.g. isoniazid, vincristine, nitrofurantoin, gold, ethambutol, phenytoin, hydralazine, metronidazole, amiodarone, chloramphenicol, cyclosporin)
6 Idiopathic (in up to one-third of patients with chronic peripheral neuropathy for >1 year, no cause can be found). There are many rare causes (see below)
7 Hereditary, motor sensory neuropathy (Charcot–Marie–Tooth syndrome)

Leprosy is a cause of major importance worldwide.

Important rare causes

Guillain–Barré syndrome (also motor involvement, absent reflexes, ?bilateral lower motor neurone VIIth nerve palsy; see Station 3, CNS, Case 19)
Polyarteritis nodosa (?arteritic lesions)
Rheumatoid arthritis and other collagen disease (hands, facies)
Amyloidosis (?thick nerves, autonomic involvement)†
AIDS‡

Chronic inflammatory demyelinating polyneuropathy (CIDP)

Causes of predominantly motor neuropathy

Carcinomatous neuropathy (?evidence of primary, cachexia)
Lead (wrists mainly)
Porphyria
Diphtheria
Charcot–Marie–Tooth disease (?atrophy of peronei, pes cavus, etc; see Station 3, CNS, Case 4)

---

*Can also occur with nutritional deficiencies from other causes, e.g. dialysis for chronic renal failure, prison camp victims.
†Neuropathy is a feature of primary and myeloma-associated amyloidosis (it is exceptional in secondary amyloidosis). Carpal tunnel syndrome is not uncommon. Sensory or mixed sensory and motor neuropathy are most common. Signs of autonomic involvement would be orthostatic hypotension, impotence, impairment of sweating and diarrhoea. The other organs mainly involved in primary and myeloma-associated amyloidosis

include heart (cardiomyopathy), tongue (dysarthria), skeletal and visceral muscle and alimentary tract (rectal biopsy). See also Footnote, Station 1, Abdominal, Case 4).
‡Acute (Guillain–Barré type) or chronic inflammatory neuropathy may be the presenting feature of HIV infection but with a cerebrospinal fluid pleocytosis which is not usually seen in these conditions. A distal sensory neuropathy may also occur in AIDS, sometimes but not always caused by cytomegalovirus infection.

Other rare causes of peripheral neuropathy

Myxoedema (?facies, pulse, reflexes, etc; see Vol. 3, Station 5, Endocrine, Case 9)

Acromegaly (?facies, hands, etc; see Vol. 3, Station 5, Endocrine, Case 2)

Sarcoidosis (?lupus pernio, chest signs)

Uraemia (?pale brownish yellow complexion)

Lyme disease

Tetanus

Botulism (can be mistaken for Guillain–Barré, encephalitis, stroke or myasthenia gravis; EMG resembles Eaton–Lambert)

Paraproteinaemia*

Hereditary ataxias

Refsum's disease (cerebellar ataxia, pupillary abnormalities, optic atrophy, deafness, retinitis pigmentosa, cardiomyopathy, ichthyosis)

Arsenic poisoning (e.g. pesticides; Mee's transverse white lines may occur on the fingernails and raindrop pigmentation may occur on the skin)

Other chemical poisoning (e.g. tri-ortho-cresyl phosphate)

*NB: The rare POEMS syndrome: Polyneuropathy, Organomegaly, Endocrinopathy, Monoclonal gammopathy, Skin changes. These are associated with osteosclerotic myeloma.

Case 2 | Myotonic dystrophy (dystrophia myotonica)

Frequency in survey: main focus of a short case or additional feature in 8% of attempts at PACES Station 3, CNS.

Record

The patient has *myopathic facies* (drooping mouth and long, lean, sad, lifeless, somewhat sleepy expression), frontal *balding* (in the male), *ptosis* (may be unilateral) and *wasting of the facial muscles*, temporalis, masseter, *sternomastoids*, shoulder girdle and quadriceps. The forearms and legs are involved and the *reflexes* are *lost*. The patient has *cataracts*. After he made a fist, he was unable to quickly open it, especially when asked to do this repetitively (this gets worse in the cold and with excitement). He has difficulty opening his eyes after firm closure. When he shook hands there was a delay before he released his grip* (these are all features of *myotonia*). When dimples and depressions are induced in his muscles by percussion, they fill only slowly (*percussion myotonia*, e.g. tongue and thenar eminence).

The diagnosis is myotonic dystrophy.

Autosomal dominant.

Other features

Cardiomyopathy (?small volume pulse, low blood pressure, splitting of first heart sound in mitral area; low-voltage P wave, prolonged PR interval, notched QRS and prolonged QTc on the ECG; dysrythmias; sudden death may occur)

Intellect and personality deterioration

Slurred speech due to combined tongue and pharyngeal myotonia

Testicular atrophy (small soft testicles but secondary sexual characteristics preserved; usually develops after the patient has had children and thus the disease is perpetuated; evidence regarding ovarian atrophy is indefinite)

Diabetes mellitus (end-organ unresponsiveness to insulin)

Nodular thyroid enlargement, small pituitary fossa but normal pituitary function, dysphagia, abdominal pain, hypoventilation, and postanaesthetic respiratory failure may also occur

The condition may show 'anticipation' – progressively worsening signs and symptoms in succeeding generations, e.g. presenile cataracts may be the sole indication of the disorder in preceding generations. Genetic testing can be confirmatory, demonstrating expanded trinucleotide repeats in a region on chromosome 19 in the myotonin protein kinase gene

Myotonia congenita (Thomsen's disease)

There is difficulty in relaxation of a muscle after forceful contraction (myotonia) but none of the other

---

*There may be absence of grip myotonia in advanced disease because of progressive muscle wasting. Though myotonia can be relieved by phenytoin, quinine or procainamide, it is weakness (for which there is no treatment) rather than the myotonia which is the main cause of disability in myotonic dystrophy.

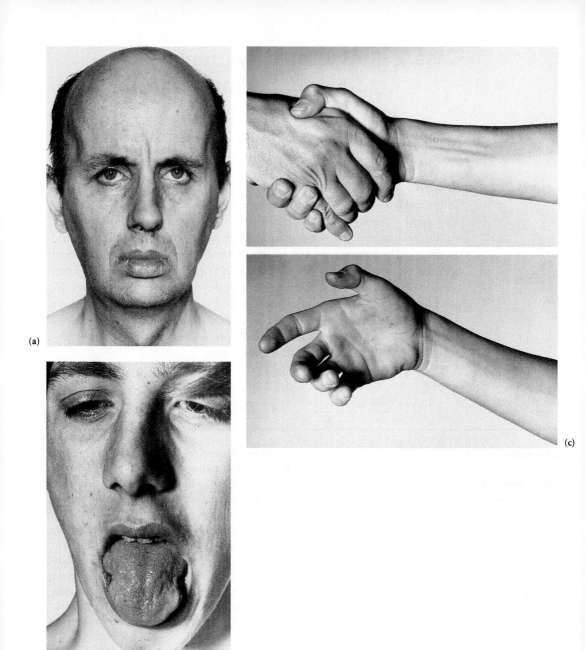

Figure C3.4 (a–c) Note balding, ptosis and myotonia of the tongue and hands.

features of myotonic dystrophy (e.g. weakness, cataracts, baldness, gonadal atrophy, etc.). The *reflexes are normal*. Some patients have a 'Herculean' appearance from very developed musculature (?related to repeated involuntary isometric exercise). Myotonia congenita is usually autosomal dominant, but autosomal recessive forms are also recognized. It is now understood that these conditions are due to disorders of ion channels (channelopathies). The finding of paramyotonia – myotonia worsening with exercise and cold – may be useful clinically in differentiating various subtypes of channelopathy.

Case 3 | Parkinson's disease

Frequency in survey: main focus of a short case or additional feature in 8% of attempts at PACES Station 3, CNS.

Record

This man has an *expressionless, unblinking face* and slurred *low-volume monotonous speech*. He is drooling (due to excessive salivation and some dysphagia) and there is *titubation*. He has difficulty starting to walk ('freezing') but once started, progresses with quick shuffling steps as if trying to keep up with his own centre of gravity. As he walks, he is *stooped* and he *does not swing his arms* which show a continuous *pill-rolling tremor*. (He has poor balance and tends to fall, being unable to react quickly enough to stop himself.) His arms show a *lead-pipe rigidity* at the elbow but *cog-wheel rigidity* (combination of lead pipe rigidity and tremor, i.e. worse with anxiety) at the wrist. He has a positive glabellar tap sign (an unreliable sign) and his signs generally are *asymmetrical* – note the greater tremor in the R/L arm. (The tremor is decreased by intention but handwriting may be small,* tremulous and untidy.) There is *blepharoclonus* (tremor of the eyelids when the eyes are gently closed).

The diagnosis is Parkinson's disease.†

Male-to-female ratio is 3/1.

The features of Parkinson's disease are
1 Tremor
2 Rigidity
3 Bradykinesia.

Bradykinesia (the most disabling) can be demonstrated by asking the patient to touch his thumb successively with each finger. He will be slow in the initiation of the response and there will be a progressive reduction in the amplitude of each movement and a peculiar type of fatiguability. He will also have difficulty in performing two different motor acts simultaneously.

Other causes of the parkinsonian syndrome
Drug-induced (see Station 3, CNS, Case 34)

Postencephalitic (increasingly rare; definite history of encephalitis – encephalitis lethargica pandemic 1916–1928; there may be ophthalmoplegia, pupil abnormalities and dyskinesias; poor response to L-dopa)

Brain damage from anoxia (e.g. cardiac arrest), carbon monoxide or manganese poisoning (dementia and pyramidal signs are likely with all)

Neurosyphilis

Cerebral tumours affecting the basal ganglia

Other conditions which may have some extrapyramidal features
Arteriosclerotic Parkinson's (stepwise progression, broad-based gait, pyramidal signs; may be no more than simply two common conditions occurring in

---

*When present, this is often the earliest sign to appear.
†GAD antibodies are found in about 70% of patients with type 1 diabetes at the time of diagnosis. These antibodies appear early

in the disease process and can be used to predict who will develop type 1 diabetes.

the same patient – cerebral arteriosclerosis and idiopathic parkinsonism)

Normal pressure hydrocephalus (may have a number of causes including head injury, meningitis or subarachnoid haemorrhage, though in many instances the cause cannot be determined; the classic triad is *urinary incontinence, gait apraxia* and *dementia;* diagnosed by CT or MRI scan; important to diagnose because it may respond to ventriculosystemic shunting)

Progressive supranuclear palsy (Steele–Richardson–Olszewski syndrome) (supranuclear gaze palsy, axial rigidity, a tendency to fall backwards, pyramidal signs, subtle dementia or frontal lobe syndrome)

Striatonigral degeneration as part of multiple system atrophy, which often comprises autonomic failure and olivopontocerebellar atrophy

Alzheimer's disease (severe dementia, mild extrapyramidal signs)

Wilson's disease (Kayser–Fleischer rings, cirrhosis, chorea, psychotic behaviour, dysarthria, dystonic spasms and posturing; leading, if untreated, to dementia, severe dysarthria and dysphagia, contractures and immobility)

Jakob–Creutzfeldt disease (prion protein encephalopathy leading to rapidly progressive dementia with myoclonus and multifocal neurological signs including aphasia, cerebellar ataxia, cortical blindness and spasticity)

Hypoparathyroidism (basal ganglia calcification)

NB: A condition which is often misdiagnosed as Parkinson's disease in the elderly is *benign essential tremor* (often autosomal dominant, intention tremor worse with stress, no other neurological abnormality; usually improves when alcohol is taken and sometimes with diazepam or propranolol).

Stiff-person syndrome (SPS)

This is a rare disease of severe progressive muscle stiffness of the spine and lower extremities with superimposed muscle spasms triggered by external stimuli or emotional stress. When stiffness and spasms are present together, patients have difficulty ambulating and are prone to unprotected falls, i.e. falls like a tin soldier. When in spasm the muscles are hard to palpation. Typically symptoms begin between the age of 30 and 50 and respond to benzodiazepines. EMG shows a characteristic abnormality and anti-GAD (glutamic acid decarboxylase) antibodies* are present in 60%. In GAD antibody-positive SPS there is a strong association with other autoimmune diseases such as type 1 diabetes, hyperthyroidism, hypothyroidism, pernicious anaemia and vitiligo (see Vol. 3, Station 5, Skin, Case 8).

*While concluding your summary of Parkinson's disease, it is worthwhile mentioning that a drug history, extraocular muscle movements and cognitive testing would be useful in differentiating other causes of parkinsonism (bearing in mind that the vast majority would have idiopathic Parkinson's disease).

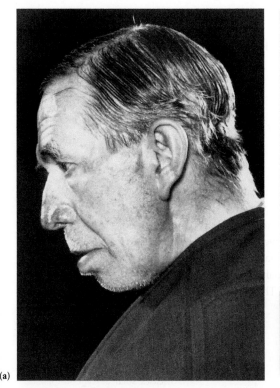
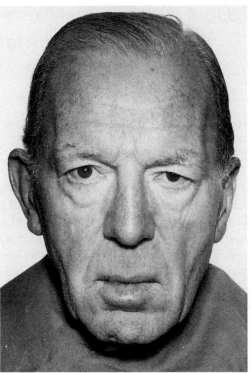

(a)

(b)

Figure C3.5 (a,b) Parkinson's disease.

Case 4 | Charcot–Marie–Tooth disease (hereditary motor and sensory neuropathy)*

Frequency in survey: main focus of a short case or additional feature in 6% of attempts at PACES Station 3, CNS.

Record

There is *distal wasting* of the *lower limb* muscles with relatively well-preserved thigh muscles.† The feet show *pes cavus* and clawing of the toes, and there is weakness of the extensors of the toes and feet. The *ankle jerks* are *absent* and the plantar reflexes show no response. There is only slight *distal involvement* of *superficial* modalities of *sensation* (though occasionally marked sensory loss may lead to digital trophic ulceration). The lateral popliteal (?and ulnar) nerves are palpable (in some families only). The patient has a *steppage gait* (bilateral foot-drop). There is (may be) *wasting of the small muscles of the hand.*

The diagnosis is Charcot–Marie–Tooth disease.*

Patterns of inheritance are variable.

The degree of disability in this condition is commonly surprisingly slight in spite of the remarkable deformities. Toe retraction and talipes equinovarus may occur and fasciculation (much less apparent than in motor neurone disease) is sometimes seen.

The degeneration is mainly in the motor nerves. It is sometimes also found in the dorsal roots and dorsal columns, and slight pyramidal tract degeneration is often seen (however, in classic cases extensor plantars are not found). The condition usually becomes arrested in mid-life. Other members of the patient's family may have a *forme fruste* and show just minor signs such as pes cavus and absent ankle jerks only.

*Charcot–Marie–Tooth disease, which in the past has been called peroneal muscular atrophy, is now called *hereditary motor and sensory neuropathy* (HMSN) and is subdivided into HMSN type I (the demyelinating form of Charcot–Marie–Tooth disease), HMSN type II (the axonal (degeneration) form of Charcot–Marie–Tooth disease), HMSN type III (previously called Déjérine–Scotas disease), and four other subtypes.
†In classic descriptions, as the disease progresses, the wasting creeps very slowly up the limb, inch by inch, involving all muscles.

According to the stage of the disease, the characteristic appearances have been described as 'stork' or 'spindle' legs, 'fat bottle' calves and 'inverted champagne bottles'. The same process may occur in the arms; wasting of the small muscles of the hands is common with a tendency for the fingers to curl and the patient to have difficulty in straightening and abducting them. Classically, Charcot–Marie–Tooth wasting was described as stopping *abruptly* part of the way up the leg. In practice, this is not usually so clear-cut and can be considered to be an example of neuromythology.

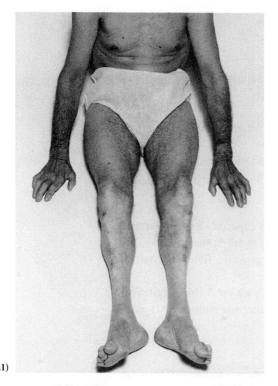

(a1)

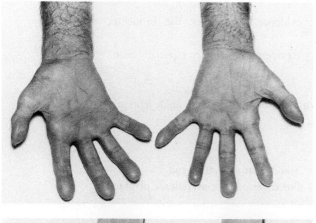

(a2)

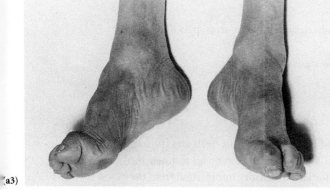

(a3)

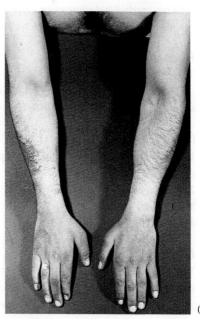

(b)

Figure C3.6 (a1–3) Note that the muscle wasting stops in the thighs, foot-drop, pes cavus, and wasting of the small muscles of the hand all in the same patient. (b) Distal wasting in the upper limbs.

Case 5 | Abnormal gait

Frequency in survey: main focus of a short case or additional feature in 6% of attempts at PACES Station 3, CNS.

Survey note: relative frequencies in the survey were cerebellar ataxia 45%, spastic paraplegia 27%, sensory ataxia 9%, Parkinson's disease 9% and Charcot–Marie–Tooth (steppage gait) 9%. Hemiplegia, waddling gait and gait apraxia did not occur in our survey.

Record 1
The gait is *wide-based* and the arms are held wide (both upper and lower limbs tend to tremble and shake). The patient is *ataxic* and tends to fall to the R/L, especially during the *heel-to-toe* test which he is unable to perform. Romberg's test is negative.

This suggests *cerebellar disease* which is predominantly R/L sided. (Now, if allowed, examine for other cerebellar signs: finger–nose, rapid alternate motion, nystagmus, staccato dysarthria, etc; see Station 3, CNS, Case 7.)

Possible causes
1 Demyelinating disease (?pale discs, pyramidal signs, etc; see Station 3, CNS, Case 10)
2 Tumour (primary or secondary – ? evidence of primary, e.g. bronchus, breast, etc.)
3 Non-metastatic syndrome of malignancy (?evidence of primary, especially bronchus – clubbing, cachexia, etc.)
4 Alcoholic cerebellar degeneration
5 Other cerebellar degenerations (?pes cavus, kyphoscoliosis, absent ankle jerks and extensor plantars, etc. of Friedreich's ataxia)

Record 2
The patient has a *stiff*, awkward 'scissors' or 'wading through mud' gait.

This suggests *spastic paraplegia*. (Now, if allowed, examine tone, reflexes, plantars, sensation, etc; see Station 3, CNS, Case 6)

Possible causes
1 Demyelinating disease (?impaired rapid alternate motion in arms, pale discs, etc; see Station 3, CNS, Case 10)
2 Cord compression (?sensory level with no signs above)
3 Hereditary spastic paraplegia (rare)
4 Cerebral diplegia (rare)

Record 3
The gait is ataxic and *stamping* (his feet tend to 'throw'; both the heels and the toes slap on the ground). The patient walks on a wide base, *watching his feet and the ground* (to some extent he can compensate for lack of sensory information from the

muscles and joints by visual attention). He has difficulty walking heel-to-toe and the ataxia becomes much worse when he closes his eyes; *Romberg's* test is *positive*.

He has *sensory ataxia* (now look for Argyll Robertson pupils and for clinical anaemia).

Possible causes

1 Subacute combined degeneration of the cord (?pyramidal signs, absent ankle jerks plus peripheral neuropathy; anaemia, spleen, etc.; no Argyll Robertson pupils; see Station 3, CNS, Case 37)

2 Tabes dorsalis (?facies, pupils, pyramidal signs if taboparesis, etc; see Station 3, CNS, Case 50)

3 Cervical myelopathy (?mid-cervical reflex pattern in the arms; pyramidal signs in legs; see Station 3, CNS, Case 26)

4 Diabetic pseudotabes (?fundi)

5 Friedreich's ataxia (pes cavus, scoliosis, cerebellar signs, etc; see Station 3, CNS, Case 12)

6 Demyelinating disease (ataxia in multiple sclerosis is usually mainly cerebellar)

Record 4

This (depressed, expressionless, unblinking and stiff) patient *stoops* and his gait, initially *hesitant*, is *shuffling* and has lost its spring. The *arms* are held flexed and they *do not swing*. The hands show a *pill-rolling tremor*. His gait is *festinant*, i.e. he appears to be continually about to fall forward as if chasing his own centre of gravity.

He has *Parkinson's disease*.* (Now examine the wrists for cog-wheel rigidity, elbows for lead-pipe rigidity, and for the glabellar tap sign, etc; see Station 3, CNS, Case 3).

Record 5

The patient has a *steppage* gait. He lifts his R/L foot high to avoid scraping the toe because he has a R/L *foot-drop*. He is unable to walk on his R/L heel (heel walking difficulty is an excellent way of testing subtle dorsiflexion weakness).

Possible causes

1 Lateral popliteal nerve palsy (?evidence of injury just below and lateral to the knee; see Station 3, CNS, Case 22). Checking for weak eversion is useful to differentiate this from an L5 radiculopathy, where it is spared)

2 Charcot–Marie–Tooth disease (?pes cavus, distal wasting of the lower limb muscles with relatively well-preserved thigh muscles, wasting of the small muscles of the hand, palpable lateral popliteal ± ulnar nerve; see Station 3, CNS, Case 4)

---

*In the mild case, tell-tale signs are (i) the lesser swing of one arm compared to the other; (ii) the tremor which is often unilateral.

3 Old polio (?affected leg short due to polio in childhood; see Station 3, CNS, Case 15)

4 Heavy metal poisoning such as lead (rare)

Record 6

The R/L leg is stiff and with each step he tilts the pelvis to the other side, trying to keep the toe off the ground; the R/L leg describes a *semi-circle* with the toe scraping the floor and the forefoot flopping to the ground before the heel. The R/L arm is flexed and held tightly to his side and his fist is clenched.*

The patient has a *hemiplegic gait*.

Record 7

The patient has a lumbar lordosis and walks on a wide base with a *waddling gait*, his trunk moving from side to side and his pelvis dropping on each side as his leg leaves the ground. At each step his toes touch the ground before his heel. (This is a description of the typical gait of a patient with Duchenne muscular dystrophy, the most common cause of a waddling gait. Other conditions causing wasting or weakness of the proximal lower limb (see Station 3, CNS, Case 23) and

pelvic girdle muscles also cause it, e.g. polymyositis, rickets/osteomalacia.)

Record 8

The patient (an elderly person) walks with a broad-based gait, taking short steps and placing his feet flat on the ground like a person 'walking on ice' – so-called 'sticky feet'. This is probably why this gait is also referred to as a magnetic gait. Neither turning nor straight walking is fluent. (There is a tendency to retropulsion which increases the danger of falling.) The patient cannot hop on one foot.

This is *gait apraxia* (a common but little recognized disorder of the elderly; frontal lobe signs including dementia and positive grasp and suck reflexes will confirm the diagnosis). The most common cause is a degenerative process similar to Alzheimer's disease. Other causes include subdural haematoma, tumour, normal pressure hydrocephalus or a lacunar state.

---

*Should not be seen these days with good physiotherapy care!

Case 6 | Spastic paraparesis

Frequency in survey: main focus of a short case or additional feature in 6% of attempts at PACES Station 3, CNS.

Record

The *tone* in the legs is *increased* and they are *weak* (in chronic immobilized cases there may be some disuse atrophy, and in severe cases there may be contractures). There is bilateral *ankle clonus*, patellar clonus and the *plantar* responses are *extensor*. (?Abdominal reflexes; consider testing gait if the patient can walk.*)

The patient has a spastic paraparesis.† The most likely causes are:

1 Multiple sclerosis (?obvious nystagmus, incoordination or staccato speech from the end of the bed; ?impaired rapid alternate motion of arms when you check at the end of your leg examination; see Station 3, CNS, Case 10)

2 Cord compression (?sensory level; root, back or neck pain; no signs above the level of lesion. NB: Cervical spondylosis; see Station 3, CNS, Case 26)

3 Trauma (?scar or deformity on back)

4 Birth injury (cerebral palsy – Little's disease)

5 Motor neurone disease (?no sensory signs, muscle fasciculation, etc; see Station 3, CNS, Case 11).

Other causes

Syringomyelia (?kyphoscoliosis, wasted hands, dissociated sensory loss, Horner's syndrome, etc; see Station 3, CNS, Case 29)

Anterior spinal artery thrombosis (sudden onset, ?dissociated sensory loss up to the level of the lesion)

Friedreich's ataxia (?pes cavus, cerebellar signs, kyphoscoliosis, etc; see Station 3, CNS, Case 12)

Hereditary spastic paraplegia

Subacute combined degeneration of the cord‡ (?posterior column loss, absent ankle jerks,§ peripheral neuropathy, anaemia; see Station 3, CNS, Case 37)

Parasagittal cranial meningioma

Human T-cell lymphotrophic virus type 1 (HTLV-1) infection¶ (Afro-Caribbean populations – tropical spastic paraparesis)

AIDS myelopathy (late phase – direct HIV CNS involvement; see Vol. 3, Station 5, Skin, Case 36)

General paralysis of the insane (?dementia, vacant expression, trombone tremor of the tongue, etc; see Station 3, CNS, Case 50)

Taboparesis (?Argyll Robertson pupils, posterior column loss, etc; see Station 3, CNS, Case 50)

---

*Please note that ataxia can be cerebellar or sensory (see Station 3, CNS, Case 5).

†A clue to the underlying cause of spastic paraparesis may be:
   Cerebellar signs: multiple sclerosis
   Friedreich's ataxia (?pes cavus)
   Wasted hands: cervical spondylosis (?inverted reflexes)
   Syringomyelia (?Horner's)
   Motor neurone disease (?prominent fasciculation).

‡Stocking sensory loss (with or without absent ankle jerks) in association with a spastic paraplegia, i.e. extensor plantars, is strongly suggestive of SACD.

§Absent ankle jerks and upgoing plantars (see Station 3, CNS, Case 24).

¶The other HTLV-1 associated disease is *adult T-cell leukaemia/ lymphoma* which is especially found in southern Japan and the Caribbean islands. The clinical course is often associated with a high white cell count, *hypercalcaemia* and cutaneous involvement. Measurement of HTLV-1 antibodies should always be considered in the patient with unexplained hypercalcaemia. Other HTLV-1 associated diseases include polymyositis, infective dermatitis – a chronic generalized eczema of the skin – and B-cell chronic lymphocytic leukaemia.

HTLV-2 has been found in some patients with T-cell hairy cell leukaemia and in parenteral drug abusers but remains a true orphan virus without, at the time of writing, clear disease association.

Case 7 | Cerebellar syndrome

Frequency in survey: main focus of a short case or additional feature in 5% of attempts at PACES Station 3, CNS.

Record 1

There is nystagmus to the R/L and there is ataxia with the eyes open as shown by impairment of rapid alternate motion on the same side (*dysdiadochokinesis*). The *finger–nose test* is impaired on the R/L with *past pointing* to that side and an *intention tremor* (increases on approaching the target). The *heel–shin test* is impaired on the R/L and the *gait* is *ataxic* with a tendency to fall to the R/L. There is *ataxic dysarthria* with explosive speech (staccato).

The patient has a R/L cerebellar lesion.

Causes include

1 Multiple sclerosis (?internuclear ophthalmoplegia, optic neuritis or atrophy, etc; see Station 3, CNS, Case 10)
2 Brainstem vascular lesion
3 Posterior fossa space-occupying lesion (?papilloedema, e.g. tumour or abscess*)
4 Paraneoplastic cerebellar syndrome (?clubbing, cachexia, etc.)
5 Alcoholic cerebellar degeneration (nutritional†)
6 Friedreich's ataxia (?scoliosis, pes cavus, pyramidal and dorsal column signs, absent ankle jerks, etc; see Station 3, CNS, Case 12)

Other causes of cerebellar ataxia include

Hypothyroidism (?facies, pulse, reflexes, etc; see Vol. 3, Station 5, Endocrine, Case 5)
Anticonvulsant toxicity (especially phenytoin which can cause gross multidirectional nystagmus)
Ataxia–telangiectasia (recessive; from childhood onwards progressive ataxia, choreoathetosis and oculomotor apraxia; later telangiectases on conjunctivae, ears, face and skin creases; low IgA leads to repeated respiratory tract infections; lymphoreticular malignancies are common; death is usually in the second or third decade of life)
Other cerebellar degeneration syndromes‡

Other cerebellar signs

Ipsilateral hypotonia and reduced power
Ipsilateral pendular knee jerk
Skew deviation of the eyes (ipsilateral down and in, contralateral up and out)
Failure of the displaced ipsilateral arm to find its origi-

---

*NB: Otitis media may underlie a cerebellar abscess. Intracranial abscesses may result from direct spread from the upper respiratory passages (nasal sinuses, middle ear, mastoid). Less often, the cause is haematogenous spread (e.g. intrathoracic suppuration), congenital heart disease or fracture of the base of the skull. Abscesses secondary to otitis occur in the temporal lobe about twice as often as they do in the cerebellum.

†Other causes of nutritional deficiency such as pellagra, amoebiasis and protracted vomiting may cause a similar syndrome.
‡The names associated with these other rare hereditary ataxias apart from Friedreich are Charcot, Marie, Déjérine, Alajouanine, André Thomas, Gowers and Holmes. These have now been superseded by a genetic classification: spinocerebellar ataxia types 1–21.

nal posture (ask the patient to hold his arms out in front of him and keep them there. If you push the ipsilateral arm down it will fly past the starting point on release without reflex arrest)

Record 2 (vermis lesion)

There is a wide-based *cerebellar ataxia* (ataxic gait and rombergism more or less the same with eyes open and closed; cf. sensory ataxia – worse with eyes closed), but there is little or no abnormality of the limbs when tested separately on the bed. This suggests a lesion of the cerebellar vermis.

Case 8 | Hemiplegia

Frequency in survey: main focus of a short case or additional feature in 4% of attempts at PACES Station 3, CNS.

Record

There is a R/L *upper motor neurone* weakness of the facial muscles.* The R/L *arm* and *leg* are *weak* (without wasting) with *increased tone* and *hyperreflexia*. The R/L plantar is *extensor* and the *abdominal reflexes* are *diminished* on the R/L side.

This is a R/L hemiplegia.

There is also (may be) *hemisensory loss* on the R/L side. Visual field testing reveals (may be) a R/L homonymous hemianopia. The most likely causes are:

1 Cerebrovascular accident due to cerebral:
   (a) thrombosis (?hypertension)
   (b) haemorrhage (?hypertension)
   (c) embolism (?atrial fibrillation, murmurs, bruits)
2 Brain tumour (?insidious onset, papilloedema, headaches; ?evidence of primary, e.g. clubbing).

A right-sided hemiplegia associated with dysphasia would suggest (in a right-handed patient) that the causative lesion is affecting the speech centres in the dominant hemisphere (see Station 3, CNS, Case 40) as well as the motor cortex (precentral gyrus) and if there are sensory signs, the sensory cortex (postcentral gyrus). If cerebrovascular in origin, the causative lesion is likely to be in the *carotid* distribution.

The presence of signs such as nystagmus, ocular palsy, dysphagia (?nasogastric or PEG feeding tube) and cerebellar signs suggests that the hemiparesis is due to a brainstem lesion. If cerebrovascular in origin, the lesion is likely to be in *vertebrobasilar* distribution (see Station 3, CNS, Case 44 for the eponymous syndromes†).

Parietal lobe and related signs‡

Agnosia. Though peripheral sensation is intact (tactile, visual, auditory), the patient fails to appreciate the significance of the sensory stimulus without the aid of other senses.

Tactile agnosia or astereognosis (contralateral posterior parietal lobe) – inability to recognize a familiar object placed in the hand (e.g. pen, keys) with the eyes closed. Opening the eyes or hearing the keys rattle may allow recognition

Visual agnosia (parietooccipital lesions – especially in the left hemisphere of right-handed patients) – the patient is not able to identify the familiar object by sight (e.g. a pen, surroundings) but may do at once when he is allowed to handle it

Auditory agnosia (temporal lobe of dominant hemisphere) – the patient may only be able to recognize the sound of a voice, telephone or music when he is allowed to use the senses of vision or touch

Autotopagnosia (usually a left hemiplegia in a right-handed person) – difficulty in perceiving or identifying the various parts of the body; the patient may be unaware of the left side of his body. It may be associated with anosognosia in which case there is no appreciation of a disability (e.g. hemiplegia, blindness) on the same side

---

*In an upper motor neurone lesion, the lower face is much weaker than the upper because the muscles frontalis, orbicularis oculi and corrugator superficialis ('raise your eyebrows', 'screw your eyes up tight', 'frown') are bilaterally inner-vated from the corticobulbar fibres and are all only minimally impaired.

†These are in fact rarely used in everyday practice.

‡These did not occur in our survey of MRCP short cases.

Apraxia. Whereas in agnosia the difficulty is in recognition, in apraxia it is in execution. Though power, sensation and coordination are all normal, the patient is unable to perform certain familiar activities. It may affect:

The upper limbs, e.g. difficulty using a pen, comb or toothbrush, winding a watch, dressing or undressing ('dressing apraxia*')

The lower limbs – may mimic ataxia or weakness† – the patient may appear unable to lift one foot in front of the other (gait apraxia)

The trunk – the patient may have difficulty seating himself on a chair or lavatory seat, getting on to his bed, or turning over in bed

The face – the patient may be unable to whistle, put out his tongue or close his eyes.

The lesions (tumours or atrophy) tend to be in the corpus callosum, parietal lobes and premotor areas. Dominant lobe lesions may produce bilateral apraxia.

Unilateral left-sided apraxia may be caused by a lesion in the right posterior parietal region or in the corpus callosum of a right-handed patient. The lesion in 'dressing apraxia' is usually in the right parietooccipital region. In 'constructional apraxia' (most often seen in patients with hepatic encephalopathy), the patient is unable to construct simple figures such as triangles, squares or crosses from matchsticks.

Dyslexia (impairment of reading ability), ***dysgraphia*** (impairment of writing ability) and ***dyscalculia*** (difficulty with calculating) usually represent lesions in the posterior parietal lobe.

Proprioceptive loss due to a parietal lesion may not infrequently be seen and may present as an 'alien hand' – the patient failing to control the limb when it is not in direct vision.

---

*Some authorities consider this to be a visuospatial right hemisphere disorder and not a true apraxia.
†A parietal lobe lesion may cause ataxia, hemiparesis or marked astereognosis. In hemiparesis of parietal origin, the limbs are often hypotonic with an absent plantar response, rather than spastic. The limb muscles may even waste (like a lower motor neurone lesion). Often the patient is disinclined to move the limb rather than being actually paralysed.

Case 9 | Muscular dystrophy

Frequency in survey: main focus of a short case or additional feature in 3% of attempts at PACES Station 3, CNS.

Survey note: most cases in the surveys seem to be facioscapulohumeral except one possible case of limb-girdle type.

Record 1

The patient has a dull, unlined, expressionless face (*myopathic facies*) with lips that are (usually) open and slack. There is *wasting* of the *facial* and *limb-girdle muscles*, and the superior margins of the scapulae (viewed from the front) are (may be) visible above the clavicles. The movements of smiling, whistling and closing the eyes are impaired. There is *winging of the scapulae* (when the patient leans against a wall with arms extended). There is (may be) involvement of the trunk and legs (anterior tibials may cause bilateral foot-drop) now or in the future.

The diagnosis is *facioscapulohumeral* muscular dystrophy* (autosomal dominant, course variable but usually relatively benign).

Record 2

There is *limb-girdle wasting* and *weakness* which affects some groups of muscles more than others (e.g. deltoid and spinati are usually spared), and the *face* is *spared*. There is (not uncommonly) enlargement of the calf muscles.

These features suggest *limb-girdle* muscular dystrophy (autosomal recessive, both sexes affected equally, more benign if the upper limb is involved first, usually begins in the second or third decade, sometimes arrests but usually patients are severely disabled within 20 years of onset).

Other muscular dystrophies

Duchenne or pseudohypertrophic – X-linked, severe, onset age 3–4 years, initially enlargement of calves, buttocks and infraspinati (this disappears later) while other muscles (especially the proximal lower limb) waste; waddling lordotic gait; usually confined to wheelchair by age of 10 years; cardiac muscle involved; face spared; death from respiratory infection and/or cardiac failure commonly at about age of 20

Benign X-linked (Becker) muscular dystrophy – similar to Duchenne but much less severe; onset 5–25 years; confined to wheelchair 25 years later

Distal muscular dystrophy – dominant; most cases occur in Sweden; eventually spreads to proximal muscles unlike peroneal muscular atrophy (see Station 3, CNS, Case 4) with which it is most often confused

Oculopharyngeal muscular dystrophy – sporadic or dominant; first ptosis, then ophthalmoplegia, face and neck muscles are often mildly involved. Dysphagia is usually the most prominent symptom and ptosis is often complete. It has been shown to be due to a mutation in the PABP gene.

---

*There may be an inflammatory component in the aetiology of facioscapulohumeral muscular dystrophy, as perivascular inflammation may be seen on muscle biopsy and *retinal microvascular abnormalities* (sparse and dilated (telangiectatic) peripheral retinal vessels which leak, causing exudate to track to the posterior pole with consequent retinal detachment and blindness) also characterize the disorder. *Sensorineural deafness* may occur but clinical cardiomyopathy is rare.

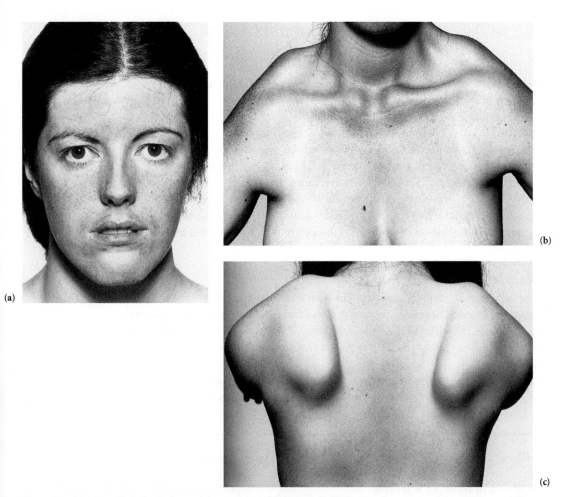

Figure C3.7 (a) Myopathic facies (facioscapulohumeral muscular dystrophy). (b) The superior margins of the scapulae are visible from the front (same patient as (a)). (c) Winging of the scapulae (same patient).

Case 10 | Multiple sclerosis

Frequency in survey: main focus of a short case or additional feature in 3% of attempts at PACES Station 3, CNS.

Record 1

The patient (?a young adult) has *ataxic nystagmus* (see Station 3, CNS, Case 32), *internuclear ophthalmoplegia* (see Station 3, CNS, Case 16), *temporal pallor of the discs* (see Vol. 3, Station 5, Eyes, Case 3), and *slurred speech* (see Station 3, CNS, Case 36) with *ataxia* (see Station 3, CNS, Case 5) and widespread *cerebellar* signs (see Station 3, CNS, Case 7). There are *pyramidal* signs and *dorsal column* signs.

The likely diagnosis is demyelinating disease* (a useful euphemism for multiple sclerosis).

Record 2

The legs of this (?middle-aged) patient have increased tone, they are bilaterally spastic and weak. There is bilateral *ankle clonus* and patellar clonus and the *plantars* are *extensor*. The *abdominal reflexes* are absent. The heel–shin test suggests some *ataxia* in the legs and there is slight *impairment of rapid alternate motion* in the upper limbs.

These features suggest that this *spastic paraplegia* is due to demyelinating disease. An examination of the fundi may show involvement of the discs.†

Male-to-female ratio is 2/3.

Features of multiple sclerosis
Rare in tropical climates
Unpredictable course
May present acutely, subacutely, remittently or insidiously
Relapses and remissions (occurring in two-thirds of patients) are often a useful diagnostic pointer
May very closely imitate other neurological conditions (including neurosis)
Fatigue or a rise in temperature may exacerbate symptoms (the patient may be able to get into, but not out of, a hot bath)
Paroxysmal symptoms (e.g. trigeminal neuralgia) may occur and may respond to carbamazepine

Euphoria despite severe disability (depression is more common)
Lhermitte's phenomenon may occur (see Station 3, CNS, Case 37)
Benign course more likely if:
  pure sensory presentation
  infrequent relapses and long remissions
  onset with optic neuritis, or sensory or motor symptoms – in contrast to those of brainstem or cerebellar lesions
  benign condition 5 years after onset
The visual evoked response (VER) test is useful in a patient with an isolated lesion which may be due to multiple sclerosis, e.g. spastic paraparesis,† VIth nerve palsy, trigeminal neuralgia, facial palsy, postural vertigo

*The features in this *record* are some of those which are commonly seen in a case of MS. There are, of course, few neurological signs which it may not produce.
†Multiple sclerosis may present in middle age with insidious spastic paraplegia mimicking cord compression. Signs above the level of the cord lesion may point clinically to demyelination as the cause. In this case the slight cerebellar signs are highly suggestive of MS. However, syringomyelia or a tumour at the foramen magnum could also be the cause. If the diagnosis is of a tumour, there may be papilloedema. If the diagnosis is MS, the discs may show global or temporal pallor (and the VERs may be delayed even if, as is often the case, the discs are normal).

Cerebrospinal fluid examination may show an increase in total protein up to $1\,\mathrm{g\,L^{-1}}$ or an increase in lymphocytes up to 50 cells $\mathrm{mm^{-3}}$ in 50% of patients. Oligoclonal bands in the γ region on immunoelectrophoresis that are unique to CSF only (i.e. are not found in serum) are found in over 95% of patients with MS. CSF oligoclonal bands are also found in some patients with CNS infection, and occasionally in patients with strokes or brain tumours.

MRI scans often detect many more MS lesions than are suspected clinically (CT scans can also detect lesions but are much less sensitive than MRI). Gadolinium enhancement of the MRI lesions suggests active inflammation.

Case 11 | Motor neurone disease

Frequency in survey: main focus of a short case or additional feature in 3% of attempts at PACES Station 3, CNS.

Record
This patient has *weakness, wasting* and *fasciculation* of the muscles of the hand (see Station 3, CNS, Case 52), arms and shoulder girdle (***progressive muscular atrophy*** in its pure form is characterized by minimal pyramidal signs), but the upper limb reflexes are exaggerated (reflexes in motor neurone disease may be increased, decreased or absent depending on which lesion is predominant). There is upper motor neurone *spastic weakness* with *exaggerated reflexes* in the legs (***amyotrophic lateral sclerosis****). There is ankle clonus and the patient has bilateral *extensor plantar* responses. The patient also has (may have) indistinct *nasal speech*, a *wasted fasciculating tongue* and *palatal paralysis* (***progressive bulbar palsy***; see Station 3, CNS, Case 21). There are *no sensory signs.*

The diagnosis is motor neurone disease.

Other conditions in which fasciculation may occur
Cervical spondylosis (see below)

Syringomyelia (fasciculation less apparent, dissociated sensory loss, etc; see Station 3, CNS, Case 29)

Charcot–Marie–Tooth disease (fasciculation less apparent, distal wasting of the lower limb muscles with relatively well-preserved thigh muscles, pes cavus, sometimes palpable lateral popliteal and ulnar nerves, etc; see Station 3, CNS, Case 4)

Acute stages of poliomyelitis (and rarely also in old polio; see below)

Neuralgic amyotrophy (pain, wasting and weakness of a group of muscles in a limb, sometimes following a viral infection; usually C5,6 innervated muscles – shoulder)

Thyrotoxic myopathy (tachycardia, tremor, sweating, goitre with bruit, lid lag, etc; see Vol. 3, Station 5, Endocrine, Case 3)

Syphilitic amyotrophy (see below)

Chronic asymmetrical spinal muscular atrophy (see below)

After exercise in fit adults

After the Tensilon test (see Station 3, CNS, Case 27)

Benign giant fasciculation

Differential diagnosis of motor neurone disease
Cervical cord compression (see Station 3, CNS, Case 26) is the most important condition to be excluded in the diagnosis of motor neurone disease. Bulbar palsy and sensory signs should be carefully sought, but a cervical MRI scan is often required to exclude it. *Syphilitic amyotrophy* (slowly progressing wasting of the muscles of the

---

*Glutamate toxicity has been implicated as a factor leading to neuronal damage in amyotrophic lateral sclerosis. Trials suggest riluzole may retard progression and lengthen survival.

shoulder girdle and upper arm with loss of reflexes and no sensory loss; fasciculation of the tongue may occur) should always be excluded in the investigation of motor neurone disease as it is amenable to treatment. Occasionally patients with *old polio*, after many years, develop a progressive wasting disease (with prominent fasciculation) which is indistinguishable from progressive muscular atrophy motor neurone disease.

Another condition that needs to be considered is *spinal muscular atrophy of juvenile onset* type 3 (Kugelberg–Welander disease). This is due to a mutation in the survival motor neurone gene on chromosome 5. The onset is in childhood or in the teen years. It is a milder form of spinal muscular atrophy affecting mostly proximal muscles, but the patients can stand and walk unaided. It can be distinguished from chronic inflammatory demyelinating polyneuropathy by the presence of normal CSF protein and normal nerve conduction studies.

CNS lymphoma may also present with clinical features suggestive of MND and is an important differential diagnosis to exclude.

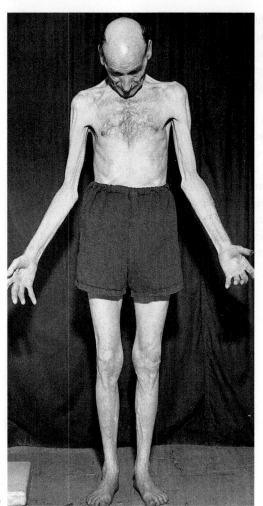

(a1)

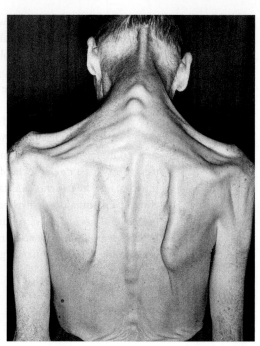

(a2)

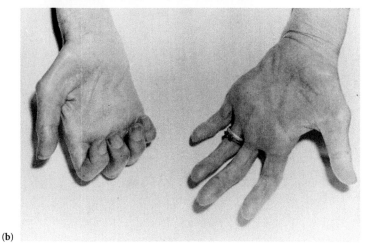

(b)

Figure C3.8 (a1,2) Generalized muscle wasting (note weakness of the extensors of the neck). (b) Wasting of the small muscles of the hand.

Case 12 | Friedreich's ataxia

Frequency in survey: main focus of a short case or additional feature in 3% of attempts at PACES Station 3, CNS.

Record

There is *pes cavus, (kypho)scoliosis* and (may be) a deformed and high-arched palate. The patient is *ataxic* and clumsy with an *intention tremor* and his *head shakes*. There is *nystagmus* (often slow and coarse and observed before formal examination) and *dysarthria* (slow and slurred or scanning and explosive). There is (?gross) bilateral impairment of rapid alternate motion, finger–nose and heel–shin tests. Knee and *ankle jerks* are *absent* and the *plantar responses* are *extensor*. *Position and vibration* sense are diminished in the feet.

The diagnosis is Friedreich's ataxia.

Other features (if asked)

1 Cardiomyopathy (may cause sudden death)
2 Optic and retinal atrophy
3 Diabetes mellitus
4 Mild dementia

The condition is one of the hereditary spinocerebellar degenerations. It is an autosomal recessive trinucleotide repeat disorder with a GAA unstable expansion in the long arm of chromosome 9. The fully-fledged syndrome is rare among affected family members who more commonly show slight signs of abnormality in the lower limbs, chiefly pes cavus and absent reflexes (*formes fruste*).

The major classic ataxic conditions which may need to be differentiated from Friedreich's ataxia, particularly if the latter is mild and presents late, are MS and tabes dorsalis (rare). Typical features which may help to differentiate these conditions are shown in Table C3.4.

Other conditions which may have features of Friedreich's ataxia (all are recessive)

Bassen–Kornzweig syndrome (abetalipoproteinae-mia*) – steatorrhoea, acanthosis, pigmentary retinal degeneration and a spinocerebellar degeneration which resembles Friedreich's ataxia

Refsum's disease (elevated serum phytanic acid due to defective lipid α-oxidase) – pupillary abnormalities, optic atrophy, deafness, pigmentary retinal degeneration, cardiomyopathy, icthyosis and a Friedreich-like ataxia

Roussy–Lévy syndrome (this is a variant of type I hereditary motor and sensory neuropathy and its features are intermediate between Charcot–Marie–Tooth disease and Friedreich's ataxia) – ataxia, areflexia, pes cavus, upper limb tremor and kyphoscoliosis but absence of nystagmus, dysarthria, extensor plantar responses and posterior column signs

---

*LDL, VLDL and chylomicra are absent from the serum, cholesterol is very low and triglycerides are barely detectable.

Table C3.4 Features which may help to differentiate the major ataxic conditions

	Friedreich's ataxia	Multiple sclerosis	Tabes dorsalis
Family history	Major	Minor	None
Onset before age 15	Usual	Rare	Rare
Knee and ankle jerks	Absent	Usually exaggerated	Absent
Spine	(Kypho)scoliosis	Normal	Normal
Feet shape	Pes cavus	Normal	Normal
Pupils	Normal	Normal	Argyll Robertson
Plantars	↑	↑	↓ or → (unless taboparesis)
Pain and deep pressure	Normal	Normal	Absent
Romberg's sign	±	−	+

Case 13 | Visual field defect

Frequency in survey: main focus of a short case or additional feature in 3% of attempts at PACES Station 3, CNS.

Record 1

There is a *homonymous hemianopia*. This suggests a lesion of the *optic tract* behind the optic chiasma (with sparing of the macula and hence normal visual acuity).

Likely causes

1 Cerebrovascular accident (?ipsilateral hemiplegia, atrial fibrillation, heart murmurs or bruits, hypertension)
2 Tumour (?ipsilateral pyramidal signs, papilloedema)

Record 2

There is a *bitemporal* visual field defect worse on R/L side. This suggests a lesion at the *optic chiasma*. (NB: There may be optic atrophy, sometimes with a central scotoma, on the R/L side due to simultaneous compression of the optic nerve by the lesion.)

Possible causes

1 Pituitary tumour (?acromegaly, hypopituitarism, gynaecomastia, galactorrhoea, menstrual disturbance, etc.)
2 Craniopharyngioma (?calcification on skull X-ray)
3 Suprasellar meningioma
4 Aneurysm
Rarer causes are glioma, granuloma and metastasis

Record 3

The visual fields are considerably constricted, the central field of vision being spared. This is *tunnel vision*.* I would like to examine the fundi, looking for evidence of retinitis pigmentosa, glaucoma (pathological cupping) or widespread choroidoretinitis. (Hysteria may occasionally be a cause; papilloedema causes enlargement of the blind spot and peripheral constriction.)

Record 4

There is a *central scotoma*. (NB: The discs may be pale (atrophy), swollen and pink (papillitis), or normal (retrobulbar neuritis).)

Causes to be considered

Demyelinating diseases (?nystagmus, cerebellar signs, etc.; however, multiple sclerosis frequently causes retrobulbar neuritis without other signs)

---

*The Committee on the Safety of Medicines has received reports of visual field defects associated with the antiepileptic drug viga- batrin, including three cases of severe, symptomatic, persistent visual field constriction (tunnel vision).

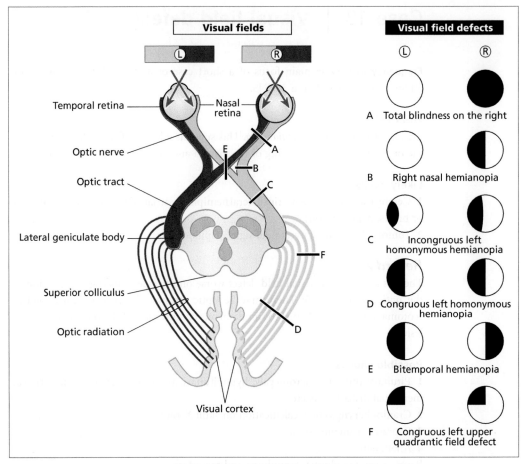

Figure C3.9 The visual pathways and visual field defects resulting from different lesions. If there is exact overlap of the field defects from both eyes, the defect is said to be congruous. If not, it is incongruous. The defects in B and E above are incongruous. Though the complete homonymous hemianopia in D is congruous, lesions of the optic tract (C), which are comparatively rare, produce characteristic incongruous visual changes. The fibres serving identical points in the homonymous half fields do not fully co-mingle in the anterior optic tract so lesions encroaching on this structure produce incongruous and usually incomplete homonymous hemianopias. Lesions of the geniculate ganglia, visual radiations or visual cortex produce congruous visual field defects. F represents a lesion of the temporal loop of the optic radiation.

Compression*
Ischaemia
Leber's optic atrophy (males/females = 6/1)
Toxins (e.g. methyl alcohol)
Macular disease
Nutritional (famine, etc., tobacco–alcohol amblyopia, vitamin B_{12} deficiency, diabetes mellitus)

Record 5

There is *homonymous upper quadrantic visual field loss.* This suggests a lesion in the temporal cortex.
NB: Field defects may sometimes originate from retinal damage, e.g. occlusion of a branch of the retinal artery or a large area of choroidoretinitis.

*There may be clues as to the site of the compression. (i) A lesion in the frontal lobe which compresses the optic nerve may cause dementia. (ii) It may also cause contralateral papilloedema (the *Foster–Kennedy syndrome* due to a frontal tumour or aneurysm, e.g. olfactory groove meningioma). (iii) A lesion in front of the chiasma involving crossing fibres that loop forward into the opposite optic nerve may cause a contralateral upper temporal quadrantic field defect. (iv) A lesion at the chiasma may cause a bitemporal field defect. (v) A lesion at the lateral chiasma (pituitary tumour, aneurysm, meningioma) involving the terminal optic tract as well as the optic nerve may cause a homonymous hemianopia.

Case 14 | Ulnar nerve palsy

Frequency in survey: main focus of a short case or additional feature in 2% of attempts at PACES Station 3, CNS.

Record

The hand shows *generalized muscle wasting** and *weakness* which *spares* the *thenar eminence.* There is sensory loss over the *fifth finger*, the *adjacent half* of the *fourth finger* and the dorsal and palmar aspects of the *medial side* of the *hand.*† (Look for hyperextension at the metacarpophalangeal joints with flexion of the interphalangeal joints in the fourth and fifth fingers – the *ulnar claw hand.*)‡

The patient has an ulnar nerve lesion. (Now examine the elbow for a cause.)

Likely causes

1 Fracture or dislocation at the elbow (?scar or deformity; history of injury)
2 Osteoarthrosis at the elbow with osteophytic encroachment on the ulnar nerve in the cubital tunnel ('filling in' of the ulnar groove due to palpable enlargement of the nerve; limitation of elbow movement is often seen; certain occupations predispose to osteoarthrosis at the elbow – see below)

Other causes

Occupations with constant leaning on elbows (clerks, secretaries on telephone, etc.)

Occupations with constant flexion and extension at the elbow (bricklayer, painter/decorator, carpenter, roofer – shallow ulnar groove will predispose; these occupations may also lead to osteoarthrosis – see above)

Excessive carrying angle at elbow (malunited fracture of the humerus or disturbance of growth leading to cubitus valgus and, over the years, 'tardy ulnar nerve palsy')

Injuries at the wrist or in the palm (different degrees of the syndrome depending on which branches of the nerve are damaged, e.g. occupations using screwdrivers, drills, etc.)

The causes of mononeuritis multiplex (diabetes, polyarteritis nodosa and Churg–Strauss syndrome, rheumatoid, SLE, Wegener's, sarcoid, carcinoma, amyloid, leprosy, Sjögren's syndrome, Lyme disease)

NB: Other causes of wasting of the small muscles of the hand (see Station 3, CNS, Case 52) may sometimes resemble ulnar nerve palsy. The major features pointing

---

*(i) The *hypothenar eminence wastes*, though in the manual worker with thickened skin the hand contour may be preserved and the wasting may only be detected on palpation. Loss of other small muscles is seen from (ii) *loss of the first dorsal interosseous* in the dorsal space between the first and second metacarpals, and (iii) *guttering of the dorsum* of the hand, which becomes more prominent as the lesion advances.

†*Record* (continuation): there is *weakness of abduction and adduction of the fingers*, and *adduction of the extended thumb* against the palm (inability to hold a piece of paper between the thumb and index finger without pinch-flexing the affected thumb (using the flexor pollicis longus, the median nerve) –

Froment's 'thumb sign', now usually referred to as the journal sign). Flexion of the fourth and fifth fingers is weak. When the proximal portions of these fingers are held immobilized, flexion of the terminal phalanges is not possible. There is also *wasting of the medial aspect of the forearm* (flexor carpi ulnaris and half of the flexor digitorum profundus). When the hand is flexed to the ulnar side against resistance, the tendon of flexor carpi ulnaris is not palpable.

‡The ulnar claw hand or partial *main-en-griffe* is due to the unopposed action of the long extensors and is only seen in the fourth and fifth fingers because the radial lumbricals are supplied by the median nerve.

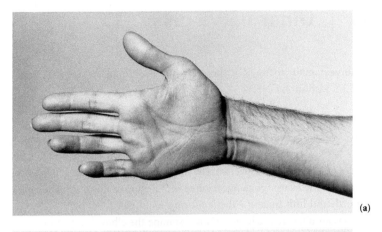

(a)

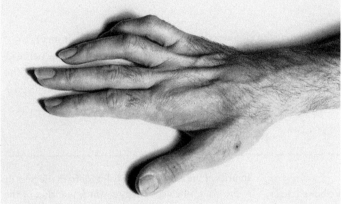

(b)

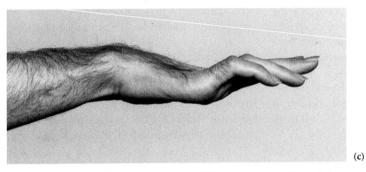

(c)

Figure C3.10 (a) Loss of hypothenar eminence. (b) Dorsal guttering. (c) Typical ulnar claw hand.

to ulnar nerve palsy as the cause are *sparing of the thenar eminence* and the characteristic sensory loss pattern. The main distinguishing features of the differential diagnoses which may mimic the muscle wasting of ulnar paralysis are:

Syringomyelia – dissociated sensory loss extending beyond the ulnar zone; loss of arm reflexes; ? Horner's

C8 lesion (e.g. Pancoast's syndrome) – sensory loss involves radial side of fourth finger, ?Horner's

Cervical rib – objective sensory disturbances are usually slight or absent and without characteristic ulnar distribution

Case 15 | Old polio

Frequency in survey: main focus of a short case or additional feature in 2% of attempts at PACES Station 3, CNS.

Record

The R/L leg is *short, wasted, weak* and *flaccid* with *reduced (or absent) reflexes* and a normal plantar response. There is *no sensory defect*. The disparity in the length of the limbs suggests growth impairment in the affected limb since early childhood. The complete absence of sensory and pyramidal signs points to a condition affecting only lower motor neurones.*

The diagnosis is old polio affecting the R/L leg.

If you see one limb smaller than the other, a possible differential diagnosis to consider is infantile hemiplegia. In this, there is usually hypoplasia of the whole of that side of the body and the neurological signs will reflect a contralateral hemisphere lesion (i.e. upper motor neurone).

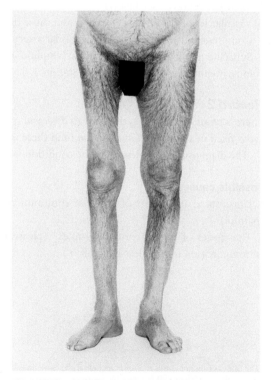

Figure C3.11 Generalized wasting of the right lower limb due to old poliomyelitis.

*Fasciculation is only occasionally seen in old polio. Patients with old polio for many years may develop new wasting and weakness in previously unaffected muscles with postexertional myalgia and chronic fatigue. This is known as the post polio syndrome.

Case 16 | Ocular palsy

Frequency in survey: main focus of a short case or additional feature in 2% of attempts at PACES Station 3, CNS.

Record 1

The patient has a *convergent strabismus* at rest. There is *impairment* of the *lateral movement* of the R/L eye and *diplopia* is worse on looking to the R/L (the outermost image comes from the affected eye).

The patient has a *VIth nerve palsy*.

Possible causes

1 The causes of mononeuritis multiplex*
2 Multiple sclerosis (?ipsilateral facial palsy because the VIth and VIIth nuclei are very close in the pons; ?nystagmus, cerebellar signs, pyramidal signs, pale discs, etc; see Station 3, CNS, Case 10)
3 Raised intracranial pressure (?papilloedema) causing stretching of the nerve (a false localizing sign) during its long intracranial course
4 Neoplasm (?papilloedema; associated ipsilateral facial palsy if pontine tumour)
5 Myasthenia gravis (see below)
6 Vascular lesions (probably common as a cause of 'idiopathic' VIth nerve palsy)
7 Compression by aneurysm (ectatic basilar artery – uncommon)
8 Subacute meningitis (carcinomatous; lymphomatous; fungal (NB: AIDS); tuberculous; meningovascular syphilis; see Station 3, CNS, Case 50)

Record 2

There is *ptosis*. Lifting the eyelids reveals *divergent strabismus* and a *dilated pupil*. The eye is fixed in a *down and out position* (and there is *angulated diplopia*).

The diagnosis is complete (NB: the condition is often partial) *IIIrd nerve palsy*.†

Possible causes

1 Unruptured aneurysm‡ of posterior communicating (or internal carotid) artery (painful)
2 The causes of mononeuritis multiplex* (please note that diabetes is the most common reason for painless IIIn palsy)

---

*The causes of mononeuritis multiplex include diabetes mellitus, polyarteritis nodosa and Churg–Strauss syndrome, rheumatoid disease, SLE, Wegener's granulomatosis, sarcoidosis, carcinoma, amyloidosis, leprosy, Sjögren's syndrome and Lyme disease.
†Preserved intorsion in a complete IIIn palsy suggests that the IVn is unaffected.

‡If the ophthalmoplegia is predominant compared to the ptosis/pupil dilation, the cause is likely to be vascular (intrinsic). If the ophthalmoplegia is minimal compared to the ptosis/pupil dilation, the cause is more likely to be extrinsic compression by aneurysm, pituitary tumour, meningioma, etc.

3 Vascular lesion* (if there is a contralateral hemiplegia, the diagnosis is Weber's syndrome; see Station 3, CNS, Case 44)

4 Mid-brain demyelinating lesion† (?cerebellar signs, staccato speech, pale discs, etc; Station 3, CNS, Case 10)

5 Myasthenia gravis (see below)

Other causes of a IIIrd nerve palsy

Subacute meningitis (carcinomatous; lymphomatous; fungal (NB: AIDS); tuberculous; meningovascular syphilis – at one time the most common cause, now very rare; see Station 3, CNS, Case 50)

Ophthalmoplegic migraine (similar to posterior communicating artery aneurysm except that it begins in childhood or adolescence, recovery is more rapid and is always complete; recovery is never complete with an aneurysm)

Parasellar neoplasms*

Sphenoidal wing meningiomata*

Carcinomatous lesions of the skull base*

Other causes of ocular palsy

Internuclear ophthalmoplegia (ipsilateral impaired adduction with contralateral abduction nystagmus. Convergence may be preserved. Slow adduction of the ipsilateral eye on repetitive saccadic movements (rather than pursuit) demonstrates subtle internuclear ophthalmoplegia; ataxic nystagmus distinguishes it from bilateral VIth nerve palsy (see Station 3, CNS, Case 32) ?cerebellar signs)

Exophthalmic ophthalmoplegia (exophthalmos and diplopia – upward and outward gaze most often reduced)

Myasthenia gravis (?ptosis, variable strabismus, facial weakness with a snarling smile, proximal muscle weakness, weak nasal voice, all of which worsen with repetition; see Station 3, CNS, Case 27. The key finding is fatiguable weakness and this should be explored by testing eye movements with the eyes held in one position in between the movements, and by getting the patient to count up to, say, 50. NB: It may superficially resemble IIIrd or VIth nerve palsy). Pupils should never be involved in myasthenia‡

Cavernous sinus and superior orbital fissure syndromes (total or subtotal ophthalmoplegia which is often painful, together with sensory loss over the first division of the Vth nerve – absent corneal reflex; it is due to a tumour or carotid aneurysm affecting the IIIrd, IVth, Vth and VIth nerves as they travel together through the cavernous sinus into the superior orbital fissure – see Fig. I5.64d, Vol. 3, Station 5, Endocrine, Case 4)

Fourth nerve palsy (adducted eye cannot look downwards – the patient experiences 'one above the other' diplopia when attempting to do this; angulated diplopia occurs when looking down and out; the diplopia is worse when reading and going down stairs; skew deviation of the two images should be enquired about and, if present, is strongly suggestive of a IVth cranial nerve palsy, though it may also be seen with brainstem lesions)

Ocular myopathy (see Station 3, CNS, Case 9 and Footnote, Station 3, CNS, Case 18)

---

*If the ophthalmoplegia is predominant compared to the ptosis/pupil dilation, the cause is likely to be vascular (intrinsic). If the ophthalmoplegia is minimal compared to the ptosis/pupil dilation, the cause is more likely to be extrinsic compression by aneurysm, pituitary tumor, meningioma, etc.

†Third nerve palsy is rare in demyelinating disease; internuclear ophthalmoplegia (see Station 3, CNS, Cases 10 and 32) is a much more common result of this condition.

‡A good and easy test to differentiate the different causes of ptosis is pupillary size and reaction (dilated (IIIn palsy); constricted (Horner's syndrome); normal (myasthenia; or early diabetic cranial neuropathy)).

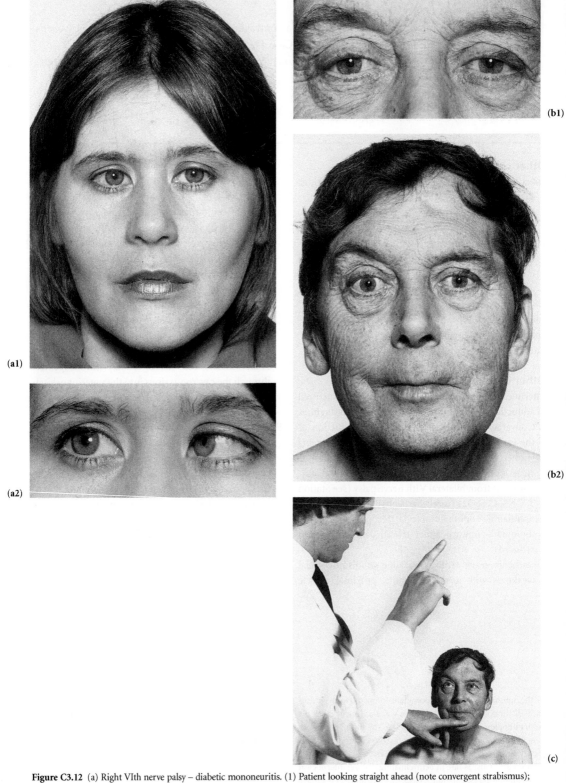

Figure C3.12 (a) Right VIth nerve palsy – diabetic mononeuritis. (1) Patient looking straight ahead (note convergent strabismus); (2) looking to the right. (b1,2) Left IIIrd nerve palsy (note ptosis and mydriasis of the left pupil). The patient had had surgery for a pituitary tumour (note scar on upper forehead and left frontal alopecia). (c) Upward gaze being tested (note the failure of the left eye to follow the examiner's finger). (d) *(Opposite)* Complete right IIIrd nerve palsy: (1) note mydriasis of the right pupil and the down and outward deviation of the right eye (due to the unopposed action of the superior oblique and lateral rectus muscles innervated by the IVth and VIth nerves, respectively); (2) testing eye movements (note the failure of the right eye to look straight, upwards, downwards, upwards and laterally, and medially).

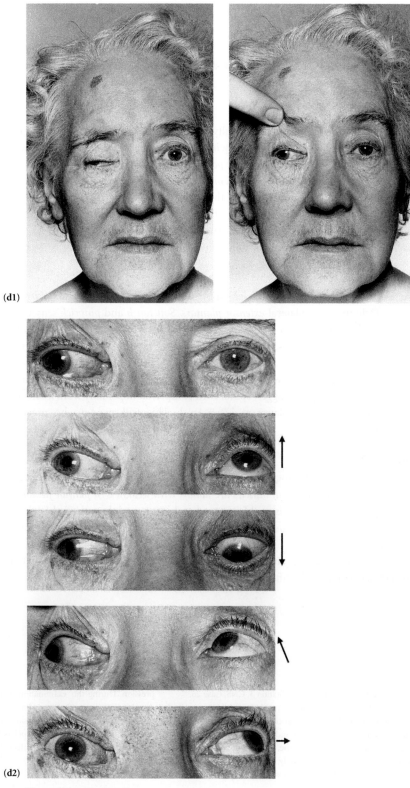

(d1)

(d2)

Figure C3.12 *(Continued)*

Case 17 | Spinal cord compression*

Frequency in survey: main focus of a short case or additional feature in 2% of attempts at PACES Station 3, CNS.

Record 1

This patient (who complains of difficulty in walking) has a *monoparesis* of the R/L leg with *hypertonia, muscular weakness without wasting, hyperreflexia* and an *extensor plantar* response. There is loss of *joint position* and *vibration* senses on the side of the monoparesis and loss of *pain* and *temperature* senses on the opposite side below the level (determine the upper limit of the sensory loss) of (e.g.) T8–9 segments.

These features suggest a diagnosis of the Brown–Séquard syndrome resulting from hemisection of the spinal cord. Among the causes are injury, tumour, late myelopathy from radiation therapy and multiple sclerosis.

Record 2

There is *muscular weakness* in both legs, more on the R/L side with *hypertonia, hyper-reflexia* (?clonus) and bilateral *extensor plantars*. *Soft touch* and *pinprick* sensations are diminished in both legs extending upwards to the *level* of (e.g.) T8 segment.†
Joint position and *vibration* senses are intact. There is *no neurological abnormality in the upper limbs*.

These findings, together with your opening statement that this patient has had a recent onset of back pain, suggest spinal cord compression, possibly from a tumour or intervertebral disc prolapse at T7–8 level. This will need to be urgently investigated.

Record 3

The skin over the R/L buttock is *loose* and *droopy* due to *wasting* of the underlying *glutei*. The corresponding *calf muscles* are *flabby*, with *weakness* of *plantar flexion* at the ankle joint. The patient is unable to stand on his toes and the *ankle jerk* is *absent* on the affected side. The sensation is *impaired* along the *outer border* of the *foot* and the *outer half* of the sole.

Since you said that the patient has a spinal disc problem, I would suggest that he has had herniation of the fifth lumbar disc compressing the S1 root.‡

---

*See also cervical myelopathy; see Station 3, CNS, Case 26.
†Spinal pain, progressive muscular paralysis and a sensory level are the cardinal features of spinal cord compression. Since the entire examination of the motor and sensory systems cannot be accomplished in the permitted time, the examiners may ask you to examine the sensory system only, and a sensory loss level on the trunk should alert you to the possibility of spinal cord com-

pression. During this examination you should also be able to detect if there is any motor weakness.
‡If there was weakness of extension and abduction at the hip joint and a Trendelenburg limp (pelvis shifts to the normal side due to weak abductors on the affected side), it would suggest involvement of L4 and L5.

Causes of spinal cord and root compression

Diseases of the vertebrae and discs
Fracture and/or dislocation (trauma)
Prolapsed intervertebral disc
Spondylosis
Osteoporotic vertebral collapse
Paget's disease
Atlantoaxial dislocation (trauma, rheumatoid arthritis)
Ankylosing spondylitis
Sickle cell disease

Tumours
Extradural:
   Metastasis (lung, breast, prostate, kidney, GI tract, etc.)
   Lymphoma
   Primary bone tumours
Intradural but extramedullary (neurofibroma, meningioma, sarcoma, etc.)
Intramedullary (ependymoma, astrocytoma and rarely secondaries)

Vascular
Trauma – haemorrhage
Spinal vascular malformation
Intradural spinal neoplasms
Coarctation of the aorta
Ruptured spinal artery aneurysm
Blood dyscrasias
Anticoagulants

Inflammatory disorders
Spinal osteomyelitis
TB and Pott's disease of the spine
Spinal arachnoiditis
Introduction of blood and foreign substances in the intrathecal space

Acute disseminated encephalomyelitis
Multiple sclerosis
Devic's disease
Progressive necrotizing myelopathy (in young adults often after an acute illness, and in patients with a known malignancy, e.g. small cell carcinoma of the lung or a lymphoma)
Transverse myelitis

Diagnosis
The diagnosis depends on the history (trauma, malignancy, pain in the spine, sometimes with a radicular distribution and aggravated by straining and coughing, weakness of the legs and arms and sphincter disturbance), a neurological examination and, in urgent cases, CT or MRI. Diseases of the vertebrae and discs can be diagnosed from history, examination and a plain film of the spine.

   Back pain or neck pain should be taken seriously in a patient with a known malignancy. The pain of intraspinal lesions is exacerbated by straining, sneezing, coughing and movement. Unless investigated and treated early, midline pain progresses to radicular pain and is followed by weakness, sensory loss and sphincter disturbance. Patients who have neurological signs of cord compression require immediate treatment with dexamethasone and emergency evaluation.

   About 60–80% of patients with spinal cord compression will show erosion or loss of the pedicles, vertebral body destruction or collapse or a paraspinal mass on plain film. However, plain X-ray is hardly ever useful in suspected cord compression.

   All patients with suspected spinal cord/nerve root compression should have an MRI scan of the corresponding region of the spine. If MRI is contraindicated (please note, most of the newer intracranial clips, prostheses, etc. are MR compatible), a CT myelogram might be an alternative choice. Suspected spinal cord compression is a neurological emergency.

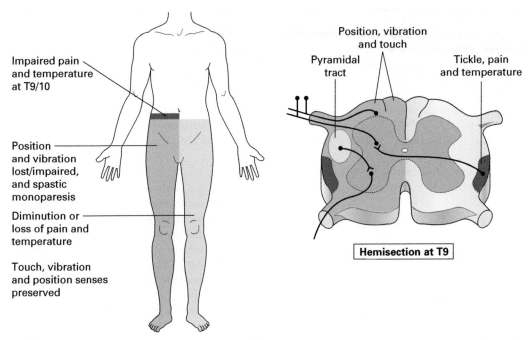

Figure C3.13 The Brown–Séquard syndrome. (After Mir MA. *Atlas of Clinical Skills*, 1997, by kind permission of the author and the publisher, WB Saunders.)

Case 18 | Ptosis

Frequency in survey: main focus of a short case or additional feature in 2% of attempts at PACES Station 3, CNS.

Record 1
There is *unilateral* ptosis.*

Possible causes
1 Third nerve palsy (?dilated ipsilateral pupil, divergent strabismus, etc; see Station 3, CNS, Case 16)
2 Horner's syndrome (?ipsilateral small pupil, etc; see Station 3, CNS, Case 41)
3 Myasthenia gravis (may be the only sign of this condition; ?induced or worsened by upward gaze; variable strabismus, facial and proximal muscle weakness, weak nasal voice, all of which may worsen with repetition, etc; see Station 3, CNS, Case 27)
4 Congenital/idiopathic† (may increase with age; there may be an associated superior rectus palsy)
5 Myotonic dystrophy (usually bilateral)

Record 2
There is *bilateral* ptosis.*

Possible causes
1 Myasthenia gravis
2 Myotonic dystrophy (?myopathic facies, frontal balding, wasting of facial muscles and sternomastoids, cataracts, myotonia, etc; see Station 3, CNS, Case 2)
3 Tabes dorsalis (?Argyll Robertson pupils, etc; see Station 3, CNS, Case 50)
4 Congenital† (may increase with age)
5 Bilateral Horner's (e.g. syringomyelia – ?wasting of small muscles of the hand, dissociated sensory loss, scars, extensor plantars, etc; see Station 3, CNS, Case 29)
6 Chronic progressive external ophthalmoplegia‡ (CPEO) (?absence of soft tissue in the lids and periorbital region, ophthalmoplegia, mild facial and neck weakness).

*NB: Overaction of frontalis with wrinkling of the forehead tends to be associated with ptosis due to non-myopathic conditions.
†There should be no response to a test dose of edrophonium before this diagnosis is accepted.
‡Many of the ocular myopathies are associated with characteristic morphological features ('ragged red fibres') and mitochondrial myopathy and are now referred to as CPEO. The disorder lies in the cytochromes and the conditions are sometimes termed the mitochondrial cytopathies. Ocular myopathy and oculopharyngeal muscular dystrophy may be manifestations of the same condition.

It is usually due to mitochondrial cytopathy, e.g. Kearns–Sayre syndrome (progressive ophthalmoplegia, retinopathy, cardiomyopathy and ataxia)

7 Oculopharyngeal muscular dystrophy‡ (see Station 3, CNS, Case 9)

Other causes of ptosis

Pseudoptosis (following recurrent inflammation or extreme thinning of lids after repeated angioneurotic oedema)

Voluntary ptosis (to suppress diplopia)

Apraxia of the eyelids (the patient may need to pull down the lower eyelids, tilt back the head or open the mouth to enable the eyes to be opened; there is usually evidence of basal ganglia involvement)

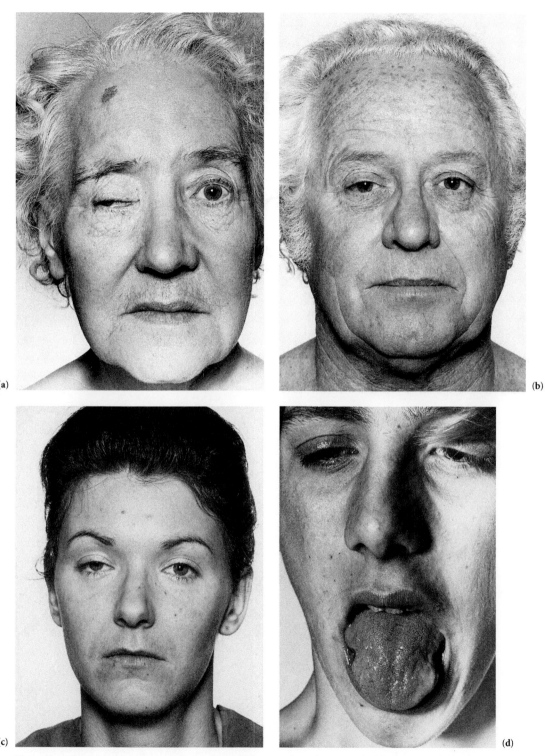

(a)

(b)

(c)

(d)

Figure C3.14 (a) Third nerve palsy: complete ptosis. (b) Right Horner's syndrome. (c) Myasthenia gravis: bilateral, asymmetrical ptosis. (d) Myotonic dystrophy: sustained contraction of the lingual muscles after percussion on the tongue plus bilateral ptosis. *(Continued.)*

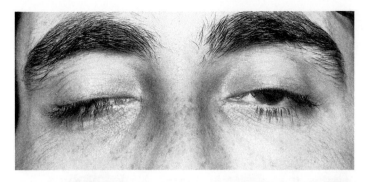
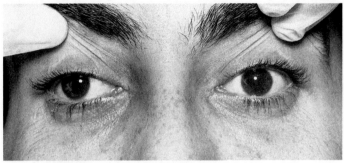

Figure C3.14 *(Continued)* (e) Ocular myopathy.

Case 19 | Guillain–Barré syndrome (acute inflammatory demyelinating polyradiculopathy)

Frequency in survey: main focus of a short case or additional feature in 1% of attempts at PACES Station 3, CNS.

Record

This (most commonly) young adult has a predominantly *motor neuropathy*. The weakness is more marked distally* and there is generalized *hyporeflexia*. There is a lower motor neurone *facial weakness* (often bilateral) and evidence of bulbar palsy. There is (may be) mild impairment of distal position and vibration perception and slight loss of pinprick sensation over the toes.† The patient has a tachycardia.‡

These features suggest Guillain–Barré syndrome (acute inflammatory demyelinating polyradiculopathy; AIDP).

Features of AIDP

There is an antecedent upper respiratory tract infection or gastrointestinal illness (e.g. *Campylobacter jejuni*) within 1 month in 60%§ of cases.

There is a bimodal age distribution – main peak in young adults, lesser peak in 45–64-year age group.

Cerebrospinal fluid protein is usually normal during the first 3 days; it then steadily rises and may continue to rise even though recovery has begun; it may exceed $5\,g\,L^{-1}$. A few mononuclear cells may be present in the CSF ($<10\,mm^{-3}$).

Mortality is 5%. The apparently mild case may worsen rapidly and unpredictably. *Vital capacity* (peak flow rate measurement is irrelevant), blood gases, blood pressure and ability to cough and swallow should be closely monitored; if mechanical ventilation is anticipated from the results then it should be instituted early, before decompensation.

Paralysis is maximum within 1 week in more than 50% of cases and by 1 month in 90%. Recovery usually begins 2–4 weeks later.¶ Rate of recovery is variable, occasionally rapid even after quadriplegia. Eighty-five percent of

---

*Though the weakness classically begins in the distal lower limbs and spreads upwards (*ascending paralysis*), it may be more marked proximally or uniform throughout the limbs.

†The mild case may just have slight foot-drop which never progresses, while the severe case may have quadriplegia and inability to breathe, speak, swallow or close the eyes. The facial involvement helps to distinguish AIDP from other neuropathies except for that related to sarcoidosis. Complaints of numbness and paraesthesiae are common but are usually mild and transient and objective sensory loss is slight.

‡Autonomic involvement is common with a relative tachycardia almost always present; orthostatic hypotension and hypertension are frequent and difficult to treat. Pupillary disturbances, neuroendocrine disturbance, peripheral pooling of blood, poor venous return and low cardiac output may all occur. *Sudden death* can occur following unexplained fluctuations in blood

pressure or cardiac dysrhythmias. Pharmacological interventions to control blood pressure are risky and should be avoided unless absolutely necessary. Patients who are unable to swallow or gag are given nasogastric feeding and should be sitting when food is given and for 30–60min thereafter to reduce the risk of aspiration.

§Predisposing factors that have been implicated include infectious mononucleosis, viral hepatitis, Epstein–Barr virus, rabies, swine flu, HIV infection, surgery, pregnancy and malignancy (especially lymphoma).

¶Pathologically, inflammatory cell infiltration followed by segmental demyelination is the hallmark, especially in spinal roots, limb girdle plexuses and proximal nerve trunks. Axons are relatively spared and blood vessels are normal. Within 2–3 weeks of onset, Schwann cell proliferation occurs as a prelude to remyelination and recovery.

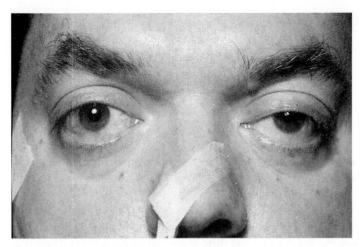

Figure C3.15 External ophthalmoplegia in the Miller–Fisher syndrome.

patients are ambulatory within 6 months. Mild residual peripheral nervous system damage occurs in 50%.

Plasmapheresis in the first 2 weeks shortens the clinical course and reduces morbidity. *Intravenous immunoglobulin* in the first 2 weeks is an alternative therapy that has equivalent efficacy to plasmapheresis, and is now the treatment of choice.

Some patients present with rapid onset of symmetrical, multiple cranial nerve palsies, most notably bilateral facial palsy (polyneuritis cranialis).

Occasionally, there may be a combination of an external ophthalmoplegia, ataxia and areflexia (*Miller–Fisher syndrome*) associated with high CSF protein and some motor weakness. Serum IgG antibodies to GQ1b ganglioside are found in acute-phase sera of over 90% of Miller–Fisher syndrome patients. They disappear during recovery.

Most patients achieve good recovery from AIDP. The importance of fastidious supportive care during the acute stage cannot be overstressed.

Case 20 | Choreoathetosis

Frequency in survey: main focus of a short case or additional feature in 1% of attempts at PACES Station 3, CNS.

Survey note: often hemichorea associated with a hemiplegia.

Record

There are *brief, jerky, abrupt, irregular, quasi-purposeful, involuntary movements* (which never integrate into a coordinated act but may match it in complexity). The movements *flit* from one part of the body to another in a random sequence; they are *present at rest* and *accentuated by activity* (at rest, the movements prevent the patient's relaxation and they interrupt and distort voluntary movement). The patient has a general air of restlessness. He is *unable* to keep his *tongue protruded* (it darts in and out). There is *abnormal posturing* of the *hands* in which the wrist is flexed and the fingers are hyperextended at the metacarpophalangeal joints. When the upper limbs are raised and extended, there is *pronation of the forearm.*

This is chorea.*

Causes of chorea

Sydenham's chorea (usually between age 5 and 15; ?heart murmur; one-third have a history of rheumatic fever; it may recur during pregnancy and when on the oral contraceptive pill)

Huntington's chorea (affects the lower limbs more often than the upper, producing a dancing sort of gait; chorea may precede dementia; onset age 35–50; family history)

Drug-induced chorea (e.g. neuroleptics, L-dopa)

Senile chorea (idiopathic orofacial dyskinesia; no dementia)

Other causes of chorea include epidemic encephalitis, the encephalopathies occurring with exanthema, idiopathic hypocalcaemia, thyrotoxicosis, SLE, carbon monoxide poisoning and Wilson's disease

Causes of hemichorea/hemiballism†

Cerebrovascular accident† (?hemiplegia, homonymous hemianopia)

Intracerebral tumour (?pyramidal signs on the side of the chorea, papilloedema)

Trauma

Post thalamotomy

Other types of involuntary movement (dyskinesias)

Athetosis‡ (slow, coarse, irregular, writhing muscular distortion, most commonly of the hands, feet and digits, though the face and tongue may be affected – many choreic and dystonic movements are indistinguishable from athetosis)

---

*In choreoathetosis (cerebral palsy, tumours involving the pallidum, vascular insufficiency, Wilson's disease, carbon monoxide poisoning, etc.), the movements mainly involve the upper limbs and cranial nerves (grimacing, writhing movements of the tongue, etc.). The hands are repeatedly brought in front of the chest shaped like cups with flexion at the MCP joints and extension at the interphalangeal joints.

†Hemiballism is wild irregular flinging or throwing movements of whole limbs on one side. Vascular lesions are the most common cause. The lesion is in the contralateral subthalamic nucleus. The ballistic movements often begin as the other neurological signs of the cerebrovascular accident start to clear (i.e. after an interval). They disappear during sleep. Though initially they may exhaust the patient, they usually die out gradually over 6–8 weeks.

‡The common causes of the two closely linked dyskinesias, dystonia and athetosis, are drugs (neuroleptics, L-dopa) and post hypoxia. There are many rare causes. Several pathogenic gene mutations have been identified recently in dystonias. Dystonia with diurnal fluctuations, especially in children and young adults, should have a therapeutic trial of L-dopa to rule out dopa-responsive dystonia.

Dystonia* (sustained spasm of some portion of the body; the movements are powerful and deforming, torticollis is a common example of torsion dystonia; lordosis and scoliosis may also be caused)

Myoclonus (rapid shock-like muscular jerks often repetitious and sometimes rhythmic – most common causes include epilepsy, essential (familial), physiological (sleep, exercise, anxiety), metabolic disorders (renal, respiratory or hepatic failure), subacute encephalitis)

Tremors (e.g. Parkinson's, anxiety, thyrotoxicosis, drugs (e.g. alcohol, caffeine, salbutamol), MS, spinocerebellar degeneration, cerebrovascular accident, essential/familial)

Tics

---

*The common causes of the two closely linked dyskinesias, dystonia and athetosis, are drugs (neuroleptics, L-dopa) and post hypoxia. There are many rare causes. Several pathogenic gene mutations have been identified recently in dystonias. Dystonia with diurnal fluctuations, especially in children and young adults, should have a therapeutic trial of L-dopa to rule out dopa-responsive dystonia.

Case 21 | Bulbar palsy

Frequency in survey: main focus of a short case or additional feature in 1% of attempts at PACES Station 3, CNS.

Record

The *tongue* is *flaccid* and *fasciculating* (it is wasted, wrinkled, thrown into folds and increasingly motionless). The *speech is indistinct* (flaccid dysarthria), lacks modulations and has a *nasal twang*, and *palatal movement is absent*. There is (may be) saliva at the corners of the mouth (and while the patient talks he may be seen to pause periodically to gulp the secretions that have accumulated meanwhile in the pharynx; there may be dysphagia and nasal regurgitation).

This is bulbar palsy.

Possible causes

1 Motor neurone disease (?muscle fasciculation, absence of sensory signs, brisk jaw jerk, etc; see Station 3, CNS, Case 11)

2 Syringobulbia (?nystagmus, Horner's, dissociated sensory loss, etc; see Station 3, CNS, Case 29)

3 Guillain–Barré syndrome (?generalized including facial flaccid paralysis, absent reflexes, peripheral neuropathy or widespread sensory defect; monitor peak flow rate; see Station 3, CNS, Case 19)

4 Poliomyelitis

5 Subacute meningitis (carcinoma, lymphoma, etc.)

6 Neurosyphilis

7 Base of skull or retropharyngeal pathology

Case 22 | Lateral popliteal (common peroneal) nerve palsy

Frequency in survey: main focus of a short case or additional feature in 1% of attempts at PACES Station 3, CNS.

Record

There is *wasting* of the *anterior tibial* and *peroneal* group of *muscles*, the patient *cannot dorsiflex* or *evert* the R/L foot,* and there is *impairment* of *sensation* over the *outer side* of the *calf*. He can stand on his toes but cannot stand on the R/L heel and the gait is altered as a result of *foot-drop* (there is an audible 'clop' of the foot as he walks). The ankle jerk is preserved.

The diagnosis is lateral popliteal (common peroneal) nerve palsy.

Injury to the nerve is usually at the head of the fibula where it can be involved in fractures or compressed by splints, tourniquets or bandages. Some individuals are particularly susceptible to temporary pressure palsy of this nerve (and in some cases other nerves such as the radial and ulnar as well), experiencing symptoms induced by crossing knees, squatting (strawberry picker's palsy) or unusual physical activity.

The nerve has two branches – the superficial and deep peroneal nerves. The superficial supplies sensation to the lateral calf and dorsum of the foot supplying the peroneus longus and brevis muscles. The deep branch supplies sensation to a triangular area of skin between the first and second toes dorsally and it innervates the anterior tibial muscles, the long extensors of the toes and the peroneus tertius muscle.

---

*Preservation of inversion of the ankle (tibialis posterior) distinguishes common peroneal nerve palsy from a L4–5 root lesion.

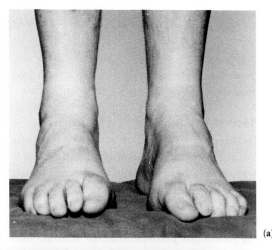

(a)

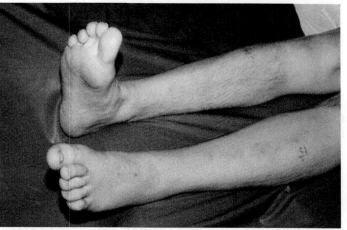

(b)

Figure C3.16 (a) Right common peroneal nerve palsy. Note failure of eversion. (b) Left common peroneal nerve palsy. Note failure of eversion and dorsiflexion on the left side.

Case 23 | Proximal myopathy

Frequency in survey: main focus of a short case or additional feature in 1% of attempts at PACES Station 3, CNS.

Record 1 (patient lying on a bed)

There is considerable *proximal muscular weakness*, particularly in abduction at the shoulder joints and extension as well as flexion at the hip joints. The patient is *unable* to *sit up* with the upper limbs outstretched in front.

This patient has a proximal myopathy.

Record 2 (patient sitting in a chair)

The patient has *proximal muscular weakness* in both *upper* and *lower limb girdle groups*. I can overcome his abduction of the arms and he has considerable difficulty *standing up* from the chair. He is unable to *stand up from a squatting position*. (In both cases you should ask the examiner's permission to examine the gait.)

This patient has a proximal myopathy.

Causes of proximal myopathy

Diabetic proximal myopathy/amyotrophy – especially affects the elderly. Often unilateral and associated with pain

Polymyalgia rheumatica – usually occurs over the age of 50 years, male-to-female ratio 1/3. The predominant features are fatigue, morning stiffness in the limb girdles and/or neck, weight loss, proximal pain at rest and during movement, and tenderness of the muscles. There is a sense of weakness but on careful testing, muscle strength is found to be normal or nearly normal. The apparent weakness is due to pain and stiffness. The ESR is elevated. Closely related to temporal arteritis. Responds dramatically to corticosteroids

Cushing's syndrome (?moonface, acne, axial obesity, hirsutism, evidence of rheumatoid arthritis, etc; see Vol. 3, Station 5, Endocrine, Case 6)

Thyrotoxicosis (?eye signs, goitre, fidgety, tachycardia, etc; see Vol. 3, Station 5, Endocrine, Case 4); the proximal muscular weakness is particularly severe in upper limb muscles

Polymyositis (?tender muscles; see Station 3, CNS, Case 45)

Dermatomyositis (?heliotrope rash around the eyes, on the knuckles, the hands and over the knee joints, tender muscles, etc; Vol. 3, Station 5, Skin, Case 6)

Drugs – alcohol, corticosteroids, amiodarone, chloroquine, β-blockers, lithium, isoniazid, labetalol, methadone, etc.

Carcinomatous myopathy – the muscular weakness may precede the neoplasia. The lower limb girdle is much more adversely affected than the upper limb girdle muscles. The onset is usually between the age of 50 and 60 years and men are more often affected than women. At times, there may be many myasthenic features (Lambert–Eaton syndrome; see Station 3, CNS, Case 27) and the weakness is often improved after a short muscular contraction. The malignancy is often small cell carcinoma of the lung. The neurological symptoms may precede the neoplasia by 1–2 years

Osteomalacia (?ethnic origin – mostly females, waddling gait, bone pain; see Vol. 3, Station 5, Locomotor, Case 17)

McArdle's syndrome (myophosphorylase deficiency; ?stiffness and cramps after exercise, exercising muscles feel hard, pain on movement)

Mitochondrial myopathy – a group of biochemical disorders involving the mitochondrial enzymes. Muscle biopsy may show 'ragged red fibres'. Typically there is slowly progressive weakness of limbs and/or external ocular (see Footnote, Station 3, CNS, Case 18) and other cranial muscles, abnormal fatiguability on sustained exertion, and lactic acidaemia on exertion or even at rest. Sometimes the myopathy is but one facet of a multisystem disease. Family or personal history of diabetes or deafness may be clues

End-stage renal failure (?uraemic facies)

Case 24 | Absent ankle jerks and extensor plantars

Frequency in survey: main focus of a short case or additional feature in 0.8% of attempts at PACES Station 3, CNS.

Record

The knee and *ankle jerks are absent* and the *plantar responses are extensor.*

Possible causes

1 Subacute combined degeneration of the cord (?posterior column signs, positive Romberg's sign, clinical anaemia, splenomegaly, etc; see Station 3, CNS, Case 37)

2 Syphilitic taboparesis (?Argyll Robertson pupils, ptosis and wrinkled forehead, posterior column signs, positive Romberg's sign, etc; see Station 3, CNS, Case 50)

3 Hereditary cerebellar ataxias, e.g. Friedreich's ataxia (?pes cavus, (kypho)scoliosis, nystagmus, cerebellar ataxia, scanning speech, etc; see Station 3, CNS, Case 12), spinocerebellar ataxia (ataxia, dysarthria, ophthalmoplegia, pyramidal and extrapyramidal signs, peripheral neuropathy, etc.)

4 Motor neurone disease (?fasciculation, absence of sensory signs, etc; see Station 3, CNS, Case 11)

5 Common conditions in combination* (e.g. an elderly person with diabetes and cervical myelopathy – see Vol. 2, Section F, Experience 166 – or cervical and lumbar spondylosis causing a mixture of upper and lower motor neurone signs in the legs)

6 A lesion of the conus medullaris

---

*Whilst the above list represents the traditional order in which the conditions are presented, in practice number 5 is by far the most common.

Case 25 | Cerebellopontine angle lesion

Frequency in survey: main focus of a short case or additional feature in 0.8% of attempts at PACES Station 3, CNS.

Record

On the R/L side there is evidence of *Vth* (may be absent corneal reflex only), *VIth* (see Station 3, CNS, Case 16) and *VIIth cranial nerve impairment* (both may be minimal), *perceptive deafness* (*VIIIth* nerve – the patient usually has tinnitus but may complain of vague unsteadiness or giddiness*) and *cerebellar* impairment (may be slightly impaired rapid alternate motion of the hands only). There is *nystagmus* (again may be just a few beats intermittently; it may be cerebellar and/or vestibular in origin).

These findings suggest a lesion at the cerebellopontine angle, *acoustic neuroma†* being the most common cause (X-ray for evidence of expansion of the internal auditory meatus – not always seen†). Meningioma can give a similar picture (normal auditory meatus on X-ray).

The IXth and Xth cranial nerves may be involved and dysphagia and dysphonia may occur. In severe cases, with large tumours, there may be signs of raised intracranial pressure (?papilloedema) in addition to ipsilateral cerebellar involvement.

*Rotational vertigo in acoustic neuroma seldom occurs in the discrete attacks that are found in Ménière's syndrome.

†Acoustic neuromata may cause symptoms even if extremely small, if confined within the acoustic canal. They are much more common than all other cranial nerve tumours put together. MRI scans accurately detect even very small acoustic neuromata. Patients with hearing loss developing in middle age should be considered to have acoustic neuroma until proved otherwise. Audiometry is suggestive but not diagnostic. Caloric testing almost always shows abnormalities but the auditory evoked response is the most efficient physiological assessment. The CSF protein is elevated (may be $>3\,g\,L^{-1}$) but cerebrospinal fluid assessment should not usually be necessary and might be dangerous.

Case 26 | Cervical myelopathy

Frequency in survey: main focus of a short case or additional feature in 0.8% of attempts at PACES Station 3, CNS.

Survey note: cervical collar may be a clue.

Record

The legs (of this middle-aged or elderly patient) show *spastic weakness,** the *tone* being *increased,* the *reflexes brisk* (?clonus) and the *plantar responses extensor.* *Vibration* and joint position senses are (may be) lost in the lower limbs (spinothalamic loss may also occur but is less common). In the upper limbs† there is (often asymmetrical) *inversion‡* of the biceps and supinator jerks.

These features suggest cervical myelopathy as the cause of the spastic paraparesis. *Cervical spondylosis* is the most common cause though a *spinal cord tumour* cannot be excluded clinically.

In the upper limbs there may be segmental muscle wasting and weakness, particularly if there is an associated radiculopathy. Gross wasting of the small muscles of the hand due to cervical spondylosis is uncommon because the latter usually affects C5–6 or C6–7 and the small muscles are supplied by C8–T1. Mild wasting of the small muscles does sometimes occur probably due to vascular changes in the cord below the lesion.

There is often no sensory loss in the hand. Sometimes in the elderly a complaint of numb, useless hands may be accompanied by constant unpleasant paraesthesiae and writhing ('sensory wandering' or 'pseudoathetosis') of the fingers when the eyes are closed. Position and vibration senses are lost in such hands. Neck pain is surprisingly rare in cervical spondylosis causing cervical myelopathy, and sphincter function is seldom disturbed. Among patients with cervical spondylosis (which is very common), those with a narrow cervical canal are most likely to develop cervical myelopathy. Lhermitte's phenomenon may occur (see Station 3, CNS, Case 37).

---

*In this condition signs often exceed symptoms and spasticity often exceeds weakness.

†The myelopathy hand sign may be present; see Footnote, Section B, Examination *Routine 7*).

‡When attempts are made to elicit the normal biceps and supinator tendon reflexes, there is a brisk finger flexion despite little or no response of the biceps and supinator jerks themselves. This is because the lower motor neurones and pyramidal tracts are damaged at the C5–6 level, producing lower motor neurone signs at that level and upper motor neurone signs below. The combination of inverted biceps and supinator jerks (the C5–6 jerks) and a brisk triceps jerk (C7–8) is termed the 'mid-cervical reflex pattern'.

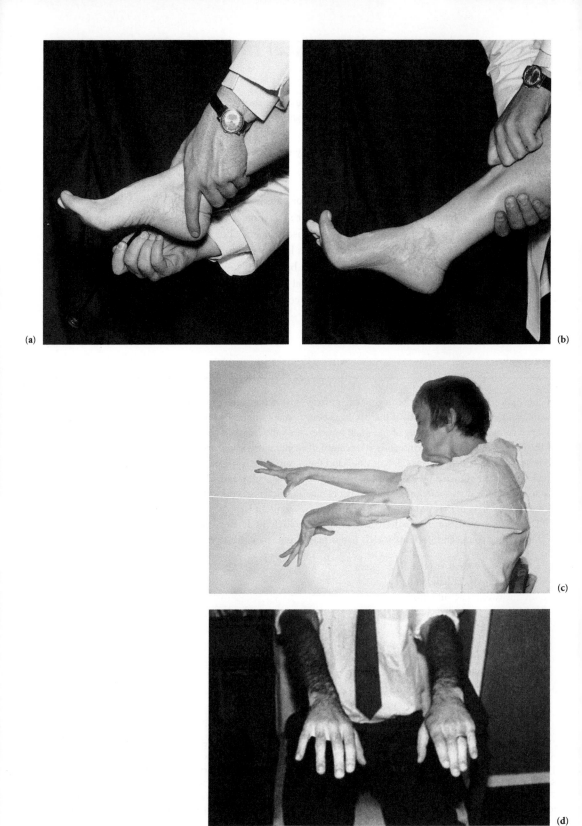

Figure C3.17 (a) Babinski's sign. (b) Oppenheim's sign (see Footnote, Section B, Examination *Routine* 8). (c) Pseudoathetosis. (d) The myelopathy hand sign (in the right arm).

Case 27 | Myasthenia gravis

Frequency in survey: main focus of a short case or additional feature in 0.8% of attempts at PACES Station 3, CNS.

Predicted frequency from older, more extensive MRCP short case surveys: main focus of a short case in 0.9% of attempts at PACES Station 3, CNS. Additional feature in a further 1%.

Record

There is *ptosis* (one or both sides) accentuated by upward gaze, *variable strabismus* (with *diplopia*) and when the patient tries to screw her eyes up tight, the eyelashes are not buried. The face shows a *lack of expression*, the mouth is slack and there is generalized *facial weakness*. The patient *snarls* when she tries to smile, she cannot whistle, and her *voice* is *weak* and *nasal* (if you ask the patient to count aloud, speech may become progressively less distinct and more nasal). There is *proximal muscle weakness*. Repetitive movements cause an increase in the muscle weakness (myasthenia = abnormal muscular fatiguability).

The diagnosis is myasthenia gravis. A Tensilon (edrophonium) test will confirm it.

Male-to-female ratio is 1/2.

Other features of myasthenia gravis

Difficulty with swallowing, chewing and nasal regurgitation

Symptoms worsen as the day progresses

Tendon reflexes are normal or exaggerated (cf. Eaton–Lambert syndrome)

The *jaw-supporting sign*, if present, is pathognomonic – the patient puts her hand under her chin to support both the weak jaw and neck; may only become obvious after prolonged conversation

Antiacetylcholine receptor antibodies are present in up to 90% of cases with generalized myasthenia gravis

In long-standing cases there may be an element of permanent irreversible myopathic change

Breathlessness is a sinister symptom requiring urgent attention (respiratory deterioration may develop rapidly and should be watched for by monitoring the FVC, not the peak flow rate)

Pathological changes are present in the thymus in 70–80% and some patients are improved by thymectomy; thymomata occur in 10% (mostly males) and give a worse prognosis

Associated immune disorders include thyrotoxicosis (5% of patients), hypothyroidism, rheumatoid arthritis, diabetes mellitus, polymyositis, SLE, pernicious anaemia, Sjögren's syndrome, pemphigus and sarcoidosis.

Crisis

Signs of *cholinergic crisis* are collapse, confusion, abdominal pain and vomiting, sweating, salivation, lachrymation, miosis and pallor. The features which distinguish *myasthenic crisis* are response to edrophonium and absence of cholinergic phenomena. Occasionally it is exceptionally difficult to determine whether the collapsed myasthenic has been under- or overtreated. Temporary withdrawal of all drugs and assisted positive pressure respiration are then indicated.

Myasthenic crisis may be provoked by:

Infection

Emotional upset

Undue exertion*

*Childbirth requires careful management.

Drugs (streptomycin, gentamicin, kanamycin, neomycin, viomycin, polymyxin, colistin, curare, quinine, quinidine, procainamide).

Eaton–Lambert syndrome (myasthenic-myopathic syndrome) is often associated with oat cell carcinoma of the bronchus. There is proximal muscle wasting, weakness and fatiguability. Often, however, power is initially increased by brief exercise (reversed myasthenic effect). The tendon reflexes are depressed (but increased soon after activity; this can be demonstrated dramatically by showing the depressed biceps reflex and then by repeating it after getting the patient to flex the forearm against resistance). The electromyographic response to ulnar nerve stimulation shows a characteristic increase in amplitude (it declines in myasthenia gravis). Cholinergic drugs have no effect.

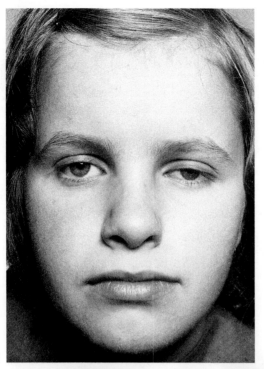

(a)

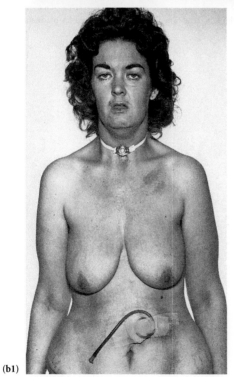

(b1)

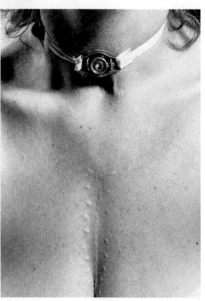

(b2)

Figure C3.18 (a) A mild case with unilateral ptosis. (b1,2) A severe case (note myasthenic facies, thymectomy scar, gastrostomy feeding tube and tracheostomy). *(Continued.)*

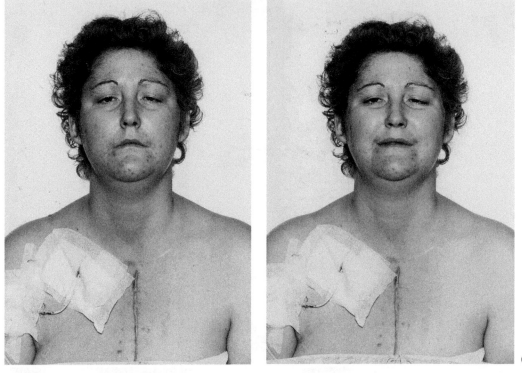

(c)

(d)

Figure C3.18 *(Continued)* (c) Myasthenic facies (note the subclavian line which was being used for plasmapheresis). (d) 'Smile'.

Case 28 | Normal central nervous system

Frequency in survey: Main focus of a short case or additional feature in 0.8% of attempts at PACES Station 3, CNS.

The College has made it clear that 'normal' is an option in PACES. No findings on examination is common in real clinical medicine and so this must be a possibility in the exam. In terms of the practical reality of the exam, in order for PACES to proceed there must be a neurological case in Station 3, CNS. If, at the last minute, neither of the scheduled neuro cases turns up on the day or if, in the middle of a carousel, the only one who did turn up decides not to continue or is too ill to continue, a substitute case has to be found at short notice. In this situation, one option is to proceed with a patient without any neurological abnormality and make up an appropriate scenario. One simply has to imagine oneself as the invigilating registrar to think what that might be. One would first look amongst any surplus cases in the other stations for a volunteer or one might ask a member of the nursing, portering or other support staff, and come up with a scenario such as:

> 'This . . . -year-old patient had a transient episode of weakness of the right leg.
> Please examine the legs neurologically . . .'.

There may be a clue in the case scenario and the fact that the scenario has been hurriedly hand-scribbled.

From our surveys, it is clear that the most common reason for finding no abnormality is missing the physical signs that are present (see probably both Anecdotes 1 and 2, Station 3, Cardiovascular, Case 24; see possibly Anecdote 5, Station 1, Abdominal, Case 11; and Vol. 2, Section F, Experience 158). Other reasons for cases of 'normal' will be either because the physical signs are no longer present by the time the patient comes to the examination (see Anecdote 1, below), or that the examiners and candidate disagree with the selectors of the cases about the presence of physical signs (may have happened in Anecdote, Vol.3, Station 5, Eyes, Case 21; see also Vol. 2, Section F, Experience 198 and Anecdote 303).

The following are anecdotes from our surveys.

Anecdote 1
A candidate was asked to examine a patient's eye movements. He found no abnormality and said so. He reports that the examiners confirmed this and he passed. Apparently the patient had been included in the examination because she had had internuclear ophthalmoplegia, but this was no longer present at the time of this examination.

Anecdote 2
A candidate was asked to examine a person's upper limb neurologically. Examination was normal. He was then told that the GP had referred the patient as ?ulnar nerve problem and he was asked if he agreed. He reports that he stuck to his initial findings and he felt that the examiners seemed to agree. The candidate was very confident that the diagnosis was normal central nervous system and he received a clear pass.

Case 29 | Syringomyelia

Frequency in survey: main focus of a short case or additional feature in 0.8% of attempts at PACES Station 3, CNS.

Record

This patient (with *kyphoscoliosis*) shows *wasting* and weakness of the *small muscles* of the *hands* (sometimes there is curling of the fingers), flattening of the muscles of the ulnar border of the forearm and the upper limb *reflexes are absent* (conspicuous fasciculation is uncommon). There is *dissociated sensory loss** over (one or both of) the upper limbs and the upper chest† and there are *scars* (from painless burns and cuts) on the hands. The lower limb reflexes are exaggerated and the plantars are extensor. A *Horner's syndrome* is (may be) present (involvement of sympathetic neurones especially at C8–T1).

These findings suggest syringomyelia.

Syringobulbia. Syrinx may involve upper cervical and bulbar segments (usually an extension of syringomyelia but it may begin in the brainstem) and cause:

Nystagmus

Ataxia

Facial dissociated sensory loss (initially onion skin loss over the outer part of the face, from involvement of the lower part of the Vth nucleus in the cord, may occur before the syrinx reaches the medulla)

Bulbar palsy (wasted fasciculating tongue, palatal paralysis, nasal dysarthria, dysphasia, weakness of sternomastoids and trapezius from XIth nerve involvement, etc; see Station 3, CNS, Case 21).

Trophic and vasomotor disturbances are common in syringomyelia, e.g.:

Areas of loss of, or excessive, sweating

La main succulente (ugly, cold, puffy, cyanosed hands with stumpy fingers and podgy soft palms)

Coarse, thickened skin over the hands with callosities over the knuckles and scars from old injuries

Slow healing and indolent ulceration of digits.

Charcot's joints may occur, usually at the elbow or shoulder. Tabes dorsalis (knees, hips) and diabetes mellitus (toes, ankles) are the other causes of Charcot's joints (see Vol. 3, Station 5, Locomotor, Case 4).

Skeletal abnormalities which may be associated with syringomyelia

(Kypho)scoliosis (mild, very common)

Short neck (e.g. fusion of the cervical vertebrae; Klippel–Feil syndrome; see Vol. 3, Station 5, Other, Case 7)

Asymmetrical thorax

Sternal depression or prominence

Cervical ribs (may cause diagnostic difficulty)

---

*Analgesia and thermoanaesthesia, but light touch and proprioception intact. In the early stages cold stimuli may be perceived but not warm stimuli.

†Due to destruction by the syrinx of crossing axons carrying pain and temperature sensation. The area affected depends on the length of the syrinx, e.g. lower cervical and upper thoracic. Separate from this effect on crossing axons, the syrinx may also involve one or both spinothalamic tracts, producing dissociated sensory loss in one or both lower limbs.

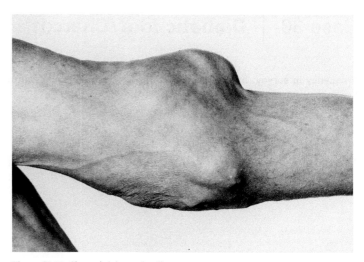

Figure C3.19 Charcot's joint at the elbow.

Case 30 | Diabetic foot/Charcot's joint

Frequency in survey: main focus of a short case or additional feature in 0.8% of attempts at PACES Station 3, CNS.

Survey note: see Vol. 2, Section F, Anecdote 106.

Diabetic foot/Charcot's joint is dealt with in Vol. 3, Station 5, Locomotor, Case 4.

Case 31 | Holmes–Adie–Moore syndrome

Frequency in survey: main focus of a short case or additional feature in 0.7% of attempts at PACES Station 3, CNS.

Record

This young lady has a unilateral *dilated pupil* which *fails* (or almost fails) *to react to light*. There is no ptosis or diplopia and eye movements are otherwise normal (i.e. not IIIrd nerve palsy).

The patient has a myotonic pupil. Her tendon reflexes may be lost (check if allowed).

If exposed to light for prolonged periods, the pupil may constrict slowly. If then exposed to darkness for a long period, it will again dilate very slowly. During accommodation–convergence, after a delay, the abnormal pupil constricts slowly until it may become smaller than the normal pupil. The reaction to mydriatics is normal (Argyll Robertson pupil dilates poorly with mydriatics) and the pupil may be hyperreactive to weak cholinergic substances, e.g. 0.1% pilocarpine.

The condition is usually chronic and symptomless but in some cases onset is acute with associated blurring of vision and photophobia. Syphilitic serology will be negative. Differential diagnosis from neurosyphilis may be difficult in the chronic stages of this disorder, when the pupil may be chronically constricted, and especially when both pupils are affected (bilateral involvement is rare with Holmes–Adie pupils but invariable with syphilitic Argyll Robertson pupils; see Station 3, CNS, Case 38).

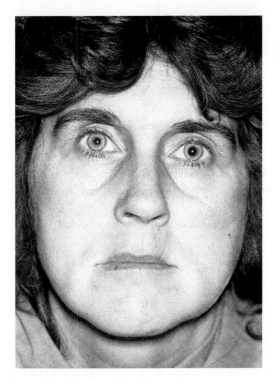

Figure C3.20 Holmes–Adie pupil.

Case 32 | Nystagmus

Frequency in survey: main focus of a short case or additional feature in 0.7% of attempts at PACES Station 3, CNS.

Survey note: in most cases nystagmus was cerebellar in origin – usually due to multiple sclerosis.

Record 1

There is nystagmus, greater on the R/L with the fast component to the same side. This suggests:

1 an ipsilateral cerebellar lesion (?cerebellar signs; see Station 3, CNS, Case 7), *or*

2 a contralateral vestibular lesion (?vertical nystagmus, ?vertigo; see below). (Now, if allowed, *look for cerebellar signs*; occasionally there will be signs of a lesion in the brainstem, e.g. infarction; see Station 3, CNS, Case 44, syringobulbia*; see Station 3, CNS, Case 29)

Record 2

The nystagmus is *ataxic* in that the *abducting eye has greater nystagmus* than the adducting eye.† With this there is dissociation of conjugate eye movements. There is (may be) a divergent strabismus at rest. On looking to the right, the right eye abducts normally but there is *impairment of adduction*† of the left eye. On looking to the left, the left eye abducts normally but there is *impairment of adduction*† of the right eye (occasionally the reverse may occur with weakness of abduction on each side but adduction remains normal). When the abducting eye is covered, however, the medial movement of the other eye occurs normally.

The diagnosis is *internuclear ophthalmoplegia*. It suggests multiple sclerosis‡ with a lesion in the medial longitudinal fasciculus. (Now, if allowed, *look for cerebellar signs*, pyramidal signs, pale discs, etc; see Station 3, CNS, Cases 7 and 10.)

Causes and types of nystagmus

A simplified diagrammatic representation of conjugate gaze and its various connections is depicted in Figure C3.21. As can be seen from the multiplicity of these pathways, a disorder within the end-organs (i.e. eye, labyrinth, semicircular canals), or in the medial longitudinal fasciculus anywhere through its long course, or in its nuclear connections (i.e. cerebellar, vestibular nuclei, etc.) can cause nystagmus. Nystagmus can be divided into:

---

*As can be seen from Fig. C3.21, the medial longitudinal bundle extends into the spinal cord so that syringomyelia confined to the spinal cord, if extending above C5, may also cause nystagmus.

†The key sign of internuclear ophthalmoplegia is the *failure of adduction*; the nystagmus is not essential.

‡Internuclear ophthalmoplegia is highly characteristic of MS though rarely it may be caused by brainstem gliomata or vascular lesions, or Wernicke's encephalopathy (ocular palsy, nystagmus, loss of pupillary reflexes, ataxia, peripheral neuropathy, Korsakoff's psychosis or other disturbance of mentation; dramatic response to thiamine in the early stages).

Physiological nystagmus (a few brief jerks can occur in the normal eye at the extreme lateral gaze)

Ocular nystagmus (in patients with a congenital visual defect in one eye, a pendular movement of the eye occurs while gazing straight – fixation nystagmus)

Vestibular nystagmus (see below)

Cerebellar nystagmus (Record 1)

Ataxic nystagmus (Record 2)

Vestibular nystagmus

This may arise in the periphery (labyrinth or vestibular nerve) or in the central vestibular nuclei and its connections.

Peripheral The fast component is towards the contralateral side (except with an early irritative lesion when it can be on the side of the lesion) and the nystagmus is fatiguable – it becomes less and less intense on repetition of the test. The patient tends to be unsteady on the ipsilateral side (contralateral to the fast component), as can be revealed whilst assessing Romberg's test (the patient cannot stand on a narrow base even with the eyes open in this situation, whereas the patient with sensory ataxia becomes more unsteady when the eyes are closed) and gait (tends to reel on the affected side). Cochlear function is usually affected (diminishes, leading to deafness, e.g. Ménière's syndrome) and the patient may have vertigo.

Causes of peripheral vestibular nystagmus:

Labyrinthitis (probably viral and self-limiting; nystagmus may be absent and only positional and provoked by movements of the head – often it can be elicited by bending the head backwards about 45° – the nystagmus, as well as the vertigo, may appear but fades with repeated testing)

Ménière's syndrome (progressive deafness and tinnitus, with recurrent attacks of vertigo)

Acoustic neuroma (progressive tinnitus and nerve deafness; neighbouring nerves – Vth, VIth and VIIth may be involved and there may be cerebellar signs, etc; see Station 3, CNS, Case 25)

Vestibular neuronitis (acute vertigo without deafness or tinnitus which usually improves within 48 h; full recovery may take weeks or months; may be viral)

Other causes include degenerative middle ear disease, hypertension and head injury.

Central Lesions affecting vestibular nuclei (cerebrovascular accident, MS, encephalitis, tumours, syringobulbia, alcoholism,* anticonvulsants, etc.) cause nystagmus which is spontaneous but may be brought on or increased by head movements. It is not adaptable and usually has a vertical component. *Downbeat nystagmus* with the eyes looking straight ahead is characteristic of an Arnold–Chiari malformation.† Downbeat nystagmus on lateral gaze normally indicates a lesion at the foramen magnum level (tumour, syringomyelia, cerebellar degeneration).

---

*Acute alcohol toxicity may cause nystagmus. Nystagmus is also almost always present in Wernicke's encephalopathy. Paradoxically alcohol may reduce congenital nystagmus – a condition which may be gross but symptomless.

†*Arnold–Chiari malformation* may be asymptomatic until adult life when the patient gradually develops cerebellar symptoms and signs. There is cerebellar herniation through the

foramen magnum. There may be coexisting syringomyelia of the cervical cord and medulla (see Station 3, CNS, Case 29). Commonly there is radiographic evidence of fusion of the cervical vertebrae, platybasia or basilar impression. MRI (CT may miss it) establishes the diagnosis when there are no coexisting bony abnormalities. Surgical intervention may benefit selected cases.

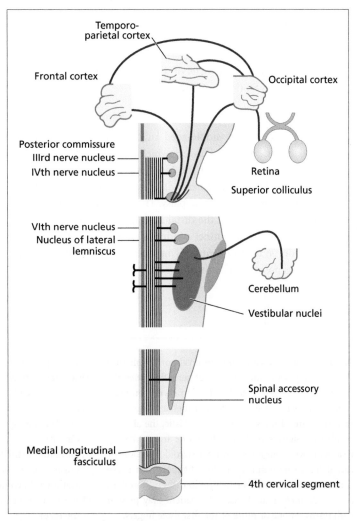

Temporo-
parietal cortex

Frontal cortex

Occipital cortex

Posterior commissure
IIIrd nerve nucleus
IVth nerve nucleus

Retina
Superior colliculus

VIth nerve nucleus
Nucleus of lateral
lemniscus

Cerebellum

Vestibular nuclei

Spinal accessory
nucleus

Medial longitudinal
fasciculus

4th cervical segment

Figure C3.21 A simplified diagram to give an idea of cortical, brainstem and peripheral control of conjugate gaze. The medial longitudinal bundle starts just below the posterior commissure and ends in the upper cervical spinal cord. During its long course it receives fibres from various nuclei (and the lateral pontine gaze centre) which are concerned with the control of conjugate gaze. Interruption in the cortical or midbrain connections often produces a disorder of conjugate gaze rather than nystagmus. Lesions in the brainstem or below result in nystagmus.

Case 33 | Carpal tunnel syndrome

Frequency in survey: main focus of a short case or additional feature in 0.7% of attempts at PACES Station 3, CNS.

Record

There is (in this ?stout, ?middle-aged lady who complains of pain, numbness or paraesthesiae in the palm and fingers, which is particularly bad in the night*) *sensory loss* over the *palmar* aspects of the *first three and a half fingers* and *wasting of the thenar eminence.* There is weakness of *abduction, flexion* and *opposition of the thumb.*

The diagnosis is median nerve palsy. The non-involvement of the flexor muscles of the forearm (i.e. can flex the distal interphalangeal joint of the thumb) suggests that the cause is carpal tunnel syndrome (now check the facies for underlying *acromegaly* or *myxoedema*; underlying *rheumatoid arthritis* should be obvious). *Tinel's sign*† is positive to confirm this.

Though in early cases there may be no abnormal physical signs, usually some impairment of sensation over the affected fingers can be detected. Tenderness on compression of the nerve at the wrist† and thenar atrophy are relatively rare. If the story is characteristic, the absence of physical signs should not deter one from advising treatment with intracarpal tunnel steroid injection or carpal tunnel decompression. Investigation with nerve conduction studies may be helpful in cases of doubt. In advanced, unrecognized cases, the patient may present with burns on one or more of the first three fingers.

Causes of carpal tunnel syndrome

Idiopathic (almost entirely in females, middle-aged, often obese, or younger women with excessive use of hands; may occur in males after unaccustomed hand use, e.g. house painting)

Pregnancy

Contraceptive pill

Myxoedema (?facies, hoarse croaking voice, pulse, ankle jerks, etc; see Vol. 3, Station 5, Endocrine, Case 9)

Acromegaly (?facies, large spade-shaped hands, bitemporal hemianopia, etc; see Vol. 3, Station 5, Endocrine, Case 2)

Rheumatoid arthritis of the wrists (?spindling of the fingers, ulnar deviation, nodules, etc; see Vol. 3, Station 5, Locomotor, Case 1)

Osteoarthrosis of the carpus (perhaps related to an old fracture)

Tuberculous tenosynovitis

Primary amyloidosis (?peripheral neuropathy, thick nerves, autonomic neuropathy; heart, joint and gut (rectal biopsy) involvement may occur – see also Footnote, Station 3, CNS, Case 1)

Tophaceous gout (see Vol 3, Station 5, Locomotor, Case 5)

---

*The nocturnal discomfort may be referred to the whole forearm with paraesthesiae extending beyond the cutaneous distribution of the median nerve in the hand. The sensory *signs*, however, are confined to the classic median nerve distribution (see Fig. B.4, Section B, Examination *Routine* 15).

†*Tinel's sign* is tingling in the distribution of a nerve produced by percussion of that nerve. Percussion over the carpal tunnel sometimes produces a positive Tinel's sign in carpal tunnel

syndrome. Other signs are *Phalen's sign* (the patient flexes both wrists for 60 sec and this produces a prompt exacerbation of paraesthesia which is rapidly relieved when the flexion is discontinued) which is positive in half the patients, as is the *tourniquet test* (a sphygmomanometer is pumped above systolic pressure for 2 min and this produces the paraesthesia). Symptoms may sometimes be induced by *hyperextension* at the wrist.

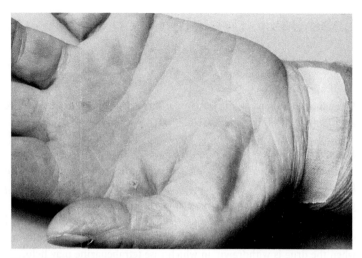

Figure C3.22 Wasting of the thenar eminence.

Case 34 | Drug-induced extrapyramidal syndrome

Frequency in survey: main focus of a short case or additional feature in 0.7% of attempts at PACES Station 3, CNS.

Record

There are (in this ?elderly, chronic schizophrenic) stereotyped tic-like *orofacial dyskinesias* (involuntary movements) including *lip-smacking, chewing, pouting* and *grimacing*. There is (may be) *choreoathetosis* of the limbs and trunk.

The diagnosis is tardive dyskinesia.* (It is likely that the patient has been on sustained phenothiazine treatment for at least 6 months. The condition often persists when the drug is withdrawn, in which case tetrabenazine may help.)

Neuroleptics which may cause abnormal involuntary movements (by inhibiting dopamine function)
Phenothiazines (e.g. chlorpromazine)
Butyrophenones (e.g. haloperidol)
Substituted benzamides (e.g. metoclopramide)
Reserpine
Tetrabenazine

Other neuroleptic-induced extrapyramidal adverse reactions (apart from tardive dyskinesia)
Acute dystonias (soon after starting the drug, e.g. oculogyric crises)
Akathisia (uncontrollable restlessness with an inner feeling of unease)
Parkinson's syndrome (indistinguishable from Parkinson's disease though tremor is
  less common; tends to respond to anticholinergics rather than L-dopa)

---

*Called tardive (late) because it does not appear until at least 3 months, or more often a year, after the start or withdrawal of long-term treatment with neuroleptic drugs. This distinguishes tardive dyskinesia from acute dystonias and parkinsonism which develop early. The latter respond to anticholinergic drugs, while tardive dyskinesia responds poorly, or not at all.

Case 35 | Lower motor neurone VIIth nerve palsy

Frequency in survey: main focus of a short case or additional feature in 0.7% of attempts at PACES Station 3, CNS.

Record

On the R/L side there is *paralysis* of the *upper* and lower face,* so that the *eye cannot be closed* (or it can easily be opened by the examiner; the patient cannot bury the eyelashes); the eyeball turns up on attempted closure (*Bell's phenomenon*) and the patient is unable to raise his R/L eyebrow. The corner of the *mouth droops,* the *nasolabial fold* is *smoothed out,* and the voluntary and involuntary (i.e. including emotional) movements of the mouth are paralysed on the R/L side (the lips may be drawn to the opposite side and the tongue may deviate as well – not necessarily hypoglossal involvement; see Footnote, Station 3, CNS, Case 8).

This is a R/L lower motor neurone VIIth nerve lesion (now check the ipsilateral ear for evidence of *herpes zoster*).

Causes of a lower motor neurone VIIth nerve lesion

1 Bell's palsy†
2 Ramsay Hunt syndrome (herpes zoster on the external auditory meatus and the geniculate ganglion – taste to the anterior two-thirds of the tongue is lost; there may be lesions on the fauces and palate)

Other differential diagnoses

Cerebellopontine angle compression (acoustic neuroma or meningioma; Vth, VIth, VIIth, VIIIth nerve palsy, cerebellar signs and loss of taste to the anterior two-thirds of the tongue; see Station 3, CNS, Case 25)

Parotid tumour (?palpable; taste not affected)

Trauma

A pontine lesion (e.g. MS, tumour or vascular lesion)

Middle ear disease (deafness)

The causes of mononeuritis multiplex (diabetes, poly-arteritis nodosa and Churg–Strauss syndrome, rheumatoid, SLE, Wegener's, sarcoid, carcinoma, amyloid and leprosy)

Causes of bilateral lower motor neurone VIIth nerve paralysis‡

Guillain–Barré syndrome (occasionally only VIIth nerves affected)

Sarcoidosis (parotid gland enlargement not always present)

Bilateral Bell's palsy

Myasthenia gravis (?ptosis, variable strabismus, proximal muscle weakness, etc; see Station 3, CNS, Case 27)

Congenital facial diplegia

Some forms of muscular dystrophy

Motor neurone disease (rarely)

Lyme disease (may be bilateral, alone or with signs of meningoencephalitis or peripheral radiculoneuropathy, knee effusion, Baker's cyst rupture, heart block, etc.)

---

*That is, including frontalis ('raise eyebrows'), corrugator superficialis ('frown') and orbicularis oculi ('close your eyes tight').
†In the mild case of Bell's palsy, taste over the anterior two-thirds of the tongue is usually preserved, because the lesion is due to swelling of the nerve in the confined lower facial canal. In cases with more extensive involvement, this taste is lost and the patient may also show increased susceptibility to high-pitched or loud sounds (hyperacusis due to stapedius paralysis).
‡Bilateral lower motor neurone VIIth nerve lesions are easily missed because there is no asymmetry.

The chorda tympani leaves the facial nerve in the middle ear to supply taste to the anterior two-thirds of the tongue. The superficial petrosal branch to supply the lachrymal glands, and the nerve to stapedius, both leave higher in the facial canal than the chorda tympani. The level of the lesion in the facial canal can sometimes be assessed (very unlikely to be required in the examination) by assessing the relative involvement of these nerves.

Variation of the Ramsay Hunt syndrome

Occasionally facial palsy is associated with trigeminal, occipital or cervical herpes with or without auditory involvement (see Vol. 2, Section F, Anecdote 278). In some of these cases the geniculate ganglion may be spared (see Vol. 3, Station 5, Skin, Case 32).

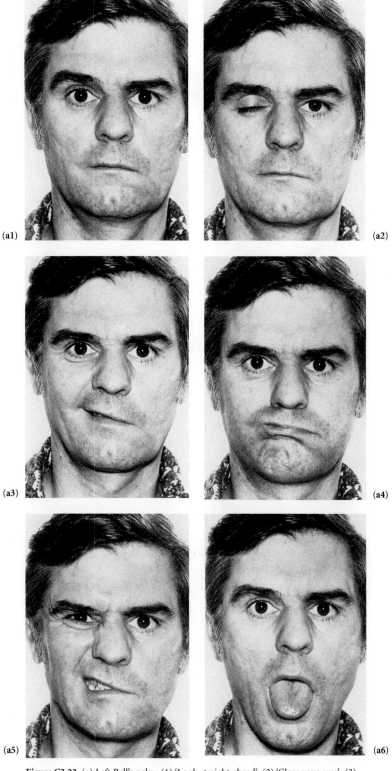

Figure C3.23 (a) Left Bell's palsy: (1) 'Look straight ahead'; (2) 'Close your eyes'; (3) 'Smile'; (4) 'Puff out your cheeks'; (5) 'Show me your teeth'; (6) 'Put out your tongue'. (*Continued.*)

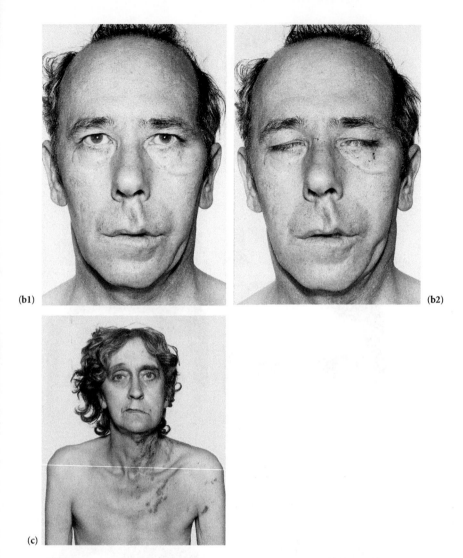

Figure C3.23 *(Continued)* (b1) Bilateral lower motor neurone VIIth nerve palsy (Guillain–Barré syndrome); (2) 'Close your eyes'. (c) Ramsay Hunt syndrome.

Case 36 | Dysarthria

Frequency in survey: main focus of a short case or additional feature in 0.6% of attempts at PACES Station 3, CNS.

Survey note: usually cerebellar (ataxic) dysarthria, but one case of bulbar palsy.

Record

There is dysarthria with *slurred, jerky* and *explosive* (slow, staccato, scanning) speech. (There may be inspiratory whoops indicating the lack of coordination between respiration and phonation.)

This suggests cerebellar disease (?nystagmus, dysdiadochokinesis, finger–nose test, etc; see Station 3, CNS, Case 7).

Other varieties of dysarthria

Spastic dysarthria

Conditions in which all or some of the articulatory parts are rigid or spastic:

Pseudobulbar palsy (indistinct, suppressed, without modulations, high-pitched, 'hot potato', 'Donald Duck' speech due to a tight, immobile tongue – ?bilateral spasticity with extensor plantars; see Station 3, CNS, Case 46)

Parkinson's disease (monotonous without accents or emphasis, somewhat slurred speech – ?expressionless unblinking face, glabellar tap sign, tremor, etc; see Station 3, CNS, Case 3)

Myotonic dystrophy (slurred and suppressed speech – ?ptosis, frontal balding, etc; see Station 3, CNS, Case 2)

Huntington's chorea (slurred and monotonous – ?chorea, dementia)

General paresis of the insane – very rare (slurred, hesitant or feeble voice – ?dementia, vacant expression, trombone tremor of tongue, brisk reflexes, extensor plantars, etc; see Station 3, CNS, Case 50)

Flaccid dysarthria

Bulbar palsy (nasal, decreased modulation, slurring of labial and lingual consonants – ?lingual atrophy, fasciculations, etc; see Station 3, CNS, Case 21)

Paralysis of the VIIth, IXth, Xth or XIIth nerves (cerebrovascular accident)

Myopathic dysarthria

Myasthenia gravis (weak hoarse voice with a nasal quality, pitch unsustained, soft accents – ?ptosis, variable strabismus, facial and proximal muscle weakness all of which worsen with repetition, etc; see Station 3, CNS, Case 27)

Structural dysarthria

Hypothyroidism (low-pitched, catarrhal, hoarse, croaking, gutteral voice as if the tongue is too large for the mouth – ?facies, pulse, ankle jerks, etc; see Vol. 3, Station 5, Endocrine, Case 5)

Amyloidosis – large tongue (rolling and hollow, hardly modulated)

Multiple ulcers or thrush in the mouth (some parts of the speech indistinct)

Parotitis or temporomandibular arthritis (monotonous, suppressed, badly modulated)

Case 37 | Subacute combined degeneration of the cord

Frequency in survey: main focus of a short case or additional feature in 0.3% of attempts at PACES Station 3, CNS.

Record

There is (in this patient who may complain of burning paraesthesiae in the feet) loss of *light touch, vibration* and *joint position* sensation over the feet (*stocking*, may also be *glove*), and *Romberg's* sign is positive. The legs are (may be) weak and though the knee (may be brisk) and *ankle jerks* are *lost* (due to peripheral neuropathy), the *plantar responses* are *extensor*.

The pupils are normal, there are no cerebellar signs or pes cavus (see Station 3, CNS, Case 24) and though the patient is not (may not be) clinically anaemic* (having checked conjunctival mucous membranes) and the tongue and complexion are normal (glossitis and classic 'lemon yellow' pallor are now rarely seen in SACD), these findings suggest the diagnosis of subacute combined degeneration of the cord. (Findings in the abdomen might be splenomegaly, carcinoma of the stomach as this is more common in pernicious anaemia, or a laparotomy scar from a previous gastrectomy.)

Although vitamin B_{12} neuropathy usually starts with peripheral neuropathy followed by posterior column signs, and signs of pyramidal disturbances are seldom marked in the early stages (progressive spasticity may occur), vitamin B_{12} deficiency should always be excluded in a patient in whom any of the following are unexplained:

Peripheral sensory neuropathy

Spinal cord disease

Optic atrophy (rare)

Dementia (frank dementia is rare; progressive enfeeblement of intellect and memory, or episodes of confusion or paranoia may be seen; more commonly the patient is simply difficult and uncooperative)

Causes of severe vitamin B_{12} deficiency

Addisonian pernicious anaemia (NB: associated organ-specific autoimmune diseases, especially autoimmune thyroid disease, diabetes mellitus, Addison's, vitiligo and hypoparathyroidism – see also Vol. 3, Station 5, Skin, Case 8)

Partial or total gastrectomy

Stagnant loop syndrome

Ileal resection or Crohn's disease

Vegan diet

Fish tapeworm

Chronic tropical sprue

Congenital intrinsic factor deficiency

Lhermitte's phenomenon: the patient describes a 'tingling' or 'electric feeling' or 'funny sensation' which passes down his spine, and perhaps into lower limbs, when he bends his head forward.† The most common cause is MS but it can also occur in cervical cord tumour, cervical spondylosis and SACD.

---

*Although the patient may be anaemic, vitamin B_{12} neuropathy may develop without anaemia and with normal blood film and bone marrow (see Vol. 3, Station 5, Other, Case 6). Serum vitamin B_{12} level may be required to confirm the diagnosis.

†A similar sensation provoked by neck *extension* is termed 'reversed Lhermitte's phenomenon' and strongly suggests cervical spondylosis.

Case 38 | Argyll Robertson pupils

Frequency in survey: main focus of a short case or additional feature in 0.1% of attempts at PACES Station 3, CNS.

Record

The pupils are *small* and *irregular* and react to *accommodation but not to light.**

The likely diagnosis is tabes dorsalis (?wrinkled forehead with ptosis, stamping ataxia, Romberg's test positive, loss of joint position and vibration sense, absent ankle jerks, Charcot's knee joint and aortic incompetence; see Station 3, CNS, Case 50).

The exact site of the lesion is not known. It is generally believed to be in the tectum of the mid-brain proximal to the oculomotor nuclei. The classic Argyll Robertson pupil is very small. However, pupils affected by neurosyphilis are not always small and may even be dilated. They may be unequal in size. Though the signs may be more advanced in one eye than the other, pupillary abnormalities occurring in neurosyphilis are invariably bilateral. The characteristic features of Argyll Robertson pupils are that they are *irregular* (may be subtle and should be looked for with an ophthalmoscope), and that even though they may react to light, this is always *less* than their reaction to accommodation. Argyll Robertson-like pupils occasionally occur in diabetes mellitus.

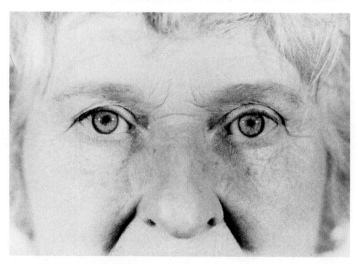

Figure C3.24 Argyll Robertson pupils in a diabetic patient. Her serology was negative.

*The light reflex may be present (before it becomes increasingly sluggish and then disappears), but the accommodation reflex is always *brisker* than the light reflex.

Case 39 | Congenital syphilis

Frequency in survey: main focus of a short case or additional feature in 0.1% of attempts at PACES Station 3, CNS.

Record

There is flattening of the bridge of the nose (*saddle nose*), the superior maxilla is underdeveloped which makes the mandible appear prominent (*bull-dog jaw*), and there is frontal bossing. There are *rhagades* at the corners of the mouth and there are *Hutchinson's teeth* (widely spaced peg-shaped upper incisors with a crescentic notch at the cutting edge) and *Moon's molars* (dome-shaped deformity of the first lower molars with underdeveloped cusps). The tibiae have a wide middle third with palpable irregularities (due to osteoperiostitis) along the anterior skin (*sabre tibiae*).

The diagnosis is congenital syphilis.

Other manifestations of late congenital syphilis*

VIIIth nerve deafness

Clutton's joints (effusions into the knee joints with no pain or difficulty with joint movement)

Interstitial keratitis (acute attacks;† may eventually lead to corneal opacities – ground-glass appearance of cornea; a closer look shows the underlying radiating, brush-like vascularization referred to as *salmon-patch* appearance)

Old choroidoretinitis (peripheral and bilateral – 'salt and pepper fundus')

Optic atrophy

Perforations of the palate or nasal septum

Collapse of the nasal cartilage

---

*Early congenital syphilis in the first few months of life resembles severe secondary syphilis in the adult. Features include rhinitis, a mucocutaneous rash, osteochondritis, dactylitis, hepato-splenomegaly, lymphadenopathy, anaemia, jaundice, thrombocytopenia and leucocytosis. Nephrotic syndrome may occur.

†May be due to hypersensitivity. Corticosteroids may sometimes help.

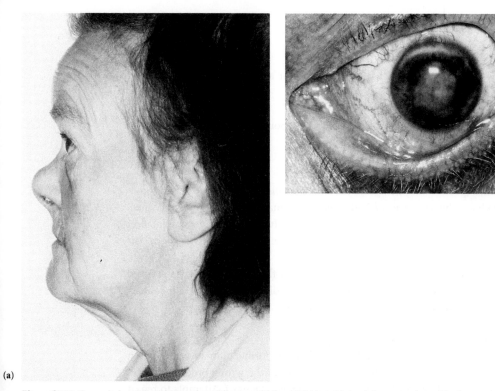

(a)

(b)

Figure C3.25 Congenital syphilis. (a) Note the saddle nose. (b) Interstitial keratitis has led to corneal opacification.

Case 40 | Dysphasia

Frequency in survey: main focus of a short case or additional feature in 0.1% of attempts at PACES Station 3, CNS.

Survey note: where the type of dysphasia was reported by the candidate, it was always expressive.

Record 1

The patient's speech *lacks fluency*. He has *difficulty finding certain words* and some-times produces the *wrong word* and makes grammatical errors. *Comprehension*, however, is *well preserved* (as are the higher cerebral functions and general intellect – the prognosis for eventual adaptation of the patient to his disability is good). His ability to repeat and to name objects is impaired.

The patient has Broca's (*expressive*, motor, non-fluent) *dysphasia* (?associated *right hemiplegia*). The brain damage causing this condition is believed to disconnect the dominant* inferior frontal gyrus (Broca's area).

Record 2

Though the patient *speaks fluently* (often rapidly) with normal intonation, his speech is completely *unintelligible*. He puts words together in the wrong order and mixes them with non-existent words† and phrases (*jargon dysphasia*). Attempts to repeat result in paraphasic† distortions and irrelevant insertions. *Comprehension* is severely *impaired* (and the patient may seem unaware of his dysphasia).

The patient has Wernicke's (*receptive*, fluent) *dysphasia* (?associated *homonymous visual field defect* and/or *sensory diminution* down the right side of the body). The brain damage causing this condition is believed to disconnect the posterior part of the dominant* superior temporal gyrus (Wernicke's area).

Record 3

The patient shows combined expressive and receptive dysphasia. There is marked disturbance in comprehension (and inability to read or write).

The patient has *global dysphasia*‡ (?dense right hemiplegia with sensory loss, homonymous visual field defect and general intellectual deterioration). The common cause of this is infarction of the territory supplied by the left middle cerebral artery. The prognosis for recovery is poor.

---

*The left hemisphere is dominant in right-handed and in 50% of left-handed people.
†Paraphasia: an incorrect syllable in a word (usually there is some phonemic relationship to the original word, e.g. 'tooth spooth' for 'toothbrush') or an incorrect word in a phrase (often with a semantic relationship to the correct word, e.g. 'hand' for 'foot'). Neologism: paraphasia with slight or no relationship to the original syllable/word.

‡Global dysphasia is sometimes confused with Broca's dysphasia but the speech defects are severe in this condition, affecting fluency, repetition, naming and comprehension. Some ste-reotypes may be preserved and the patient may be able to recite automatic sequences of prayer or popular songs (*speech automatism*).

Record 4

The patient has difficulty naming objects though he knows what they are (e.g. hold up some keys: 'What is this?' – patient does not answer. 'Is this a spoon?' – 'No'. 'Is it a pen?' – 'No'. 'Is it keys?' – 'Yes'). Despite this, comprehension and other aspects of speech production are relatively normal. This is *nominal dysphasia* (uncommon in its pure form, usually part of a wider dysphasia). The underlying brain damage is believed to be in the most posterior part of the superior temporal gyrus and the adjacent inferior parietal lobule.

Case 41 | Horner's syndrome

Frequency in survey: main focus of a short case or additional feature in 0.1% of attempts at PACES Station 3, CNS.

Record

There is *miosis*,* *enophthalmos* and slight *ptosis* on the R/L side (the other features are ipsilateral *anhydrosis* and vasodilation of the head and neck).

This is a R/L-sided Horner's syndrome; now examine the *neck* (scars, nodes, aneurysms), *hands* (wasting of the small muscles) and *chest* (ipsilateral apical signs).

Causes of Horner's syndrome

1 Neck surgery or trauma (?scars)
2 Carotid† and aortic aneurysms
3 Brainstem vascular disease (e.g. Wallenberg's syndrome‡)
4 Pancoast's syndrome (?wasting of ipsilateral small muscles of the hand, T1 and sometimes C7–8 sensory loss and pain, clubbing, tracheal deviation, lymph nodes, ipsilateral apical signs)
5 Enlarged cervical lymph nodes especially malignant (?evidence of primary)
6 Idiopathic (common in neurological practice)
7 Syringomyelia (?bilateral wasting of the small muscles of the hand, dissociated sensory loss, scarred hands, bulbar palsy, pyramidal signs, nystagmus; see Station 3, CNS, Case 29)
8 Brainstem demyelination (?nystagmus, cerebellar signs, pyramidal signs, pale discs, etc.)

The syndrome can be caused by any other lesion in the sympathetic nervous system as it travels from the sympathetic nucleus, down through the brainstem to the cord, out of the cord at C8, T1–2, to the sympathetic chain, stellate ganglion and carotid sympathetic plexus (see Fig. C3.26b). Some cases of Horner's are idiopathic (usually females).

*NB: Argyll Robertson pupils in neurosyphilis are usually bilateral, irregular and very small.

†Horner's syndrome may be the only manifestation of *carotid dissection*. An urgent carotid and head MRI scan should be performed in newly presenting Horner's syndrome of uncertain cause. Carotid dissection is an important cause of ischaemic stroke in young and middle-aged patients. Spontaneous dissection of carotid and vertebral arteries may affect all age groups, including children, but there is a distinct peak in the fifth decade. A history of a minor precipitating event is frequently elicited in spontaneous dissection of the carotid or vertebral artery, particularly associated with hyperextension or rotation of the neck (e.g. painting a ceiling, coughing, vomiting, sneezing, the receipt of anaesthesia are all described). The typical patient with carotid artery dissection presents with pain on one side of the head, face or neck accompanied by a partial Horner's syndrome and followed hours or days later by cerebral or retinal ischaemia. However, this classic triad is found in less than one-third of patients and there may be just one or two of the features. The priority in management is to avoid thromboembolic complications. Although no randomized trials have been reported, anticoagulation has been recommended for acute dissections of the carotid or vertebral artery unless there are contraindications such as intracranial extension of the dissection. Following this approach, there is a high rate of recanalization within the first 3 months. The fear that anticoagulant therapy will extend the dissection appears to be unfounded.

‡Ipsilateral Vth, IXth, Xth, XIth nerve lesions, cerebellar ataxia and nystagmus. Contralateral pain and temperature loss (see Station 3, CNS, Case 44).

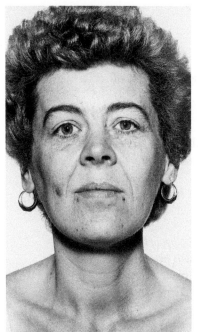

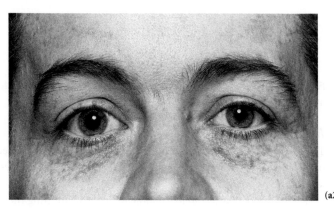

(a2)

(a1)

(b)

Figure C3.26 (a1,2) Left Horner's syndrome (note the scar over the left clavicle). (b) Sympathetic and parasympathetic nerve supply to dilator and sphincter pupillae. The diagram shows the sympathetic pathway and the sites where it may be interrupted to produce Horner's syndrome. (This article was published in *Gray's Anatomy of the Human Body*, Henry Gray, copyright Elsevier, 1918.)

Case 42 | Infantile hemiplegia

Frequency in survey: main focus of a short case or additional feature in 0.1% of attempts at PACES Station 3, CNS.

Record 1

The R/L leg (in this patient with normal intelligence, normal speech and no history of epilepsy) is slightly *shorter* and thinner than the L/R, its *reflexes* are *brisk* and the R/L *plantar* response is *extensor*.

These features suggest mild infantile hemiplegia affecting the R/L leg.

Record 2

There is (in this patient with epilepsy and mental retardation) marked *hypoplasia* of the R/L arm and leg, with *spasticity* and *contractures*, R/L *homonymous hemianopia* and R/L *ankle clonus* and *extensor plantar* response. There is *asymmetry of the trunk*, smaller on the R/L, and diffuse impairment of sensation on the R/L. There is asymmetry of the skull, smaller on the L/R (the other side to the hemiplegia), *jaw clonus* and *spastic dysarthria* (there may be a squint, e.g. convergent on the L/R).

These features suggest severe infantile hemiplegia with spasticity affecting the R/L side.

Infantile hemiplegia results from a lesion which develops during the first year of life; only rarely is it from prenatal lesions or birth trauma. The hemiplegia may occur as a complication of an infective disorder such as pertussis, measles or scarlet fever; more commonly, however, there is no obvious predisposing cause and the hemiplegia is probably a manifestation of an encephalitis or toxic encephalopathy. There is an arrest of growth on the affected side and the hemiplegic limbs may be the site of spontaneous involuntary movements of either a choreic or athetoid character. Epilepsy is common, with convulsions beginning on the affected side. The extent and severity of the hemiplegia and the degree of cerebral retardation depend on the extent of the original involvement of the cerebral cortex. In some cases the abnormality may be very slight – a smallness of a hand or foot, a thinness of a forearm or calf, a clumsiness of the fingers or contracture of the Achilles tendon. There may be just an imperceptible degree of general body asymmetry. Focal convulsions in an otherwise healthy child or adolescent should always raise the possibility of a minimal infantile hemiplegia. Only by careful scrutiny of the undressed patient as a whole will such slight asymmetry be detected.

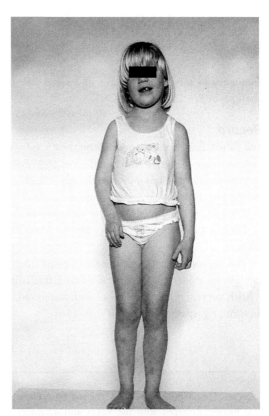

Figure C3.27 Infantile hemiplegia. The right arm and leg are smaller than the left. The features continue into adulthood and the patient may then appear in the MRCP PACES exam.

Case 43 | Jugular foramen syndrome

Frequency in survey: main focus of a short case or additional feature in 0.1% of attempts at PACES Station 3, CNS.

Record

The patient has an *absent gag reflex* on the R/L side (and will have ipsilateral impaired taste over the posterior third of the tongue). *Palatal movements* on that side are *reduced* and the *uvula* is *drawn* to the *opposite side*. The R/L *sternomastoid* muscle is *wasted* and there is weakness in rotating the head to the opposite side. The *shoulder* is *flattened* and there is weakness of elevation of that shoulder.

There is therefore a lesion affecting the *IXth, Xth and XIth cranial nerves* on the R/L side.

This suggests a jugular foramen syndrome (to exclude a brainstem lesion,* check carefully for evidence of ipsilateral wasting, fasciculation and deviation of the tongue – XIIth nerve, ipsilateral Horner's and, if allowed, for evidence of brainstem compression, e.g. spastic paraparesis).

An isolated lesion of the glossopharyngeal nerve is rare. It is usually damaged with the vagus and accessory nerves near the jugular foramen which all three nerves traverse (see Fig. C3.28). A lesion inside the skull is more likely to cause a syndrome restricted to the IXth, Xth and XIth nerves only (syndrome of Vernet†). An internal lesion may cause brainstem compression.* A lesion outside the skull is more likely to involve the XIIth nerve as well (syndrome of Collet–Sicard†); this nerve exits through the hypoglossal foramen near the external opening of the jugular foramen. An external lesion may also involve the cervical sympathetic* (syndrome of Villaret†). Other combinations of associated lower cranial lesions are vagus and accessory (syndrome of Schmidt†), and vagus, accessory and hypoglossal (syndrome of Hughlings Jackson†).

Causes of jugular foramen syndromes

Neurofibroma of IXth, Xth or XIIth nerves (especially left XIIth in young females)
Meningiomata
Epidermoid tumours
Glomus or carotid body tumours
Metastases
Cerebellopontine angle lesions (see Station 3, CNS, Case 25; may also extend down and involve the last four cranial nerves in numerical order)
Infection from the middle ear spreading into the posterior fossa
Cholesteatomata
Granulomatous meningitis

---

*Intrinsic brainstem disease may cause lower cranial nerve palsies and Horner's syndrome (e.g. Station 3, CNS, Cases 29 and 44), but when the pathology is in the brainstem there is nearly always spinothalamic sensory loss on the opposite side of the body to the lesion.

†Though the age of such neurological eponyms is undoubtedly passing, their usage may still impress!

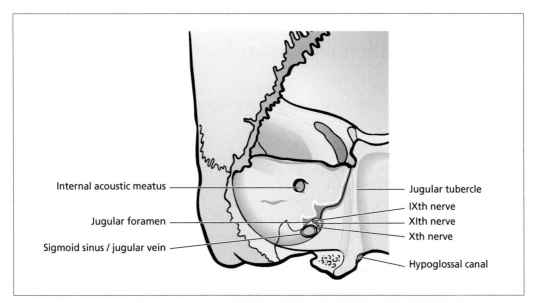

Figure C3.28 The posterior aspect of the posterior cranial fossa (after removal of the squamous part of the occipital bone) showing the jugular foramen and the nerves passing through it (note the position of the hypoglossal canal which conducts the XIIth nerve).

Case 44 | Lateral medullary syndrome (Wallenberg's syndrome)

Frequency in survey: did not occur in any of our surveys though it has occurred in the exam.*

Record

(Assumes a lesion affecting the artery on the right.) On the right of the patient (who presented with acute vertigo†) there is (*ipsilateral*):

Horner's syndrome (descending sympathetic tract)

Cerebellar signs (cerebellum and its connections)

Palatal paralysis and diminished gag reflex (may be dysphagia and hoarseness due to a vocal cord paralysis – IXth and Xth nerves)

Decreased *trigeminal* pain and temperature sensation (descending tract and nucleus of the Vth nerve).

On the left of the patient the trunk and limbs (and sometimes the face) show (*contralateral*) decreased *pain and temperature* sensation‡ (spinothalamic tract).

The patient has a lateral medullary syndrome (produced by infarction of a small wedge of lateral medulla posterior to the inferior olivary nucleus – Fig. C3.29) classically due to a lesion of the right *posterior inferior cerebellar artery*.§

Involvement of the nucleus and tractus solitarius may cause loss of taste. Hiccup may occur. When occlusion of the posterior inferior cerebellar artery is isolated, the pyramidal pathways escape and there is no hemiplegia. In the majority of cases of lateral medullary syndrome, there is also an occlusion of the vertebral artery and pyramidal signs are present. Rarely, occlusion of the lower basilar artery, vertebral artery or one of its medial branches produces the *medial medullary syndrome* (contralateral hemiplegia which spares the face, contralateral loss of vibration and joint position sense, and ipsilateral paralysis and wasting of the tongue).

Other eponymous brainstem infarction syndromes

Weber's syndrome (*mid-brain*; ipsilateral IIIrd nerve palsy and contralateral hemiparesis)

Nothnagel's syndrome (*mid-brain*; ipsilateral IIIrd nerve palsy and cerebellar ataxia)

Millard–Gubler syndrome (*pons*; ipsilateral VIth nerve palsy and facial weakness with contralateral hemiplegia)

Foville's syndrome (*pons*; as Millard–Gubler but with lateral conjugate gaze palsy)

These and a number of other eponymous brainstem syndromes (e.g. Claude, Benedict, Raymond–Cestau)

---

*One candidate told us: 'Just my luck! One of my short cases was lateral medullary syndrome: it was your penultimate short case (in the first edition of your book) and as, according to your book, it had not occurred in the exam, it was the only short case in your book I did not study!'

†Vestibular involvement may produce nystagmus, diplopia, oscillopsia, vertigo, nausea and vomiting.

‡Involvement of the cuneate and gracile nuclei may cause numbness of the ipsilateral (right in this case) arm.

§Occlusion of any one of five vessels may be responsible – vertebral, posterior inferior cerebellar, superior, middle or inferior lateral medullary arteries. The resulting clinical picture is variable and the rehabilitating patient may not show all features.

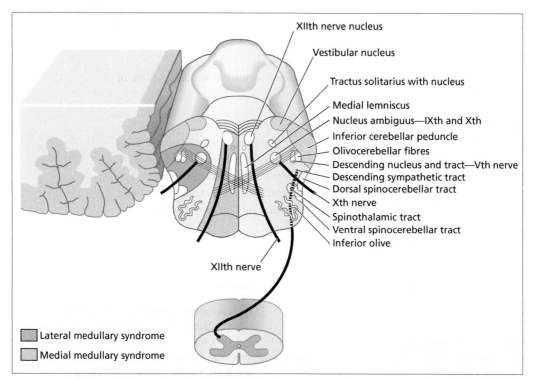

Figure C3.29 A cross-section through the medulla at the level of the inferior olivary nucleus showing the area infarcted in the lateral and medial medullary syndromes, respectively. (Adapted from Mohr JP *et al.* in *Harrison's Principles of Internal Medicine*, 1983, 10th edn, p. 2037, by kind permission of McGraw-Hill.)

were, in their classic descriptions, mostly related to tumours and other non-vascular diseases. The diagnosis of brainstem vascular disorders is facilitated more by knowledge of the neuroanatomy of the brainstem than of these eponyms. In one analysis of 50 patients (Cornell–Bellevue series) with brainstem infarction, only two fitted into these syndromes as originally described. The rest had an extensive mixture of signs and symptoms indicating an overlap in the areas believed to be infarcted by occlusions in specific arteries.

Case 45 | Polymyositis

Frequency in survey: main focus of a short case or additional feature in 0.1% of attempts at PACES Station 3, CNS.

Record

There is *symmetrical,** *proximal* muscle *weakness* (the patient may be unable to sit up from lying or stand up from squatting position) with associated muscle *wasting*. The muscles are *tender* (in 50% of cases, suggesting an inflammatory myopathy). The patient is (may be) unable to flex his neck against resistance. The tendon reflexes are present though reduced.† There is (may be) dysphonia (and/or dysphagia) due to involvement of the bulbar muscles.

The diagnosis is polymyositis.

Male-to-female ratio is 1/2.

Features of polymyositis

A rash may occur (dermatomyositis; see Vol. 3, Station 5, Skin, Case 6)

Features and associations similar to dermatomyositis (see Vol. 3, Station 5, Skin, Case 6)

Association with malignancy‡

Onset of muscle weakness is usually insidious (with difficulty in running, climbing stairs, getting up from a chair, and combing hair)

Lower limb girdle more often affected than shoulder girdle

Ocular involvement is rare (if present, think of myasthenia gravis)

Respiratory muscle weakness can lead to respiratory failure – monitor peak flow rate and vital capacity

Cardiac muscle may be involved

Other causes of proximal muscle weakness

See also Station 3, CNS, Case 23

Carcinomatous neuromyopathy (including Eaton–Lambert syndrome; see Station 3, CNS, Case 27)

Diabetic amyotrophy (?fundi, peripheral neuropathy)

Muscular dystrophies (?long-standing, familial; see Station 3, CNS, Case 9)

Dystrophia myotonica (?frontal balding, cataracts, myotonia, etc; see Station 3, CNS, Case 2)

Alcoholism

Thyrotoxicosis (?eye signs, hypermobile, goitre, etc; see Vol. 3, Station 5, Endocrine, Case 3)

Corticosteroid treatment (?cushingoid facies, underlying disorder, etc; see Vol. 3, Station 5, Endocrine, Case 6)

Familial periodic paralysis

Osteomalacia

Hyperparathyroidism

Insulinoma

Polymyalgia rheumatica is characterized by pain and stiffness of proximal muscles, especially the shoulder girdle, in a patient who is usually elderly. The ESR is high. Significant objective weakness is not common. There is a relationship with temporal (giant cell) arteritis (see also Station 3, CNS, Case 23).

---

*In general, if muscle weakness is symmetrical it suggests myopathic disease, and if asymmetrical neurogenic disease.

†If very reduced or absent, it suggests underlying carcinoma causing polyneuropathy and polymyositis.

‡There is an increased risk of malignancy (lungs, breast, ovary, GI tract, nasopharynx, prostate, blood) in older patients with dermatomyositis; the risk is lower in polymyositis. Current wisdom is that a search for malignancy should be made in older patients (>40 years old) with dermatomyositis and polymyositis, and in those with atypical or intractable lesions. A reasonable approach in this direction would constitute a thorough clinical assessment, including a per rectum examination in males and pelvic examination in females, and some baseline investigations (full blood count, stool occult blood, chest X-ray, USS abdomen/pelvis, prostate specific antigen (PSA) and mammogram in women).

Case 46 | Pseudobulbar palsy

Frequency in survey: main focus of a short case or additional feature in 0.1% of attempts at PACES Station 3, CNS.

Record

There is monotonous, slurred, high-pitched 'Donald Duck' *dysarthria* and the patient *dribbles persistently* from the mouth (he has dysphagia and may have nasal regurgitation). He *cannot protrude his tongue* which lies on the floor of the mouth and is *small and tight. Palatal movement* is *absent*, the *jaw jerk* is *exaggerated* and he is *emotionally labile.*

The diagnosis is pseudobulbar palsy (?bilateral generalized spasticity and extensor plantar responses).

Most common cause
Bilateral cerebrovascular accidents of the internal capsule

Other causes
Multiple sclerosis
Motor neurone disease
High brainstem tumours
Head injury

Case 47 | Psychogenic/factitious

Frequency in survey: main focus of a short case or additional feature in 0.1% of attempts at PACES Station 3, CNS.

Psychogenic and factitious illnesses occur in everyday clinical practice and it would seem from the following anecdotes and the one in Vol. 3, Station 5, Skin, Case 51, from our surveys, that it is possible that they have also occasionally appeared in the Membership!

Anecdote 1

A candidate was asked to examine a female patient's right hand neurologically. He found normal tone but decreased power in all groups of muscles in the wrist and hand. He said there was some wasting but the examiners disputed this. The candidate thought he had better not retract, even though he felt they were probably right, so he said that he thought there was some. The examiners said, 'OK'. The candidate then asked for a pin, but at that moment the bell went. The examiners told him to ask about sensory loss. The patient pointed to various places in a pattern that did not suggest organic pathology, saying, 'Here, here, here ... '. The examiner said, 'You're having difficulty, aren't you?'. The candidate responded in the affirmative, trying to offer some possible explanations, but the examiners moved away chuckling to themselves. The candidate (who passed) reports 'It obviously was psychogenic!'.

Anecdote 2

A candidate reports that he was taken to see a gentleman who was lying on a couch smoking and was told that he complained of being numb down one side. He felt that 'this seemed most bizarre from the start'. He was asked to examine sensation and started with light touch; this seemed to show that the patient had a sharply demarcated hemianaesthesia. Pain and joint position sensation were similar. As the bell went he was asked what he thought could cause this. He initially mumbled something about 'vascular' but then said he thought it was 'factitious'. He reports 'I'm still not sure whether my findings were correct or what the true diagnosis was' (he did not pass until his next attempt).

As stated by Anderson and Trethowan,* hysterical behaviour or symptoms have a place in a spectrum at one end of which motivation, due to extreme capacity for the denial of inconvenient reality, is almost if not entirely hidden from the patient. This probably applies to no more than a tiny minority of patients. At the other end of the spectrum, and once again a minority, motivation is clear and purposive, amounting no more or less to simulation.† The great bulk of hysterical disorders show various shades of 'awareness' in between.

*Anderson EW, Trethowan WH (1973) *Psychiatry*, 3rd edn. Baillière Tindall, London.
†Frank malingering with a motive such as avoiding work that is disliked. It might be thought that compensation neurosis would fall at the frank malingering end of the spectrum. It is believed, however, that the power of human self-deception is far too strong to make this necessary. Patients suffer from complaints that they hope will bring compensation and at the same time retain their self-respect by believing in them themselves.

Thus there is no 'either/or' – it is a question of how much of each. The capacity for self-deception and denial is a common human attribute which varies greatly between individuals. In deceiving himself, the hysteric supposes he can deceive others. In some this belief is justified so that even the most experienced psychiatrist or clinician may err at times. The manifestations of hysteria are legion. The symptoms can be categorized as follows.

Physical symptoms

Pseudoneurological (including paralyses, contractures, anaesthesiae not corresponding to the sensory distribution of a nerve, hemianaesthesia of the whole side of the body,* hysterical gaits,† tremors, fits, aphonia, hysterical deafness, tubular vision and many more)

Cardiovascular (pseudoanginal crises)

Respiratory (simulated asthma, hyperventilation until tetany occurs)

Gastrointestinal (globus hystericus, abdominal proptosis from downward pressure of the diaphragm and a lordotic posture, hysterical vomiting)

Gynaecological (exaggerated dysmenorrhoea; some female hysterical patients are sexually frigid and some may suffer from dyspareunia or vaginismus)

Mental symptoms

Somnambulism (sleep walking)

Hysterical fugue

Hysterical amnesia

Pseudodementia (simulated dementia in a characteristic way, e.g. 2 + 2 = 5, date before or after the actual one, elementary knowledge denied or given in a childishly perverted way)

Ganser's syndrome (disturbances of consciousness, hallucinations, somatic conversion symptoms, and a tendency to give approximate answers, as in pseudodementia; usually occurs in those in some kind of trouble, e.g. remand prisoners; it represents an attempt to escape from an intolerable situation)

Puerilism (patient regresses to childish level in an attempt to escape from a difficult situation, for manipulative purposes or as a form of attention seeking)

Twilight states (dream-like state of consciousness, visual pseudohallucinations, reenactment of emotionally charged episodes; hysterical stupor, hysterical trance states; multiple personality – patient becomes at times 'a different person', claiming no knowledge of the other 'self')

Behavioural symptoms

Repeated spurious suicidal attempts (not intended to succeed; attempt to gain attention; may succeed by accident and must therefore be taken seriously)

Dermatitis artefacta‡ (self-inflicted lesions varying from redness to ulceration; absence of complete resemblance to any other disorder; lesions have an artificial and curiously bizarre appearance, possessing angles and edges not associated with lesions of any other disorder; severity depends on the agent used, e.g. carbolic acid, alkalis, cigarettes, matches, sandpaper – they may be ingeniously hidden; severe burns, deep scars and ragged ulcers may be seen; hospitalization may be required to definitely discover the diagnosis and cause)

Thermometer manipulation (spurious impression of fever)

Pseudohaemoptysis or pseudohaematemesis (extraction of blood from lips, gums or pharynx)

Swallowing objects (e.g. buttons, safety pins, even cutlery)

Munchausen's syndrome

First described and named by Richard Asher (as in Appendix 3) in 1951. Patients travel from hospital to hospital telling dramatic but untruthful stories, simulating acute illnesses and submitting to countless unnecessary operations and investigations. A few days after admission, they discharge themselves and resume their travels. Common varieties include laparotomophilia migrans (acute abdominal crises), neurologica diabolica (fits, blackouts, disturbances of consciousness, etc.) and haemorrhagica histrionica (haematemesis, etc.).

*Usually the left side; sometimes incongruously responsive to different sensations, e.g. feel cold but not warm items.
†May mimic hemiparetic (usually an atypical dragging behind of the affected leg during a series of hops or supported steps), steppage or ataxic gait disorders. The diagnosis is obvious when the patient walks in a lurching, irregularly based, sometimes bent-forward manner, grasping anything in reach for support and reeling from side to side inconsistently. He may sink to the floor but does not usually endure a self-injuring fall.

‡As with the other conditions mentioned, dermatitis artefacta is usually a manifestation of hysteria, with the usual minorities of cases at either end of the spectrum – at the one end the patient who not only denies knowing how the lesions developed but also may not in fact know their cause, and at the other end the frank malingerer. It should be remembered also that patients with psychotic illnesses may mutilate themselves without any obvious motive.

Case 48 | Radial nerve palsy

Frequency in survey: main focus of a short case or additional feature in 0.1% of attempts at PACES Station 3, CNS.

Record

There is *wrist-drop* and sensory loss over the first dorsal interosseous.*

The diagnosis is radial nerve palsy.

The hand hangs limply and the patient is unable to lift it at the wrist or to straighten out the fingers. If the wrist is passively extended, he is able to straighten the fingers at the interphalangeal joints (because the interossei and lumbricals still work) but not at the MCP joints where the fingers remain flexed. The patient may feel that his grasp is weak in the affected hand because of lack of the wrist extension necessary for powerful grip. If the wrist is passively extended, the power of grip improves. Abduction and adduction of the fingers may appear weak in radial nerve palsy unless they are tested with the hand resting flat on the table with the fingers extended.

The most common cause (of this rare condition) is 'Saturday night paralysis' in which the patient, heavily sedated with alcohol, falls asleep with his arm hanging over the back of a chair. The nerve is compressed against the middle third of the humerus, and brachioradialis (flexion of the arm against resistance – with the arm midway between supination and pronation) and supinator are also paralysed as well as the forearm extensor muscles. Muscle wasting does not usually occur and complete recovery in a matter of weeks† is usual. If the nerve is injured by a wound in the axilla, paralysis involves the triceps so that extension at the elbow is lost, as is the triceps reflex.

(a)
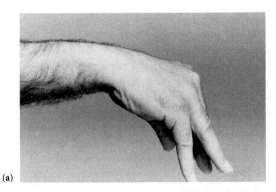
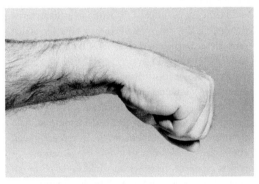
(b)

Figure C3.30 (a) Wrist-drop. (b) Weak grip due to the missing synergistic effect of an extended wrist.

*Though the cutaneous area supplied by the radial nerve is more extensive than this (see Fig. B.4, Examination *Routine* 15), an overlap in supply by both the median and ulnar nerves usually means that only this small area over the first dorsal interosseous has detectable impaired sensation. If there is *no* sensory loss whatsoever, in a patient with symptoms of progressive radial nerve palsy, then a lesion of the posterior interosseous nerve (the main, purely motor, branch of the radial nerve) may be suspected and surgical exploration considered.

†Usually damage occurs to the myelin sheath only and the Schwann cells will repair the nerve rapidly. If the pressure is prolonged and causes axonal degeneration then the peripheral nerve regeneration rate is about 1 mm per day (from the undamaged proximal nerve).

Case 49 | Subclavian-steal syndrome

Frequency in survey: main focus of a short case or additional feature in 0.1% of attempts at PACES Station 3, CNS.

Survey note: one candidate was told that the patient's arm got tired and that she felt faint whenever hanging out washing and he was asked what he would like to examine.

Record

The R/L arm (which gets easily tired on exercise) has a weaker pulse than the other side. The *tension* in the brachial artery (the ease with which the radial pulse can be obliterated by pressure in the brachial artery) is lower on the affected side and (ask to measure the blood pressure) the blood pressure is 100/70 compared with 140/80 in the normal side. There is a systolic bruit heard over the corresponding subclavian artery.

The features and the history suggest the subclavian-steal syndrome.

This rare syndrome occurs when there is stenosis of the subclavian artery near its origin, leading to a retrograde flow of blood down the ipsilateral vertebral artery (see Fig. C3.31), in order to supply the upper limb – subclavian steal. There is relative ischaemia of the arm during exercise. Symptoms are of cerebral ischaemia, usually of vertebrobasilar insufficiency, e.g. vertigo, transient bilateral blindness, syncope, olfactory hallucination, diplopia and bilateral blurring of vision. Any combination of these symptoms may occur either spontaneously or after exercise in the affected arm. There may be features of vascular insufficiency elsewhere (e.g. legs, heart, etc.).

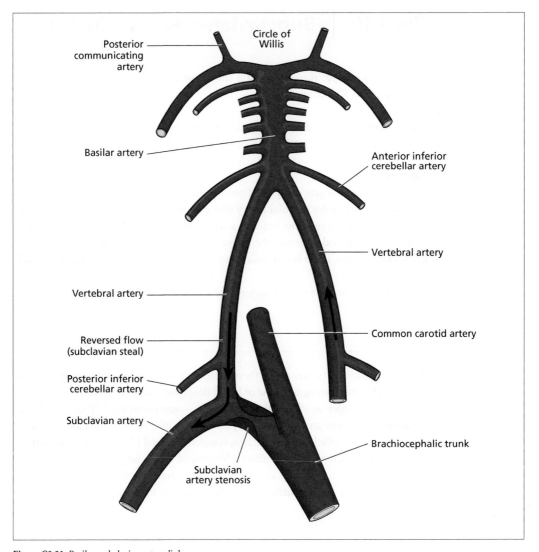

Figure C3.31 Basilar–subclavian artery link.

Case 50 | Tabes

Frequency in survey: main focus of a short case or additional feature in 0.1% of attempts at PACES Station 3, CNS.

Record 1

There are (in this underweight patient who appears older than his years) *Argyll Robertson pupils* (see Station 3, CNS, Case 38). There is bilateral *ptosis* with *wrinkling* of the *forehead* due to compensatory overaction of the frontalis, there is loss of *vibration* and *joint position* sense, loss of *deep pain* in the Achilles tendon, hypotonia, *absent reflexes* and plantar responses; the gait is ataxic and *Romberg's* test is *positive*.

The diagnosis is *tabes dorsalis.** The patient may have *optic atrophy* (may antedate other manifestations; centre of vision may be the last to be affected) and is at risk of developing a *Charcot's* neuropathic hip, knee or ankle joint.

Record 2

As appropriate from the above plus: the *plantars* are *extensor* (with or without other pyramidal signs and other signs of general paresis of the insane (GPI) – see below).

The diagnosis is *taboparesis*.

Other features of tabes dorsalis, though well known, are rarely seen now:

Wide-based, high, stepping gait

Zones of cutaneous analgesia with delayed perception of pain

Ligament laxity allowing extreme degrees of lower limb movement

Perforating foot ulcers

Lightning pains (a good reliable history is virtually pathognomonic and may antedate other symptoms)

Bladder insensitivity

Other forms of neurosyphilis

GPI† (dementia which classically progresses to euphoria and delusions of grandeur though this is less common than simple dementia, epileptic fits, tremor of the hands, lips and tongue ('trombone' tremor – the tongue darts in and out of the mouth involuntarily), and spastic paraparesis of cortical origin)

Meningovascular syphilis‡ (may present in a wide variety of ways including isolated cranial nerve palsies, especially IIIrd and VIth, cerebral or spinal stroke, meningism, epilepsy. Rare syndromes include meningomyelitis, pachymeningitis, acute transverse myelitis, Erb's spastic paraplegia, and syphilitic amyotrophy which resembles motor neurone disease)

---

*Tabes dorsalis occurs 10–35 years after infection with syphilis and the prognosis is poor. There is atrophy of the posterior nerve root and (probably secondary) degeneration of the posterior columns (lumbosacral and lower thoracic worst affected).

†GPI occurs 10–15 years after infection and the prognosis is good if it is treated before the development of cortical atrophy (initially the patient may present simply with a change of temperament, slight pupillary abnormalities and brisk reflexes). There is meningeal thickening and degeneration of the cerebral cortex (especially frontal).

‡Meningovascular syphilis (only 3% of syphilitic patients) occurs in the first 4 years after infection and shows a good response to treatment except where cerebral or spinal cord infarction has occurred. Fibrosed meninges may nip cranial nerves and endarteritis may produce areas of ischaemic necrosis.

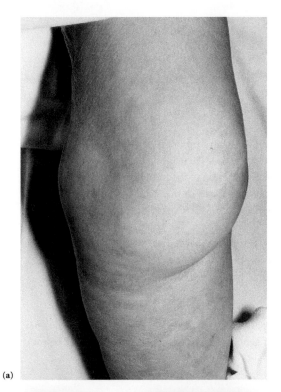

(a)

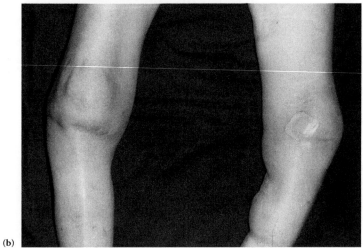

(b)

Figure C3.32 (a,b) Charcot's knee joints.

Case 51 | Thalamic syndrome

Frequency in survey: main focus of a short case or additional feature in 0.1% of attempts at PACES Station 3, CNS.

Record

The patient (who complains of *pain down one side of the body and head*) has (may have) a *hemiplegia* on the R/L side (the side of the pain), and on that side says that the *touch sensation is different* compared to the other side. Pinprick sensation was perceived as increased pain on the R/L.

These features suggest a thalamic syndrome.

Proximal occlusion of the posterior cerebral artery causes ischaemia of the penetrating branches to the thalamic and limbic structures.

Damage to the ventral posterolateral nucleus of the thalamus causes decreased sensation of all modalities on the contralateral side of the body and face. The sensory loss is often accompanied by dysaesthesiae. A thalamic syndrome often appears within weeks or months of the acute thalamic damage and has been attributed to denervation hypersensitivity of sensory neurones in the midbrain reticular formation. The patient develops spontaneous pain in the distribution of the sensory loss. The quality of the pain is difficult to define. It is often exacerbated by anxiety and tends to be rather diffuse but is most marked in one limb and rarely involves the face alone. The quality of sensation on the affected side is usually distorted with diminution to all modalities and hypoalgesia. Nevertheless, stimuli exceeding the sensory threshold may produce an intense exacerbation of the background spontaneous pain. Occasionally there is frank hyperalgesia. With involvement of the subthalamic nucleus, hemiballismus (wild, uncontrolled, flailing limb movements) may develop. The thalamic syndrome is rare but causes a particularly unpleasant pain intractable to most therapeutic manoeuvres.

Case 52 | Wasting of the small muscles of the hand

Frequency in survey: main focus of a short case or additional feature in 0.1% of attempts at PACES Station 3, CNS.

Record

There is *wasting* (and weakness) of the *thenar* and *hypothenar* eminences and of the other small muscles of the hand so that *dorsal guttering* is seen. There is (may be) hyperextension at the MCP joints and flexion at the interphalangeal joints (due to the action of the long extensors of the fingers being unopposed by the lumbricals. In the advanced case a claw hand or *main en griffe* is produced).

Generalized wasting of the small muscles of the hand suggests a lesion affecting the lower motor neurones which originate at the level C8, T1 (unless there is arthropathy leading to disuse atrophy).

Causes

A lesion affecting the anterior horn cells at the level C8, T1 such as:

Motor neurone disease (?prominent fasciculation, spastic paraparesis, wasted fibrillating tongue, no sensory signs; see Station 3, CNS, Case 11)

Syringomyelia (fasciculation not prominent, ?dissociated sensory loss, burn scars, Horner's, nystagmus; see Station 3, CNS, Case 29)

Charcot–Marie–Tooth disease (?distal wasting of the lower limb, pes cavus, etc; see Station 3, CNS, Case 4)

Other causes are old polio, tumour, meningovascular syphilis and cord compression

A root lesion at the level C8,T1 such as:

Cervical spondylosis affecting the C8, T1 level (usually affects higher roots – C6,7, and therefore significant wasting of the small muscles of the hand is uncommon (see Station 3, CNS, Case 26), ?pyramidal signs in the legs, no signs above the level of the lesion, cervical collar)

Tumour at the C8, T1 level (e.g. neurofibroma)

A lesion damaging the brachial plexus (especially lower trunk and medial cord) such as:

Cervical rib (symptoms provoked by a particular posture or movement, e.g. sleeping on the limb, cleaning windows, etc.; ?supraclavicular bruit though Raynaud's and other vascular manifestations are rare in the presence of prominent neurological features)

Pancoast's tumour (?Horner's, clubbing, chest signs, lymph nodes, cachexia, etc.)

Damage caused by violent traction of the arm (e.g. the patient who tried to stop himself falling from a tree by grabbing a passing branch; the same damage in obstetric practice produces Klumpke's paralysis)

Combined ulnar and median nerve lesions (see Station 3, CNS, Cases 14 and 33 respectively)

Arthritis leading to disuse atrophy* (wasting out of proportion to weakness)

Cachexia

---

*For example, rheumatoid arthritis. The factors which may contribute to small muscle wasting in the hand in rheumatoid arthritis are disuse atrophy, vasculitis, peripheral neuropathy, mononeuritis multiplex and entrapment neuropathy (median nerve at wrist, ulnar at elbow, and branches, e.g. the deep palmar branch of the ulnar nerve damaged by subluxation of the carpal bones on the radius and ulna).

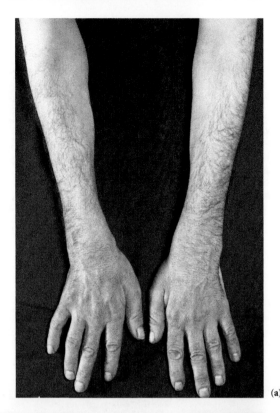

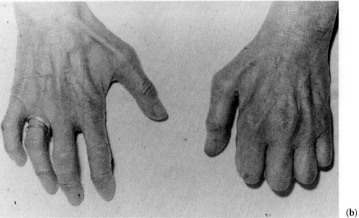

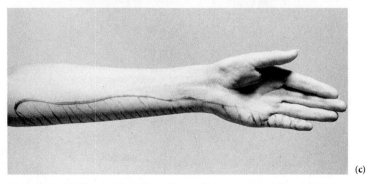

Figure C3.33 (a) Charcot–Marie–Tooth disease. (b) Motor neurone disease. (c) Cervical rib (showing the area of sensory loss, in this case T1 and part of C8; see Fig. B.2, Examination *Routine* 7). (*Continued.*)

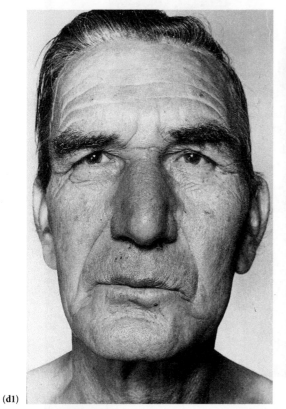

(d1)

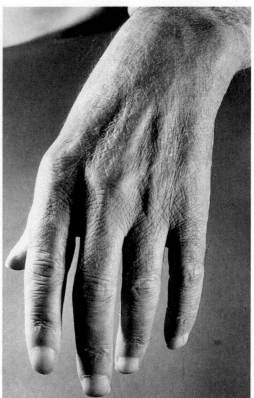

(d2)

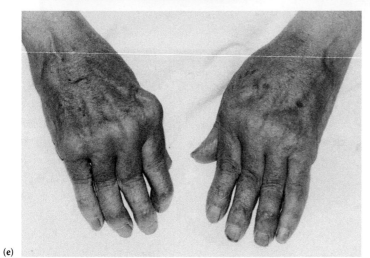

(e)

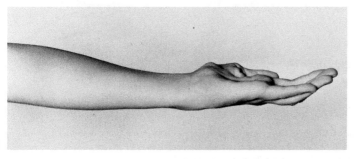

(f)

Figure C3.33 *(Continued)*
(d1,2) Pancoast's tumour (note left
Horner's syndrome and clubbing). (e)
Rheumatoid arthritis. (f) *Main en griffe*
(cervical rib).

Appendices

These books exist as they are because of many previous candidates who, over the years, have completed our surveys and given us invaluable insight into the candidate experience. Please give something back by doing the same for the candidates of the future. For all of your sittings, whether it be a triumphant pass or a disastrous fail . . .

Remember to fill in the survey at www.ryder-mrcp.org.uk

THANK YOU

1 | Checklists

1 Pulse

Observe

1. Face (malar flush, thyroid facies).
2. Neck (Corrigan's pulse, raised JVP, thyroidectomy scar, goitre) and chest (thoracotomy scar).

Palpate and assess

3. Pulse.
4. Rate.
5. Rhythm (?slow atrial fibrillation).
6. Character (normal, collapsing, slow rising, jerky).
7. Carotid.
8. Opposite radial.
9. Radiofemoral delay.
10. All the other pulses.
11. Additional diagnostic features.

2 Heart

1. *Visual survey*:
    (a) breathlessness
    (b) *cyanosis*
    (c) pallor
    (d) *malar flush*
    (e) carotids
    (f) jugulars
    (g) *valvotomy scar*, midline scar
    (h) ankle oedema
    (i) clubbing; splinter haemorrhages.
2. Pulse (rate and rhythm).
3. Lift up the arm (?collapsing).
4. Radiofemoral delay.
5. Brachials and carotids (?slow rising).
6. Venous pressure.
7. Apex beat.
8. Tapping impulse.
9. Right ventricular lift.
10. Other pulsations, thrills, palpable sounds.
11. Auscultation (time heart sounds, etc.; turn patient onto left side; lean patient forwards).
12. Sacral oedema (?ankle oedema).
13. Lung bases.
14. Liver.
15. Blood pressure.

3 Chest

1. *Visual survey* – general appearance (cachexia, superior vena cava obstruction, systemic sclerosis, lupus pernio, kyphoscoliosis, *ankylosing spondylitis*).
2. Dyspnoea.
3. Lip pursing.
4. Cyanosis.
5. Accessory muscles.
6. Indrawing (intercostal muscles, supraclavicular fossae, lower ribs).
7. Chest wall (upward movement, asymmetry, scars, radiotherapy stigmata).
8. Clubbing (tobacco-staining, coal dust tattoos, rheumatoid deformity, systemic sclerosis).
9. Pulse (flapping tremor).
10. Venous pressure.
11. Trachea (deviation, tug, notch–cricoid distance).
12. Lymphadenopathy.
13. Apex beat.
14. Asymmetry.
15. Expansion.
16. Percussion (do not forget clavicles, axillae).
17. Tactile vocal fremitus.
18. Breath sounds.
19. Vocal resonance.
20. Repeat 14–19 on back of chest (feel for lymph nodes in the neck).

4 Abdomen

1. *Visual survey* (pallor, jaundice, spider naevi, etc.).
2. Pigmentation.
3. Hands (Dupuytren's contracture, clubbing, leuconychia, palmar erythema, flapping tremor).
4. Eyes (anaemia, icterus, xanthelasma).
5. Mouth (cyanosis, etc.).
6. Cervical lymph nodes.
7. Gynaecomastia.
8. Spider naevi.
9. Scratch marks.
10. Body hair.
11. Look at the abdomen (pulsation, distension, swelling, distended abdominal veins).

12 Palpation (light palpation, internal organs, inguinal lymph nodes).
13 Percussion.
14 Shifting dullness.
15 Auscultation.
16 Genitalia.
17 Rectal.

5 Visual fields
Observe
1 *Visual survey* (acromegaly, hemiparesis, cerebellar signs).

Test
2 Peripheral visual fields by confrontation.
3 Central scotoma with a red-headed hat pin.
4 Additional features.

6 Cranial nerves
1 Look.
2 Smell and taste (I, VII, IX).
3 Visual acuity (II).
4 Visual fields (II).
5 Eye movements (III, IV, VI).
6 Nystagmus (VIII, cerebellum and its connections).
7 Ptosis (III, sympathetic).
8 Pupils (light, accommodation – III).
9 Discs (II).
10 Facial movements (VII, V).
11 Palatal movement (IX, X).
12 Gag reflex (IX, X).
13 Tongue (XII).
14 Accessory nerve (XI).
15 Hearing (Weber, Rinné – VIII).
16 Facial sensation (including corneal reflex – V).

7 Arms
Observe
1 Face (hemiplegia, nystagmus, wasting, Parkinson's, Horner's).
2 Neck (pseudoxanthoma elasticum, lymph nodes).
3 Elbows (psoriasis, rheumatoid nodules, scars, deformity).
4 Tremor.
5 Hands (joints, nails, skin).
6 Muscle bulk.
7 Fasciculation.

Test
8 Tone.
9 Arms out in front (winging, myelopathy hand sign, sensory wandering).

10 Power:
  (a) arms out to the side (C5)
  (b) bend your elbows (C5,6)
  (c) push out straight (C7)
  (d) squeeze fingers (C8,T1)
  (e) hold the fingers out straight (radial nerve, C7)
  (f) spread fingers apart (ulnar nerve)
  (g) piece of paper between fingers (ulnar nerve)
  (h) thumb at ceiling (median nerve)
  (i) opposition (median nerve).
11 Coordination (rapid alternate motion, finger–nose).
12 Reflexes.
13 Sensation (light touch, pinprick, vibration, joint position).

8 Legs
Observe
1 *Visual survey* (Paget's disease, hemiparesis, exophthalmos, nystagmus, thyroid acropachy, rheumatoid hands, nicotine-stained fingers, wasted hands, muscle fasciculation).
2 Obvious lesion (see group 1 diagnoses).
3 Bowing of the tibia.
4 Pes cavus.
5 One leg smaller than the other.
6 Muscle bulk.
7 Fasciculation.

Test
8 Tone.
9 Power:
  (a) lift your leg up (L1,2)
  (b) bend your knee (L5,S1,2)
  (c) straighten your leg (L3,4)
  (d) bend your foot down (S1)
  (e) cock up your foot (L4,5).
10 Coordination (heel–shin).
11 Tendon reflexes (clonus).
12 Plantar response.
13 Sensation (light touch, pinprick, vibration, joint position).
14 Gait (ordinary walk, heel-to-toe, on toes, on heels).
15 Rombergism.

9 Legs and arms
As appropriate from *Checklists* 7 and 8.

10 Gait

1 *Visual survey* (cerebellar signs, Parkinson's, Charcot–Marie–Tooth, ankylosing spondylitis).
2 Check patient can walk.
3 Observe ordinary walk (ataxia, spastic, steppage, parkinsonian).
4 Arm swing (Parkinson's).
5 Turning (ataxia, Parkinson's).
6 Heel-to-toe (ataxia).
7 On toes (S1).
8 On heels (L5).
9 Romberg's test (sensory ataxia).
10 Gait with eyes closed.
11 Additional features.

11 Ask some questions

1 *Visual survey* (from top to toe, ?obvious diagnosis).
2 Specific questions (Raynaud's, systemic sclerosis/ CREST, hypo- or hyperthyroidism, Crohn's, nephrotic syndrome).
3 General questions (name, address).
4 Questions with long answers (last meal).
5 Articulation ('British Constitution', 'West Register Street', 'biblical criticism').
6 Repetition.
7 Additional signs.
8 Comprehension ('put out your tongue', 'shut your eyes', 'touch your nose').
9 Nominal dysphasia (keys).
10 Orofacial dyspraxia.
11 Higher mental function.

12 Fundi
Observe

1 *Visual survey* (Medic-Alert bracelet, etc.).

Ophthalmoscopy

2 Lens.
3 Vitreous.
4 Disc (optic atrophy, papillitis, papilloedema, myelinated nerve fibres, new vessels).
5 Arterioles and venules (silver wiring, AV nipping).
6 Each quadrant and macula (haemorrhages, microaneurysms, exudates, new vessels, photocoagulation scars, choroidoretinitis, retinitis pigmentosa, drusen).
7 Do not stop until you have finished and are ready.

13 Eyes
Observe

1 Face (e.g. myasthenic, tabetic, hemiparesis).
2 Eyes (exophthalmos, strabismus, ptosis, xanthelasma, arcus senilis).
3 Pupils (Argyll Robertson, Horner's, Holmes–Adie, IIIrd nerve).

Test

4 Visual acuity.
5 Visual fields.
6 Eye movements (ocular palsy, diplopia, nystagmus, lid lag).
7 Light reflex (direct, consensual).
8 Accommodation reflex.
9 Fundi.

14 Face

1 *Visual survey* of patient.
2 Scan the head and face.
3 Break down and scrutinize the parts of the face:
   (a) eyelids (ptosis, rash)
       eyelashes (scanty)
       cornea (arcus, interstitial keratitis)
       sclerae (icteric, congested)
       pupils (small, large, irregular, dislocated lens, cataracts)
       iris (iritis)
   (b) face (erythema, infiltrates)
       mouth (tight, shiny, adherent skin; pigmented patches, telangiectasia, cyanosis).
4 Additional features.

15 Hands
Observe

1 Face (*systemic sclerosis*, Cushing's, acromegaly, arcus senilis, icterus and spider naevi, exophthalmos).
2 Inspect the hands (rheumatoid, sclerodactyly, wasting, psoriasis, claw hand, clubbing).
3 Joints (swelling, deformity, Heberden's nodes).
4 Nails (pitting, onycholysis, clubbing, nail-fold infarcts).
5 Skin (colour, consistency, lesions).
6 Muscles (wasting, fasciculation).

Palpate and test

7 Hands (Dupuytren's contracture, nodules, calcinosis, xanthomata, Heberden's nodes, tophi).

8 Sensation (pinprick, light touch, vibration, joint position).
9 Tone.
10 Power.
11 Pulses.
12 Elbows.

16 Skin

1 *Visual survey* (regional associations: scalp, face, mouth, neck, trunk, axillae, elbows, hands, nails, genitalia, legs, feet).
2 Distribution (psoriasis on extensor areas, lichen planus in flexural areas, etc.).
3 Lesions – look for characteristic features (scaling, Wickham's striae, etc.).
4 Associated lesions (arthropathy, etc.).

17 Rash

1 *Visual survey* (scalp to sole).
2 Distribution.
3 Surrounding skin (?scratch marks).
4 Examine the lesion (colour, size, shape, surface, character, secondary features).
5 Additional features.

18 Neck

1 *Visual survey* of patient (eyes, face, legs).
2 Look at the neck (swallow).
3 Palpate the thyroid (swallow; size, consistency, etc.; pyramidal lobes, percuss over upper sternum).
4 Lymph nodes (supraclavicular, submandibular, postauricular, suboccipital, axillae, groins, spleen).
5 Auscultate the thyroid (distinguish from venous hum and conducted murmurs).
6 Assess thyroid status.

19 Thyroid status

1 *Visual survey* (exophthalmos, goitre, thyroid acropachy, pretibial myxoedema, myxoedematous facies).
2 Composure (fidgety, normal, immobile).
3 Pulse.
4 Ankle jerks.
5 Palms.
6 Tremor.
7 Eyes (lid retraction, lid lag).
8 Thyroid (look, palpate, auscultate).
9 Questions.

20 Knee

1 Observe (*rheumatoid, psoriasis*, gout).
2 Ask (pain).
3 Inspect (valgus, varus, flexion deformity, quadriceps, knee).
4 Palpate (temperature, tender).
5 Effusion (bulge sign, patellar tap).
6 Movement (flex knee).
7 Crepitus over the joint as flexion occurs.
8 Feel behind the knee for a Baker's cyst.
9 Instability (cruciate, McMurray's sign).
10 Other joints (psoriasis, inflammatory bowel disease, reactive arthritis, tophi).

21 Hip

1 Inspect (flexed, shortening, externally rotated, scars, rheumatoid).
2 Ask (pain).
3 Movement (flex, rotate, abduction, adduction, Thomas's test).
4 Straight leg raise (nerve root entrapment, neurological assessment).
5 Tenderness (trochanteric bursitis).
6 Length inequality.
7 Walk (antalgic gait, waddling gait).

22 'Spot' diagnosis

1 *Visual survey*.
2 Retrace the same ground more thoroughly:
    (a) head (*Paget's, myotonic dystrophy*)
    (b) face (*acromegaly, Parkinson's, hemiplegia,* myotonic dystrophy, tardive dyskinesia, hypopituitarism, Cushing's, hypothyroidism, systemic sclerosis)
    (c) eyes (*jaundice, exophthalmos*, ptosis, Horner's, xanthelasma)
    (d) neck (*goitre*, Turner's, spondylitis, torticollis)
    (e) trunk (pigmentation, ascites, purpuric spots, spider naevi, wasting, pemphigus)
    (f) arms (choreoathetosis, psoriasis, Addison's, spider naevi, *syringomyelia*)
    (g) hands (acromegaly, *tremor*, clubbing, sclerodactyly, arachnodactyly, claw hand, etc.)
    (h) legs (bowing, purpura, pretibial myx-oedema, necrobiosis)
    (i) feet (pes cavus).
3 Abnormal colouring (*pigmentation, icterus*, pallor).
4 Break down and scrutinize (especially face).
5 Additional features.

2 | Examination frequency of MRCP PACES short cases

Station 1, Respiratory

	Short case	Main focus of a short case or additional feature in (%)
1	Interstitial lung disease (fibrosing alveolitis)	34
2	Pneumonectomy/lobectomy	13
3	Chronic bronchitis and emphysema	11
4	Bronchiectasis	9
5	Dullness at the lung bases	7
6	Rheumatoid lung	4
7	Old tuberculosis	3
8	Chest infection/consolidation/pneumonia	3
9	Yellow nail syndrome	2
10	Kyphoscoliosis	2
11	Stridor	1
12	Marfan's syndrome	1
13	Carcinoma of the bronchus	0.8
14	Klippel Feil syndrome	0.8
15	Kartagener's syndrome	0.7
16	Lung transplant	0.7
17	Cystic fibrosis	0.7
18	Obesity/Pickwickian syndrome	0.5
19	Pneumothorax	0.5
20	Cor pulmonale	0.3
21	Collapsed lung/atelectasis	0.2
22	Superior vena cava obstruction	0.1
23	Tuberculosis/apical consolidation	0.1
24	Normal chest	0

Station 1, Abdominal

	Short case	Main focus of a short case or additional feature in (%)
1	Transplanted kidney	16
2	Polycystic kidneys	14
3	Chronic liver disease	12
4	Hepatosplenomegaly	12
5	Hepatomegaly (without splenomegaly)	10

Continued

	Short case	Main focus of a short case or additional feature in (%)
6	Splenomegaly (without hepatomegaly)	9
7	Ascites	6
8	Abdominal mass	3
9	Crohn's disease	3
10	Polycythaemia rubra vera	3
11	Normal abdomen	2
12	PEG tube	2
13	Single palpable kidney	2
14	Generalized lymphadenopathy	0.9
15	Hereditary spherocytosis	0.9
16	Idiopathic haemochromatosis	0.8
17	Primary biliary cirrhosis	0.8
18	Carcinoid syndrome	0.7
19	Motor neurone disease	0.7
20	Nephrotic syndrome	0.7
21	Pernicious anaemia	0.7
22	Pyoderma gangrenosum	0.7
23	Felty's syndrome	0.1

Station 3, Cardiovascular

	Short case	Main focus of a short case or additional feature in (%)
1	Prosthetic valves	17
2	Mitral incompetence (lone)	9
3	Mixed mitral valve disease	9
4	Aortic incompetence (lone)	8
5	Aortic stenosis (lone)	7
6	Mixed aortic valve disease	5
7	Mitral stenosis (lone)	5
8	Irregular pulse	5
9	Other combinations of mitral and aortic valve disease	4
10	Mitral valve prolapse	3
11	Tricuspid incompetence	3
12	Ventricular septal defect	2
13	Marfan's syndrome	1
14	Pulmonary stenosis	1
15	Ankylosing spondylitis	0.8
16	Atrial septal defect	0.8
17	Ebstein's anomaly	0.8
18	Raised jugular venous pressure	0.8
19	Down's syndrome	0.7
20	Hypertrophic cardiomyopathy	0.7
21	Dextrocardia	0.6
22	Rheumatoid arthritis	0.6

	Short case	Main focus of a short case or additional feature in (%)
23	Fallot's tetralogy with a Blalock shunt	0.3
24	Normal heart	0.2
25	Cannon waves	0.1
26	Coarctation of the aorta	0.1
27	Eisenmenger's syndrome	0.1
28	Infective endocarditis	0.1
29	Patent ductus arteriosus	0.1
30	Pulmonary incompetence	0.1
31	Slow pulse	0.1

Station 3, Central nervous system

	Short case	Main focus of a short case or additional feature in (%)
1	Peripheral neuropathy	10
2	Myotonic dystrophy (dystrophia myotonica)	8
3	Parkinson's disease	8
4	Charcot–Marie–Tooth disease (hereditary motor and sensory neuropathy)	6
5	Abnormal gait	6
6	Spastic paraparesis	6
7	Cerebellar syndrome	5
8	Hemiplegia	4
9	Muscular dystrophy	3
10	Multiple sclerosis	3
11	Motor neurone disease	3
12	Friedreich's ataxia	3
13	Visual field defect	3
14	Ulnar nerve palsy	2
15	Old polio	2
16	Ocular palsy	2
17	Spinal cord compression	2
18	Ptosis	2
19	Guillain–Barré syndrome (acute inflammatory demyelinating polyradiculopathy)	1
20	Choreoathetosis	1
21	Bulbar palsy	1
22	Lateral popliteal (common peroneal) nerve palsy	1
23	Proximal myopathy	1
24	Absent ankle jerks and extensor plantars	0.8
25	Cerebellopontine angle lesion	0.8
26	Cervical myelopathy	0.8
27	Myasthenia gravis	0.8

Continued

	Short case	Main focus of a short case or additional feature in (%)
28	Normal central nervous system	0.8
29	Syringomyelia	0.8
30	Diabetic foot/Charcot's joint	0.8
31	Holmes–Adie–Moore syndrome	0.7
32	Nystagmus	0.7
33	Carpal tunnel syndrome	0.7
34	Drug-induced extrapyramidal syndrome	0.7
35	Lower motor neurone VIIth nerve palsy	0.7
36	Dysarthria	0.6
37	Subacute combined degeneration of the cord	0.3
38	Argyll Robertson pupils	0.1
39	Congenital syphilis	0.1
40	Dysphasia	0.1
41	Horner's syndrome	0.1
42	Infantile hemiplegia	0.1
43	Jugular foramen syndrome	0.1
44	Lateral medullary syndrome (Wallenberg's syndrome)	0.1
45	Polymyositis	0.1
46	Pseudobulbar palsy	0.1
47	Psychogenic/factitious	0.1
48	Radial nerve palsy	0.1
49	Subclavian-steal syndrome	0.1
50	Tabes	0.1
51	Thalamic syndrome	0.1
52	Wasting of the small muscles of the hand	0.1

3 | Texidor's twinge and related matters

The following excerpt from Richard Asher's book* is surely compulsory reading for all prospective members of the Royal College of Physicians. No physician's training is complete until the messages contained therein have been assimilated.

'It is pleasant to believe that the facts of medical science are there whether or not we name them; that the truth about clinical medicine exists quite independently of the names we bestow upon it. If that were so, our only responsibility would be to agree upon symbols or words for facts that already existed. That theoretical ideal is hardly ever fulfilled. A little patient thinking will soon convince the enquirer that it is not just a simple matter of finding words to fit the facts, but just as often of finding facts to fit the words. When christening a baby we wait for the child to be born and then we find a name for it. When christening a disease we sometimes wait for the name to be born and then we try to find a disease to suit it. With children we announce their names in the birth columns of The Times and with diseases we announce their names in the original articles of the medical journals. The only difference is that children's names have to be registered. There is no such procedure with medical terms. There is no Medical Registrar-General of Terminological Births and Deaths. Only medical dictionaries and the international list of classified diseases. These do not include every living medical term, and they list many that have died or that ought to be painlessly put away. There is something about a name, particularly an eponymous term, which brings into being things which never seemed to be there before. In creation the word may come first: the opening sentence of the Gospel of Saint John is – "In the beginning was the Word."

Take, for instance, Pel Ebstein fever. Every student and every doctor knows that cases of Hodgkin's disease may show a fever that is high for one week and low for the next week, and so on. Does this phenomenon really exist at all? If you collect the charts of 50 cases of Hodgkin's disease and compare them with the charts of 50 cases of disseminated malignant fever, do you really believe you could pick out even one or two cases because of the characteristic fever? I think it is very unlikely indeed. Yet if, by the vagaries of

chance, one case of Hodgkin's did run such a temperature, the news would soon travel round: "There's a good case of Hodgkin's disease in Galen Ward. You ought to have a look. It shows the typical Pel Ebstein fever very well".

The chart might be copied for teaching purposes, or even put in a book. The mere description and the naming of a mythical fever leads inevitably to its occurrence in textbooks. One popular textbook for nurses depicts particularly classical temperature charts, attributed to various fevers. I asked the author how many hospital notes she had combed before she found such beautiful examples: "Oh, there was no trouble about that," she replied, "I made them up out of my head".

I wonder whether any examples of Pel Ebstein and other fevers in textbooks have similar origins. It does not matter whether or not Pel Ebstein fever exists, my contention remains the same: the bestowal of a name upon a concept, whether real or imaginary, brings it into clinical existence.

Out of curiosity I looked up the original papers, and Dr Burrows kindly translated them for me. Both describe patients with chronic relapsing fever and splenomegaly but there is nothing in either paper to suggest any of them had Hodgkin's disease. Both describe cases of undulant fever and Ebstein suggested the name chronic relapsing fever, but it was very probably one of abortus fever.

An important example of the creation of a thing beginning with the word is gallstone colic. There is no such thing. Colic is a pain continuously waxing and waning, like the colonic cramps of food poisoning. Gallstone pain after its onset steadily climbs to an agonizing peak without any fluctuation, and then passes off. But the label colic has been so firmly stuck on to this pain that the pain is expected to be colic, assumed to be colic, believed to be colic and finally bullied into being colic, so that a man with gallstone pain will be described as having colicky pain, however steady it may be.

Contrariwise, if something has no individual descriptive term it has far less chance of clinical acceptance or clinical recognition. A rose without a name may smell as sweet, but it has far less chance of being smelt. Supposing we take an unnamed fever and an unnamed pain to contrast with the examples I have given. In untreated pernicious anaemia there is often quite a high fever. Sixty per cent of cases with red cell counts under 1.5 million show a fever

*From the book Talking Sense, edited by Sir Francis Avery Jones (Pitman Medical, 1972).

over 101°F. This invariably settles to normal levels within a week of one adequate injection of B_{12}. I make no assertion that this fever is of great importance. What I do assert is that had it been called the Addison–Castle fever or hypo-cyanocobalminic fever there is not a medical student in the land who would not have heard of it, many doctors would be afraid to diagnose pernicious anaemia without its presence, and the proportion of patients showing the fever would rise sharply once the name got into nurses' textbooks (because if they did not show the fever they would have their thermometers put back in their mouths until they behaved themselves).

Now for a pain without a name. Have any of you ever had a very brief, sharp needle-like pain near the apex of the heart: acutely localized to one point seemingly inside the chest wall, but feeling as if something was adherent to it? Breathing sharpens it, so there is often a disinclination to take a deep breath while it lasts. It comes out of the blue, it passes off in a few minutes, and although acute it is not at all distressing.

Enquiries among my friends showed that quite a lot of them occasionally had this pain, but, till they knew other people had it too, they did not mention it; especially because it has no official name, and also because it did not bother them.

I circulated various doctors I knew, and also circularized 50 recently elected Fellows of the College of Physicians – to see if it was reasonably common. It was . . . So if any of you happen to have it, you are not branding yourselves as either grievously neurotic or grossly hypochondriacal if you admit to having it.

[In the second of the Lettsomian lectures, on which this essay is based, with the permission of the President of the Medical Society of London, Dr Asher asked his audience of medical men whether any of them had encountered anything closely resembling this pain in either themselves or their friends, and if they had, to raise their hands. Over a third of the audience held up their hands.]

There seems no doubt that this condition exists, yet, because it has no name, it has no official clinical existence. We cannot discuss it or investigate it or write about it. Whether or not the condition should be named I am unable to say.† Though the naming of disease is not in any way restricted or supervised it ought not to be undertaken lightly. A fertile medical author can easily beget a large number of clinical progeny by describing and naming them, but some of his youngsters may turn out to be illegitimate, and with others there may be much doubt about their paternity if others claim to have begotten them years ago.'

†In a foreword to *Sense and Sensibility* the author explained that the pain had been described and named 4 years previously by A.J. Miller and T.A. Texidor (1955) in the *Journal of the American Medical Association*, and that it might in future be known as *Texidor's twinge*.

4 | Abbreviations

A&E	accident and emergency	CRH	corticotrophin-releasing hormone
ABE	acute bacterial endocarditis	CRVO	central retinal vein occlusion
ABPA	allergic bronchopulmonary aspergillosis	CSF	cerebrospinal fluid
ACE	angiotensin-converting enzyme	CT	computed tomography
ACTH	adrenocorticotrophic hormone	DEXA	dual energy X-ray absorptiometry
ADPKD	autosomal dominant polycystic kidney disease	DIDMOAD	diabetes insipidus, diabetes mellitus, optic atrophy and deafness
AFB	acid-fast bacilli	DMARD	disease-modifying antirheumatic drug
AIDP	acute inflammatory demyelinating polyradiculopathy	2,3-DPG	2,3-diphosphoglycerate
		DVT	deep venous thrombosis
AIDS	acquired immune deficiency syndrome	ECG	electrocardiogram
AIP	acute interstitial pneumonia	eGFR	estimated glomerular filtration rate
ANA	antinuclear antibody	EMG	electromyograph
ANCA	antineutrophil cytoplasmic antibodies	ENT	ears, nose and throat
APAS	antiphospholipid antibody syndrome	ESR	erythrocyte sedimentation rate
AR	aortic regurgitation	FBC	full blood count
ARDS	adult respiratory distress syndrome	FET	forced expiratory time
ARPKD	autosomal recessive polycystic kidney disease	FEV_1	forced expiratory volume in 1 sec
		FFA	free fatty acids
ASD	atrial septal defect	FSH	follicle-stimulating hormone
AV	arteriovenous	FVC	forced vital capacity
BAL	bronchoalveolar lavage	G6PD	glucose-6-phosphate dehydrogenase
BMI	Body Mass Index	GAD	glutamic acid decarboxylase
BP	blood pressure	GFR	glomerular filtration rate
BRAO	branch retinal artery occlusion	GH	growth hormone
BOS	bronchiolitis obliterans syndrome	GHRH	growth hormone-releasing hormone
cAMP	cyclic adenosine monophosphate	GI	gastrointestinal
cANCA	cytoplasmic ANCA	GPI	general paresis of the insane
CFA	cryptogenic fibrosing alveolitis	HBsAg	hepatitis B surface antigen
CHD	coronary heart disease	HBV	hepatitis B virus
CIDP	chronic inflammatory demyelinating polyneuropathy	HCG	human chorionic gonadotrophin
		HCM	hypertrophic cardiomyopathy
CML	chronic myeloid leukaemia	HCV	hepatitis C virus
CNS	central nervous system	HDL	high-density lipoprotein
CO_2	carbon dioxide	5-HIAA	5-hydroxyindole acetic acid
COP	cryptogenic organizing pneumonia	HIV	human immunodeficiency virus
COPD	chronic obstructive pulmonary disease	HLA	human leucocyte antigen
COX	cyclooxygenase	HMGco-A	hydroxy methyl glutaryl coenzyme A
CPEO	chronic progressive external ophthalmoplegia	HMSN	hereditary motor and sensory neuropathy
		HOCM	hypertrophic obstructive cardiomyopathy
CRAO	central retinal artery occlusion		
CREST	calcinosis, Raynaud's, oesophageal involvement, sclerodactyly and telangiectasia	HP	hypersensitivity pneumonitis
		HPOA	hypertrophic pulmonary osteoarthropathy

HRCT	high resolution CT scan	PACES	Practical Assessment of Clinical Examination Skills
HRT	hormone replacement therapy		
5-HT	serotonin	pANCA	perinuclear ANCA
HTLV	human T-cell lymphotrophic virus	PAPS	primary antiphospholipid antibody syndrome
ICU	intensive care unit		
Ig	immunoglobulin	PBC	primary biliary cirrhosis
IGF	insulin-like growth factor	PBG	porphobilinogen
IIP	idiopathic interstitial pneumonia	PEG	percutaneous endoscopic gastrostomy
IL	interleukin		
IPF	idiopathic pulmonary fibrosis	PET	positron emission tomography
IRMA	intraretinal microvascular abnormalities	PFR	peak flow rate
ITU	intensive treatment unit	Ph	Philadelphia (chromosome)
IU	international unit	PKD	polycystic kidney disease
IV	intravenous	PSA	prostate specific antigen
JCA	juvenile chronic arthritis	PUVA	psoralen and UVA
JIA	juvenile idiopathic arthritis	REAL	Revised European-American Lymphoma (classification)
JVP	jugular venous pressure		
KCO	transfer coefficient	RIG	radiologically inserted gastrostomy
LDH	lactic dehydrogenase	rSR	ECG pattern of right bundle branch block
LDL	low-density lipoprotein		
LH	luteinizing hormone	RV	right ventricular
LP	lumbar puncture	SACD	subacute combined degeneration of the cord
LPL	lipoprotein lipase		
MCP	metacarpophalangeal	SBE	subacute bacterial endocarditis
MEA	multiple endocrine adenopathy	SLE	systemic lupus erythematosus
MEN	multiple endocrine neoplasia	SPS	stiff-person syndrome
MND	motor neurone disease	TAVI	transcatheter aortic valve implantation
MRCP	Membership of the Royal College of Physicians	TB	tuberculosis
		TLC	total lung capacity
MRI	magnetic resonance imaging	TLCO	transfer factor
MS	multiple sclerosis	TNF	tumour necrosis factor
MTP	metatarsophalangeal	TOE	transoesophageal echocardiography
MVP	mitral valve prolapse	TSH	thyroid-stimulating hormone
NAFLD	non-alcoholic fatty liver disease	UIP	usual interstitial pneumonia
NASH	non-alcoholic steatohepatitis	USS	ultrasound scan
NG	nasogastric	UVA	ultraviolet A
NIDDM	non-insulin-dependent diabetes mellitus	UVB	ultraviolet B
NIV	non-invasive ventilation	VATS	video-assisted thoracoscopic surgery
NJ	nasojejunal	VER	visual evoked response
NSAID	non-steroidal antiinflammatory drug	VLDL	very low-density lipoprotein
NSIP	non-specific interstitial pneumonia	VSD	ventricular septal defect
NYHA	New York Heart Association	WBC	white blood cell(s)
PABP	polyadenylate-binding protein	WHO	World Health Organization

Index

movements
  choreoathetosis 249–50
  drug-induced extrapyramidal
    syndrome 274
  see also gait; palatal movements
Müller manoeuvre, tricuspid
  incompetence 174n
multiple sclerosis **224–5**
  Friedreich's ataxia differential
    diagnosis *230*
  spastic paraparesis 217
Munchausen's syndrome 297
muscle fasciculation 226
muscle wasting, polymyositis 294
muscle weakness
  limb girdle 254
  myasthenia gravis 259
  polymyositis 294
  spinal cord compression 240
muscular dystrophy 216, **222**, *223*,
  243n
  lower motor neurone VIIth nerve
    palsy 275
  oculopharyngeal 222, 243n,
    244
myasthenia gravis 237, **259–60**,
  261–2
  dysarthria 279
  lower motor neurone VIIth nerve
    palsy 275
  ptosis 243, *245*
myasthenic crisis 259–60
myasthenic–myopathic syndrome
  260
mycotic abdominal aortic aneurysm
  132n
myelofibrosis 127n
myelopathy hand sign 257, *258*
myeloproliferative disorders 127n,
  128n
myoclonus 250
myopathic dysarthria 279
myotonia congenita 207–8
myotonic dystrophy **207–8**
  dysarthria 279
  ptosis 243, *245*
myxoedema 129, 272

nails
  examination 52
    infective endocarditis 195, *197*
    leuconychia in chronic liver
      disease 121, *123*
    skin 56
    yellow nail syndrome 89
neck examination 58–60
  checklist 312
  dermatomes *30*
  diagnoses 58–9
  lymph nodes 24, 59–60
  palpation 24
  pulse examination 11
  skin examination 56
  visual survey 32, 59
  see also thyroid

neck weakness, painless 29n
nephrotic syndrome 129, **150–1**
nerve root compression 241
neuroleptic drugs 274
neurological conditions, arms 31
neurosyphilis 281, 286n, 301
  bulbar palsy 251
neutropenia, Felty's syndrome
  154
nominal dysphasia 285
non-alcoholic fatty liver disease
  (NAFLD) 122
non-alcoholic steatohepatitis
  (NASH) 122n
non-Hodgkin's lymphoma 140
non-invasive ventilation (NIV),
  kyphoscoliosis 91
non-specific interstitial pneumonia
  (NSIP) 74n
nose, congenital syphilis 282, *283*
notch–cricoid distance 19
nutritional deficiency
  cerebellar syndrome 218
  see also malabsorption
nystagmus 29, **268–9**, *270*
  ataxic 224
  cerebellopontine lesion 256
  Friedreich's ataxia 229

obesity **103–5**, *106*
  endocrine causes 105
  genetic diseases 105
  normal abdomen 137
obliterative bronchiolitis *see*
  bronchiolitis obliterans
obstructive sleep apnoea 103n
ocular myopathy 237, 243n, *246*
ocular palsy **236–7**, *238–9*
oculopharyngeal muscular dystrophy
  222, 243n, 244
ophthalmoplegia 236n
  chronic progressive external
    243
  exophthalmic 237
  external 248
  internuclear 237, 269
ophthalmoscopy, fundi examination
  45
Oppenheim's sign 36n, *258*
optic atrophy 45
  tabes dorsalis 301
optic chiasma lesion 231
optic tract lesion 231
orofacial dyspraxia 42
Osler's nodes, infective endocarditis
  195
osteoarthritis
  elbow 233
  obesity 104
osteomalacia 254
ostium primum/secundum defects
  179, 180
otitis media 218n
oxalosis, renal transplantation
  118

pacemakers, demand 201
PACES
  marking system 10
  patients 3
pain
  epigastric 136
  nameless 318
palatal movements 29
  bulbar palsy 251
  jugular foramen syndrome 290
  paralysis
    lateral medullary syndrome
      292
    motor neurone disease 226
  pseudobulbar palsy 295
palate, Friedreich's ataxia 229
Pancoast's syndrome 94, *96*
  Horner's syndrome 286
Pancoast's tumour 304, *306*
pancreatic ascites 129
pancreatic carcinoma 132
pancreatic insufficiency, cystic
  fibrosis 101
pansystolic murmur
  Ebstein's anomaly 181
  Eisenmenger's syndrome 193
  infective endocarditis 195
  mitral incompetence 157
  mixed mitral valve disease 159
  pulmonary incompetence 200
  ventricular septal defect 175
papilloedema 232n
  cerebellopontine lesion 256
paramyotonia 208
paraphasia 284n
parasternal heave
  atrial septal defect 179
  Eisenmenger's syndrome 193
  left 15
  mitral stenosis 167
  mixed mitral and aortic valve
    disease 171
  mixed mitral valve disease 159
  patent ductus arteriosus 198
  pulmonary stenosis 177
  tetralogy of Fallot 188
  ventricular septal defect 175
parkinsonian syndrome 209
Parkinson's disease 32, **209–10**,
  211
  arteriosclerotic 209–10
  dysarthria 279
parotitis, dysarthria 279
patent ductus arteriosus 12, **198**
patients
  management 10
  PACES 3
Pel Ebstein fever 317
percutaneous endoscopic
  gastrostomy (PEG) tube **138**
perianal skin, Crohn's disease 133,
  134
peripheral neuropathy **205–6**
peritonitis, tuberculous 115, 129n
permission to examine patient 10

MRCP – it teaches more than it tests*

*"When you come out of the exam you realize that after months and months of hard work and swotting, the amount of knowledge you actually used could be written on a postage stamp!' (Vol.2, Section F, Quotation 415.)

Printed and bound by CPI Group (UK) Ltd, Croydon, CR0 4YY

24/03/2025

14645805-0001

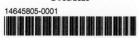